FOOD NUTRITION, SCIENCE AND TECHNOLOGY

FOOD NUTRITION, SCIENCE AND TECHNOLOGY

Neelam Singh
Dr. I. S. Singh

WOODHEAD PUBLISHING INDIA PVT LTD

New Delhi

Published by Woodhead Publishing India Pvt. Ltd.
Woodhead Publishing India Pvt. Ltd.,
303, Vardaan House, 7/28, Ansari Road,
Daryaganj, New Delhi - 110002, India
www.woodheadpublishingindia.com

First published 2018, Woodhead Publishing India Pvt. Ltd.

Woodhead Publishing India Pvt. Ltd. ISBN: 978-93-85059-43-8
Woodhead Publishing India Pvt. Ltd. e-ISBN: 978-93-85059-93-3

Typeset by Allen Smalley, Chennai

Printed and bound in India by Replika Press Pvt. Ltd.

Contents

Author Details

DETAILS OF NEELAM SINGH (FIRST AUTHOR)

- MSc. in Food and Nutrition from Karnataka State University, India.
- Post bachelorette student in Dietetics at Oregon State University (USA) 2016-2018.
- Lifestyle health coach on CDC's Diabetes Prevention Program at Providence Hospital Orenco, USA.
- Volunteered as a nutrition educator at Providence Hospital, Milwaukie, Oregon, USA.
- Has years of experience as a dietitian in India. Worked at Manipal hospital, nationwide primary health care, healthcare magic, Dringo, VLCC, as a dietitian.
- Was one of the co-founding members of the new start-up company which provides healthy diet like heart healthy, diabetic food, etc.
- Worked as a consultant dietitian and involved in educating groups, companies on different aspects of nutrition and nutrition-related health issues.
- Conducted wellness programs at several places such as old age homes, clinics, and multinational companies.
- Appeared on national radio (India) on healthy eating as well as written articles for the newspapers on health-related issues.

DETAILS OF DR. I.S. SINGH (SECOND AUTHOR)

- MS from University of California, Davis and Ph.D.
- Received advance Training in Food Technology at CFTRI Mysore.
- Has more than 45 years of experience in teaching, research, and extension in the field of post-harvest technology in various universities.
- Served in the capacity of professor post-harvest technology, and Prof. and Head Department of Food Science and Technology and Project Director, N.D. University of Agriculture and Technology Faizabad.
- Life member of 7 professional societies.
- Participated in 38 National and 16 International Symposium and conference.

- Guided 33 post graduate students in field of post harvest technology.
- Published 7 book, 106 research papers and 18 research bulletins.
- Recipient of 9 National Awards including Dr. Rajendra Prasad Award for out standing contribution/excellence in field of post harvest technology.

Foreword

World is moving fast and food industry is expanding with number of newer food products covering packaged food and fast foods. Hence, it becomes important to sensitize consumer and food industry personnel for nutrition, health and hygiene so that food and food products are conducive to good health. In the ever-changing consumer market, attitudes towards food and food safety have altered drastically in recent years. The health conscious population demands more nutritious and safe food. Adoption of recent technologies is likely to increase the availability of more fresh and processed foods. Changes are also seen in packaging, storage and value addition.

Excellent efforts have been made by the authors of this book to compile scientific information and by providing a rich source of information on food nutrition, food science and food technology. It will cater to the needs of not only the students but also to teachers, researchers, extension workers and processors. I appreciate the efforts made by Neelam Singh and Dr. I.S. Singh in bringing out this useful publication.

Prof. Panjab Singh
President
National Academy of Agricultural Sciences
New Delhi

Preface

Food is the basic necessity of life and vital for human existence. Nutrition helps growth and development, resists infection and prevents malnutrition and diseases. Hence, the knowledge of nutrition is of immense importance for one and all. Food science helps to understand the methods of storing and preserving foods for maintaining quality and preventing spoilage. It is concerned with the fundamental scientific facts about foods. Food technology deals or involved in the processing of edible raw materials into safe food products. The growth potential of food processing industries is enormous due to demand for semi-processed and processed food. Food processing is an important sector of the economy to reduce post-harvest losses, increase income, providing employment opportunities, diversify rural economy and to earn foreign exchange.

Information on food, nutrition, science, and technology is not available collectively at a single source. The literature on these aspects is scattered at diverse sources. Hence, efforts have been made to compile the latest scientific information on food nutrition, science, and technology for a better understanding of each division.

The book addresses comprehensive picture on three aspects of food. Part I - Food nutrition, which covers fundamental of food and nutrition, macronutrients, micronutrients, nutritive value of plant and animal based food and dietary allowance in the normal life cycle and various diseases. Part II - Food science which includes food sources, nutritional benefits maximization, food selection, food storage, food enzymes, food additives, food preservation techniques, food quality evaluation and food packaging. Part III - Food technology which deals processing techniques of various products of cereals, pulses, nuts and oilseeds, fats and oil, fruits, vegetables, spices, mushrooms, sugar cane, tea, coffee, milk, meat, poultry and fish, processing waste utilization and food safety.

We express our sincere gratitude to Mr. Prabhat K. Singh (Vice President, Intel Corporation) for his continuous encouragement and inspiration to author this book. His insightful and thought-provoking discussions on the topics went a long way in improving the quality of this work. We would also like to thank Dr. Anita Singh (Ph.D., Home Sciences) for giving critical suggestions and providing computer facilities in preparation of this manuscript. We all also express our sincere thanks to Woodhead Publishing India Pvt. Ltd., New Delhi for publishing this book.

Neelam Singh
I. S. Singh

Part I
Food Nutrition

1

Fundamentals of food and nutrition science

Food is vital for human existence. Food is defined as any nourishing substance that is eaten, drunk or otherwise taken into the body to sustain life. Food is the raw material from which our body is made. Food supplies nutrients to perform important functions in the body. The food we eat is digested and used for growth and development. Foods provide energy for doing work. Foods are classified on the basis of origin such as plant and animal, function and chemical composition. Plant-based foods are cereals, pulses, oil seeds and nuts, fruits and vegetables, spices and herbs and sugars. Animal-based foods are milk and milk products, eggs, fish and meat and meat products. Functional foods are energy yielding, bodybuilding and protective foods. Chemical composition includes carbohydrates, protein, fats, water, vitamins, minerals, etc.

1.1 Function of food

Food that we eat contains nutrients. There are over 40 essential nutrients, which are furnished by the food. These nutrients can be classified into six major categories. These are proteins, carbohydrates, water, fats, vitamins and minerals. The chief function of the food is to supply energy to meet physiological needs and to maintain the body in good health, but it serves other functions also. The functions of food have been broadly divided into three categories.

- Physiological function
- Social function
- Psychological function

1.1.1 Physiological function

It refers to the role of food in maintaining certain specific body functions which are discussed in the following sections.

1.1.1.1 Supplies energy

Food gives us energy. The body needs a constant supply of energy to carry out the voluntary and involuntary activities. Voluntary activities include physical activities like sitting walking, playing, performing household and professional tasks. The involuntary process includes activities performed within the body, such as beating of heart, contraction of the intestine, expansion, contraction of the lungs, etc. Besides this, energy also required for metabolism or digestion of food and regulation of body temperature. Energy is mainly provided to our body through carbohydrates and fats present in the food called body fuels.

1.1.1.2 Bodybuilding

Food provides materials for tissue building, growth and body repair which is mainly supplied through foods like proteins and minerals. The muscles, bones and different parts of the body are built up and maintained by the proteins provided by the food. Minerals like calcium, iron and phosphorus affect the formation of blood and skeleton tissue or bones.

1.1.1.3 Protective function

The protective function of food refers to the role in preventing infection by ensuring proper functioning of the body systems responsible for fighting infections. For example, consumption of vitamin A and vitamin C rich food help in building resistance in the body to fight against invading organisms.

1.1.1.4 Regulatory function

It refers to the role of food in regulating the activities of the body, such as the beating of the heart, maintenance of body temperature and contraction of muscles, control of water balance, clotting of blood, removal of waste products from the body, etc. Each of these processes is controlled. Our body temperature, for example, is maintained at 98.4°F or 37°C. Similarly, the rate at which the heart beats is also maintained. For any of these processes, one or the other nutrients is responsible. For example, vitamins of the B groups are an integral part of the enzymes and are responsible for metabolizing food and thus release energy. Vitamin K is an essential factor in clotting of blood. Vitamins, minerals, proteins and water contribute substantially to both protective and regulatory functions.

1.1.2 Social function

Food and eating have significant social meaning. It has been a part of our community, social, cultural and religious life. Food has been used as an expression of love, friendship, and social acceptance. Special foods are distributed as a benediction in the religious functions in homes, temples and churches. Feasts are given at specific stages of life, such as birth, naming ceremony, birthdays, marriages, etc. Most of the religious festivals also call for feasts and feeding of specific segments of the population. Certain menus are associated with most of these feasts in each region. Here the menu plays an important role, and the nutritive value of it is not given much emphasis. Further, people of a given religious community share a common eating pattern. Culture influences the difference in the habitual consumption of certain foods and in traditions of preparation, and in certain cases can lead to restrictions such as the exclusion of meat and milk from the diet.

Thus, food is much more, than a substance supplying nutrients for health. It is the sum of social, cultural, traditional and emotional means of communication.

1.1.3 Psychological function

Foods also satisfy the emotional needs of human beings. These include a sense of security, love and attention. People grow in a particular culture with its own unique food habits of that culture and caste. Traditional habits are characterized by certain foods, which are pleasing to persons in a particular culture. Familiar foods make people feel secure, and foods which are unfamiliar, even a nutritionally balanced meal may not be satisfying to the individual.

Food is also used as a weapon, when an insecure child refuses to eat, thereby drawing the attention of the parents especially the mother. On the contrary, food also serves as a reward. When parents' wishes to reward child, they buy sweet or an ice cream, which evokes pleasant feelings in the mind of the child for that particular food.

Food also serves as a coping mechanism to deal with emotional feelings such as stress, boredom or anxiety, even to prolong feelings of joy, some people eat more and some eat less than normal when experiencing such conditions.

1.2 Food nutrients

A nutrient is a component in foods that an organism uses to survive and grow. Nutrients are substances that provide energy for physical activities, digestion and regulation of body temperature. It also provides materials for the growth and repair of the body, and for keeping the immune system healthy. If these nutrients are not present in our food in sufficient amount, could lead to ill health and in severe cases, death. The human body requires a wide range of nutrients to stay healthy such as 'macronutrients' and micronutrients. Macronutrient is a major nutritional component present in relatively large quantities, such as carbohydrates, protein, fat and water. Micronutrients are present in relatively small amounts, such as vitamins and minerals.

Many other non-nutritive components also present in food such as colours (natural and synthetic), flavours, additives, dietary fibre, phytochemicals, flavonoids and various contaminants such as pesticides which have a significant impact on health, whether beneficial or toxic. For example, most dietary fibre is not absorbed by the human digestive tract but is important in maintaining the bulk of a bowel movement to avoid constipation. Some food additives cause harmful side effects. Therefore, food is a mixture of nutrients and non-nutrients.

The character of food gets altered during processing and cooking. The chemical nature of food is changed by storage, preservation and cooking. Food chemicals can interact among themselves within the body. For example, the availability of iron in the body from plant sources depends on the amount of vitamin C present in the food eaten. The way in which carbohydrate is absorbed from the bowel depends to some extent on the presence of dietary fibre, even though the fibre itself is not absorbed. Preservation of meat requires nitrites, which give them its characteristic pink colour. Cooking can cause changes in the colour, flavour, texture and nutritional value of foods.

The size of food particles can also affect the extent to which nutrients are digested and made ready for absorption by the body. For example, eating a whole apple has a nutritional value different from drinking an apple juice. Nutrients can be more easily absorbed from peanut butter (paste) than from the peanuts eaten whole. The smaller and finer the texture, the more easily it gets digested.

Most of the nutrients can be stored to a lesser or greater extent in our bodies. The macronutrients that provide energy are stored in the liver and muscles in the form of a carbohydrate called glycogen, and fat is stored in fatty tissues or adipose tissue in the form of triglycerides.

Micronutrients such as fat-soluble vitamins like vitamins A tend to be stored in the liver and do not need to be replenished everyday. However, water-soluble vitamins like vitamin C, and most of the vitamin B are excreted in the urine and need to be replenished everyday. Some nutrients, for example, calcium and phosphorus, are stored in bone. Thus, some nutrients are stored internally, while others are required more or less continuously. Poor health can be caused by a lack of required nutrients or, in some cases, too much of a required nutrient. For example, both salt and water (both absolutely required) will cause illness or even death in excessive amounts. Through balanced diet, body obtains the fuel and nutrients it needs to accomplish various bodily tasks.

1.2.1 Function of nutrients

The chief functions of various nutrients are given in Table 1.1.

Table 1.1. Main functions of nutrients.

Nutrients	Main function
Carbohydrates	Provide energy needed by our body
Fat	Concentrate source of energy, carriers of fat-soluble vitamins and source of essential fatty acids
Protein	Bodybuilding of new tissue and its maintenance and repair
Water	Necessary for utilization of food material in the body, elimination of food waste and maintenance of body temperature
Vitamins	Fat- and water-soluble vitamins are needed for growth and normal function of body
Minerals	Necessary for bodybuilding bones, teeth and structural part of soft tissue
Fibre	Essential component of our diet helps in constipation

1.3 Nutraceutical

Nutraceutical word consists of nutrition and pharmaceuticals. It means that food extracts can be used as preventing drugs or food supplement. Phytochemical present in food stuff prevent diseases. The major phytonutrients that have nutraceutical properties are phenolics, terpenes, phytosterols and thiols.

Phenolic is a large group of phytonutrients which has great importance in preventive medicine. Phenols have protective action against oxidative change of tissue and inflammation. Coloured grapes, barriers and brinjal are rich in phenols. The major subclasses of phenolic group are flavonoids (phytochemicals), flavonols (anthocyanidins) and isoflavones (genistein, daidzein).

Terpenes are a largest class of phytonutrients. They are found in soya products, green vegetables and grains.

Phytosterole is another major class of phytonutrients found in all plants. The rich sources which have nutraceutical functions are yam and pumpkin seeds.

Thiol is a major sulphur-containing class of phytonutrients. The food sources of thiol are garlic, onion, mustard and cruciferous vegetables. The important subclasses of thiol are glucosinolates, allylic sulphides, indoles and tocopherols.

1.4 Food groups

Grouping of foods on the basis of nutrients provided by them is known as food groups. Foods are classified into different groups for the convenience of planning diets. These food groups are basic 4, basic 5 and basic 7 which have been given in Table 1.2.

Table 1.2. Food groups and their nutrients.

Food group	Nutrient
Basic 4	
1. Milk and milk products and animal foods	Protein, calcium and B vitamins
2. Oil fats, nuts and oil seeds	Energy and protein
3. Vegetables and fruits	Vitamins, minerals and fibre
4. Cereals, millets and pulses	Energy, protein and B vitamins
Basic 5 - ICMR	
1. Cereals, grain and products: Rice, wheat, maize , ragi, bajra, jwar, rice flakes, puffed rice	Energy, protein, thiamine, riboflavin, folic acid, iron and fibre
2. Pulses and legumes: Bengal gram, black gram, cow peas, dried peas, kidney bean (rajma) and soya bean	Energy, protein, thiamine, riboflavin, folic acid, calcium, iron and fibre
3. Milk and milk products: Milk, curd skimmed milk, cheese, chicken, liver, fish, eggs and meat	Protein, fats, riboflavin and calcium
4. Fruits and vegetables	
• Mango, guava, tomato, papaya, orange, sweet lime, watermelon	Carotenoids, ascorbic acid, riboflavin, folic acid, iron and fibre
• Green leafy vegetables: Amaranth, spinach, drumstick leaves, coriander leaves, fenugreek leaves	Riboflavin, folic acid, calcium, fibre, iron, carotenoids
• Other vegetables: Carrot, onion, brinjal, okra, beans, capsicum, drumstick, cauliflower	Carotenoids, folic acid, calcium and fibre
5. Fats and sugar:	
• Fats: Butter, ghee, cooking oils, hydrozenated fat	Energy, essential fatty acid and fat-soluble vitamins
• Sugar and jaggery	Energy and iron
Basic 7	
1. Orange, grapefruit, tomato, cabbage	Ascorbic acids
2. Green and yellow vegetables	Carotenoids, ascorbic acid and iron
3. Potatoes and other vegetables	Vitamins, minerals and fibre
4. Milk and milk products	Protein, calcium, phosphorus and vitamins
5. Meat, poultry, fish and eggs	Protein, phosphorus, iron and B vitamins
6. Bread, flour and cereals	Carbohydrates, thiamine, niacin, riboflavin, iron and fibre
7. Butter/fortified margarine	Vitamin A and fat

1.5 Nutrition and health

Nutrition is the science that deals with food and nourishment, especially in humans. According to World Health Organization (WHO), 'Nutrition is the intake of food, considered in relation to the body's dietary needs'. The most comprehensive definition of nutrition is given by the American Medical Association's Council on Food and Nutrition which states 'The science of food, the nutrients and other substances therein, their action, interaction, and balance in relation to health and disease and the processes by which the organism ingests, digests, absorbs, transports, utilizes and excretes food substances'.

Nutrition is essential for our health and well-being of patients. Nutrition helps growth and development, prevents malnutrition, resists infection and prevents diseases.

1.5.1 Nutritional status

Nutritional status is the state of our body as results of consumed foods and their use by the body. Nutritional status can be assessed by various methods which are as follows.

- Dietary and nutritional intake examination
- Anthropometric measurements
- Biochemical evaluation of nutrients or their metabolism in body fluids and tissue
- Clinical assessment
- Study of vital statistics
- Assessment of ecological factors

Assessment of nutritional status helps to identify the possible occurrence, nature and extent of impairment, if any of nutritional status which may range from deficiency to excess so that appropriate dietary interventions can be initiated.

Nutritional status can be good or poor. Good nutrition is also known as optimum nutrition or adequate nutrition. It can be described as an adequate, well-balanced diet combined with regular physical activity. Poor nutrition leads to reduced immunity, increased susceptibility to disease, impaired physical and mental development, and reduced productivity. Poor nutritional status may be due to the result of poor food selection, irregular meal times, work, sleep and elimination. The characteristics of good and poor nutritional status are given in Table 1.3.

Table 1.3. Characteristics of good and poor nutrition.

Good nutritional status	Poor nutritional status
Good natural personality	Irritable personality
A well-developed body with normal weight for height	Undersized poorly developed body with abnormal weight
Healthy skin	Pale skin
Well-developed and firm muscle	Muscle small and flabby
Clear eyes	Dull eyes
Good layer of subcutaneous fat	Very little or much subcutaneous fat
Good appetite	Poor appetite
Excellent general health evident by stamina for work, sound regular sleep and resistance to disease	Lack of vigour and susceptibility to infection

1.5.2 Nutritional problems

Nutritional problems occur in India are as follows:

1. Anaemia: Adolescent girls and pregnant women
2. Stillbirth: Birth of dead baby
3. Low birth weight: <2.5 kg
4. Kwashiorkor: Children 1–4 years of age
5. Stunted growth: Abnormal growth in terms of height and weight
6. Under weight: Adult 50%
7. Over weight: Obese in school children
8. Diabetes: Above the age of 50 years
9. Hypertension: Both male and female adults suffer more in urban area
10. Cardiac problem: More in males
11. Cancer: More in females
12. Cataract: Vitamin A and vitamin C deficiencies
13. Night blindness: Vitamin A deficiency after 50 years
14. Goitre: Iodine deficiency more in females

1.5.3 Malnutrition

Malnutrition is the result of deficiency or excess or imbalance of nutrients. The term malnutrition also covers the terms undernutrition, over nutrition, imbalance and specific deficiency. Undernutrition is the state of an insufficient supply of essential nutrients. Over nutrition refers to an excessive intake of one or more nutrients which creates a stress in the body function. Imbalance is the pathological state resulting from a disproportion of essential nutrients. Specific deficiency is the pathological state resulting from absolute lacking of an individual nutrient. The causes of malnutrition are:

- Social factor such as literacy, ignorance and income
- Over population due to increased birth rate
- Cultural factors such as religion, traditional children rearing practices and traditional cooking and eating habit
- Agriculture such as poor soil, lack of rains, attack of insects and pests and inadequate storage facility for various foods

1.5.4 Dietetics

Dietetics is a branch of nutrition that deals with the study of diets in health and disease. Diet means whatever we eat and drink each day. Diet includes the normal diet we consume and the diet people consume in group. Diet can be modified and used for ill person as part of their therapy. Types of diet used in hospitals are clear fluid diet, full fluid diet, soft diet and normal diet.

1.5.5 Therapeutic nutrition

Diet in diseases is called therapeutic nutrition or diet therapy. Diet therapy refers to the use of diet in the case of sick and also in the prevention of disease and maintenance of health. The purposes of therapeutic diet are:

- Deficiency correction which may occur
- Maintaining good nutritional status
- Ascertaining body's ability to metabolize the nutrients
- Changing body weight whenever necessary

Factors affecting in planning of therapeutic diets are duration of the disease, disease condition which need a change in the diet, dietary factors which should be observed and tolerance of patient for food by mouth.

1.5.6 Health

The definition of health proposed by the WHO is 'Health is a state of complete phvsical, mental and social well-being and not merely the absence of disease or infirmity'. The essential dimensions or requisites of health include:

- Fulfilment of optimum growth and development that reflex the full expression of one's genetic potential
- Structural integrity and functional efficiency maintenance of the body tissue essential for an active and productive life

- Ability to resists infections, effect of environmental toxins and pollution and retarding or preventing the degenerative diseases like cancer
- Ability to retard or withstand ageing process with minimal functional impairment
- Ability to live in harmony with others or social well-being
- Mental health

1.6 Food digestion, absorption and utilization

The use of food in the body involves three processes which are digestion, absorption and utilization of nutrients.

Digestive System

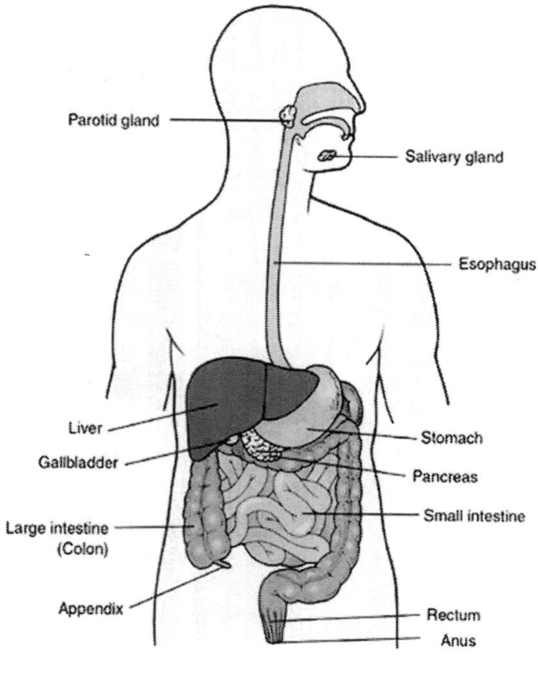

1.6.1 Food digestion

Digestion involves the mixing of food, its movement through the digestive tract and the chemical breakdown of the large molecules of food into smaller molecules.

1.6.2 Mouth

The processes of digestion begin in the mouth where the food is broken down into smaller pieces by the chewing action of the teeth and moistened by saliva. Saliva contains the starch (carbohydrate)-digesting enzyme amylase which breaks down starch into smaller molecules. It also helps to lubricate the food particles for easier swallowing.

1.6.3 Stomach

Chewed food in the mouth is swallowed and passes into the stomach through a long tube called oesophagus that extends from the bottom of the throat to the top of the stomach. The lining of the stomach secretes acidic gastric juice, which contains hydrochloric acid and pepsin, an enzyme that acts on protein and brings about their partial digestion. Peristaltic movements of the stomach wall mix and churn the food with the gastric juices, which further break up the food particles and convert it into a thin soup-like consistency.

1.6.4 Small intestine

Partially digested food from the stomach is pushed along the small intestine by muscle contractions called peristaltic waves. Here most of the digestion takes place. The small intestine contains intestinal juice secreted from the intestine, pancreatic juices from the pancreas and bile from the liver. Both intestinal and pancreatic juices contain enzymes. Partially digested food is mixed with digestive enzymes, bile and pancreatic juices. Digestive enzymes present in the small intestine are trypsin, pancreatic lipase and pancreatic amylase. Trypsin helps in the breakdown of protein, pancreatic lipase helps in the breakdown of fat and pancreatic amylase helps in the breakdown of carbohydrates. Bile aids in the digestion and absorption of fats in the small intestine. Nutrients are absorbed here through the intestinal wall into the bloodstream.

1.6.5 Large intestine

The food which is not absorbed in the small intestine along with water moves on into the large intestine. Here most of the extra water is reabsorbed and the remaining waste material is stored as faeces before being removed by defecation.

1.6.6 Factors affecting digestion

The factors that affect digestion process are

- Food conditions: Cooked foods are more digestible than raw foods.
- Psychological factors: Accepted or liked food increases secretion of saliva and stomach juice due to smell and taste, whereas unliked food depresses the secretion, resulting in poor digestion.
- Sound teeth to bite helps digestion, whereas options of molars and incisors affect the ability to grind hence, poor digestion.
- Sufficient water supply increases the efficient enzymatic break down and helps digestion.
- Adequate fibre helps to normal movement.
- Normal secretion of enzymes and presence of friendly bacteria in the intestinal tract helps digestion.
- Relaxed body permits normal digestion, whereas in stress or tense person upset the digestion process.

1.6.7 Food absorption

Absorption of food is the movement of digested food or nutrients across the intestinal wall to the bloodstream. Digested food particles are primarily absorbed in the small intestine. The inner lining of the intestine is covered with many finger-like projections called villi. The villi greatly increase the intestinal surface area available for absorbing digested material. Within each villus (singular for villi) is blood capillaries and a lymph capillary called lacteal. Digested food molecules are absorbed through the walls of the villus into both the capillaries (amino acids and carbohydrates) and the lacteals (lipids). The absorbed substances are transported via the blood vessels to different parts of the body where they are used to build complex substances such as the proteins required by our body.

1.6.8 Food utilization

Cell is the basic or functional unit of life. Therefore, a large number of the chemical reactions in the cell utilize the nutrients absorbed to produce materials needed for our existence.

1.7 Balanced diet

A balanced diet contains different types of food in such quantity and proportion that meets the needs of all nutrients adequately with a small provision for extra nutrients as a margin of safety. The safety margin is added to cover factors such as period of low intake/leanness/conditions of stress, variation of requirement from individual to individual and cooking losses.

1.7.1 Planning of balance diet

Balanced diet are planned based on recommended dietary intakes using various food groups is never generalized and suitable for all individuals. Firstly, balance diet are individual specific for given age and sex. Secondly, balanced diet is always region specific according to the availability of food in the region. Thirdly, balanced diets are income specific or depending on income.

1.7.2 Steps involved in planning of balance diet

- Identify individual with specific characteristic such as age, sex, activity level, income, socio-economic background, religion and region.
- Consulting recommended dietary intake for protein and energy.
- Determine total amount of specific groups such as energy yielding (cereals, routes and tubers, fats and oil, sugar and jaggery), bodybuilding (milk and milk products, meat, fish, egg and pulses) and regulatory/ protective (fruit and vegetables including green leafy vegetables).
- Decide on number of meals to be taken or consumed.
- Distribute total amounts between decided number of meals.
- Decide on items and its amount within each group for each meal.
- Check days diet for inclusion of specific food group in the amounts decided.

1.7.3 Use of recommended dietary allowance in planning balance diet

The recommended dietary allowances (RDAs) or intakes (RDIs) are the amount of a nutrient to be actually consumed to meet the requirements of the body. RDAs are, hence, based on requirements. The requirement for a specific nutrient is the minimum amount that needs to be consumed to prevent deficiency symptoms and to maintain normal levels of nutrient in the body. The RDAs are basically the requirement + a safety margin.

1.7.4 Salient features of RDA/RDIs

- RDA/RDIs are set high enough to meet the needs of almost all healthy people.
- RDAs do not apply to those people who are suffering from diseases that affect the nutrient needs.
- RDA for adults is based on age, sex, body size and activity level.
- RDA is expressed in kilo calories, gram, milligram and microgram.

- RDA for energy of adult men and women is based on activity level.
- RDA for protein is based on body weight (1 g/kg body weight).
- RDAs for energy and protein are given as additional intake in expectant and lactating due to physiological stress.
- RDA for vitamin A is given in terms of retinol or in terms of β-carotene.
- RDAs for thiamine, riboflavin and niacin are energy dependent. These three vitamins play role in release of energy from carbohydrate, fat and proteins.
- RDAs for thiamine, riboflavin and niacin are 0.5, 0.6 and 6.6 mg/1000 kcal, respectively.
- RDAs for energy, protein, iron, thiamine, riboflavin and niacin in infants are expressed as per kilogram body weight.
- The quantity of different foods to be consumed will depend on the RDA.

World is moving fast and food industry is expanding with number of newer food products, convenience food (packaged food partially precooked) and fast food (ready to eat foods) which are available most of the time of the day are being added everyday. Thus it becomes important to sensitized consumer and food industry personal for nutrition, health and hygiene or sanitation so that food and food products are conductive to good health.

2
Macro nutrients: Carbohydrate and water

2.1 Carbohydrates

Carbohydrates are formed in the plants from carbon dioxide of the atmosphere and water by photosynthesis in sunlight. Thus, solar energy is stored as chemical energy in the form of carbohydrates (starch and sugar). Carbohydrates contain the elements carbon, hydrogen and oxygen. Each gram of carbohydrate consumed gives 4 kcal of energy to the body. Carbohydrates are found in the form of starch, sugar and fibre.

Starch is present mainly in cereals such as wheat, rice, jowar, bajra, ragi and in tuber and root vegetables like potato, tapioca, sweet potato, yam and *Colocasia*. Pulses also contain substantial amounts of carbohydrates but they are more important in our diet as a source of protein.

Sugars are high in fruits like mango, banana, chiku and root vegetables like beetroot and in cane sugar or cube sugar and other sweeteners like jaggery, honey, etc.

Fibre refers to number of indigestible carbohydrates like cellulose present in plant foods.

2.1.1 Classification

Carbohydrates are classified into four major groups. These are monosaccharide, disaccharides, oligosaccharides and polysaccharides.

2.1.1.1 Monosaccharide (simple sugars)

The word monosaccharide is derived from coupling of two words where mono means 'one' and saccharide means 'sugar'. Monosaccharide can also be called simple sugar because it cannot be hydrolyzed further into a simple form. These are the only sugars that can be absorbed and utilized by the body. In monosaccharide, the number of carbons usually ranges from three to seven. Depending on the number of carbons in the sugar, simple sugar also may be subdivided into biose (glycolic aldehyde), triose (three carbons), tetrose (four carbons), pentose (five carbons) and hexose (six carbons).

The common single digestible sugars of importance in nutrition are discussed as follows.

1. Glucose: Present in honey, fruits, corn syrup, sweet grapes, sweet corn; hydrolysis of starch and cane sugar
2. Fructose: Found in honey, ripe fruits and some vegetables
3. Galactose: It is found in milk; synthesized in the body to make lactose

2.1.1.2 Disaccharides (2-sugar units)

Disaccharides are carbohydrates which can be hydrolyzed into two units of monosaccharides. In other words, a disaccharide is composed of two monosaccharides, that is, two sugar molecules. Disaccharides are also digestible. These are sucrose, maltose and lactose.

1. Sucrose (glucose + fructose): Hydrolyzed to glucose and fructose. Found in cane and beet sugar, maple syrup, molasses and sorghum.
2. Maltose (two glucose units): Hydrolyzed to two molecules of glucose. Present in malted products and germinating cereals; an intermediate product of starch digestion.
3. Lactose: Hydrolyzed to glucose and galactose. Found in milk and milk products.

2.1.1.3 Oligosaccharides

Oligosaccharides yield 2–8 monosaccharide molecules on hydrolysis. Raffinose, stachyose and scorodose, blood group antigens are the examples.

2.1.1.4 Polysaccharides (more than 10 sugar units)

Polysaccharides, also known as complex carbohydrates, are made up of many ('poly' means many) glucose molecules. The polysaccharides are of two types digestible and indigestible.

Digestible polysaccharides

1. Starch: It is the major storage form of carbohydrates in plants which consists of long chains of glucose (a monosaccharide) molecules. It is present in many plant-based food sources such as cereal grains, unriped fruits, vegetables, legumes and tubers.
2. Glycogen (animal starch): The stored form of glucose (monosaccharide) present in animals. Energy store within the body, stored within muscles and the liver and brain. It is present in meat products and seafoods; often called animal starch.

Indigestible polysaccharides

1. Cellulose and hemicellulose: It consists of long chains of glucose (a monosaccharide) molecules. Cellulose forms the chief constituents of the structure of cell wall of plants. Present in skins of fruits, an outer covering of seeds, stalk and leaves of vegetables. It is highly insoluble and resistant to hydrolysis. This is not attacked by digestive enzymes in human beings; hence, passes through the digestive tract. Cellulose is consumed but not digested. It is an important source of 'roughage' or dietary fibre in the diet which reduces constipation.
2. Pectin: It is present in various fruits. Pectin forms a gel in water and has used for setting jam and making various sweet foods.
3. Gums and mucilage: It is found in plant secretion, seed and exudates.

2.1.2 Functions of carbohydrates

2.1.2.1 Primary source of energy for body function

The main function of carbohydrate is to supply energy for the body processes. One gram of carbohydrate provides approximately 4 kcal. Carbohydrates supply a greater part of the energy in the diet more than 50-70% of the total calories in the diet. Some of the carbohydrates are immediately utilized by the tissues and the remaining is stored as glycogen in the liver and muscles and some are stored as adipose tissues for future energy needs.

2.1.2.2 Protein-sparing action

Carbohydrates are mainly utilized by the body for fulfilling the energy needs, thus sparing protein for tissue building and repairing. An insufficient amount of carbohydrates in the diet forces the body to break down proteins for releasing energy instead of using them for the body's growth and development. So, this function of carbohydrates of sparing protein for its primary purpose of bodybuilding and repair of tissues is termed as protein-sparing action.

2.1.2.3 Essential for utilization of fat

Some amount of carbohydrate is needed for the proper utilization of fat in the body. Presence of carbohydrate in the diet prevents the body from breaking down too much fat for energy. Excessive fat breakdown can lead to the accumulation of by-product of fat metabolism, known as ketones. The ketones interfere with the normal functioning of various body processes.

2.1.2.4 Provide energy storage

It also acts as reserve fuel supply in the form of glycogen, stored in muscle and liver. Excess of carbohydrate in the diet is converted into fat and stored in adipose tissues. These are reserve energy material of the body.

2.1.2.5 Constituents of some tissue cells

Carbohydrates are components of nervous tissue, heart valve, cartilage, bones and skin.

2.1.2.6 Imparting flavour and sweetness to foods

Carbohydrate foods add flavour, variety and the diet. Since they are non-irritant, easily digestible when cooked and are consumed as a staple food of human beings.

2.1.3 Dietary requirement

The recommended dietary allowances for energy are given in Table 2.1.

Table 2.1. Daily allowances of energy.

Group	Particulars	Body weight (kg)	Net energy (kcal)
Men	Sedentary work		2320
	Moderate work	60	2730
	Hard work		3490
Women	Sedentary work		1900
	Moderate work	55	2230
	Hard work		2850
	Expectants		+350
	Lactating		
	0–6 months	50	+600
	6–12 months	50	+520
Infants	0–6 months	5.4	92/kg/d
	6–12 months	8.4	80/kg/d
Children	1–3 years	12.9	1060
	4–6 years	18.0	1330
	7–9 years	25.1	1690
Boys	10–12 years	34.3	2190
Girls	10–12 years	35.0	2010
Boys	13–15 years	47.6	2750
Girls	13–15 years	46.6	2330
Boys	16–18 years	55.4	3020
Girls	16–18 years	52.1	2440

The percentage of calories derived from carbohydrates should be at least 40% in well-balanced diet. Carbohydrates calories in the diet also depend on availability of fat and economic condition of the people. Carbohydrates when consumed in excess, they are converted into fat and stored in the body. Carbohydrate deficiency in the diet generally does not occur.

2.1.4 Dietary sources

Foods rich in carbohydrate and energy content are given Table 2.2.

Table 2.2. Carbohydrate and energy content of various foods.

Food sources	Carbohydrate, g/100 g	Energy value (kcal)	Food sources	Carbohydrate, g/100 g	Energy value (kcal)
Cane sugar	99.4	398	Red gram dal	57.6	335
Jaggery	95.0	383	Tapioca	38.1	157
Honey	79.5	319	Sweet potato	28.2	120
Rice milled	78.2	345	Banana	27.2	116
Jwar	72.6	349	Ground nut	26.1	567
Wheat flour	69.4	341	Yam	26.0	111
Bajra	67.5	361	Custard apple	23.5	104
Maze	66.2	342	Potato	22.6	97
Oat	62.8	374	Cashew nut	22.3	596
Bengal gram whole	60.9	360	Chiku	21.4	98
Rajma	60.6	346	*Colocasia*	21.3	97
Field bean dry	60.1	347	Jack fruit	19.8	88
Green gram dal	59.9	348	Coconut dry	18.4	667
Black gram dal	59.6	347	Mango	16.9	74

Foods rich in carbohydrates are cane sugar, jiggery, honey, cereals, pulses and root and tuber vegetables. Fruits such as custard apple, chiku and banana are the fair source of carbohydrates.

2.1.5 Digestion and absorption

Digestion of carbohydrate involves the breakdown of starch and sugar into their simplest unit called glucose. Dietary fibre, which is also a type of carbohydrate found in whole grains, fruits and vegetables, cannot be broken down, digested or absorbed by human beings because stomach and intestine lack the enzymes necessary to digest the fibre (Fig. 2.1).

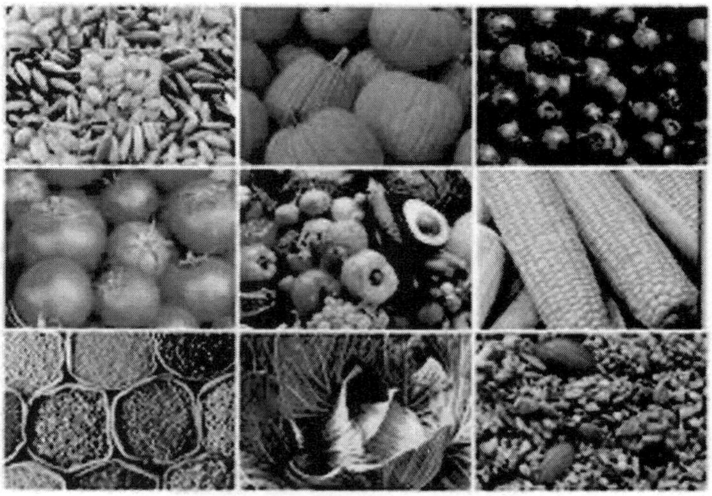

Figure 2.1. Carbohydrate rich food

2.1.5.1 Mouth

The digestion of carbohydrate begins in the mouth. The chewing of food also called mastication breaks food into fine particles. Salivary glands in the mouth secrete saliva, which helps to moisten the food. Saliva also contains an enzyme called amylase (also called ptyalin), which begins the process of breaking of cooked starch into smaller units called dextrose and maltose. However, time available for this enzyme to break down the starch in the mouth is too short to allow any significant amount of conversion to take place. The longer one chews the food, the more the digestion of starch (Fig. 2.2).

2.1.5.2 Stomach

After the carbohydrate food is chewed into smaller pieces and mixed with salivary amylase and other salivary juices, it is swallowed and passed through the oesophagus. The mixture enters the stomach where it is known as chyme. There is no further digestion of chyme, as the stomach produces acid, which destroys bacteria in the food and stops the action of the salivary amylase. There are no carbohydrate-digesting enzymes in the stomach.

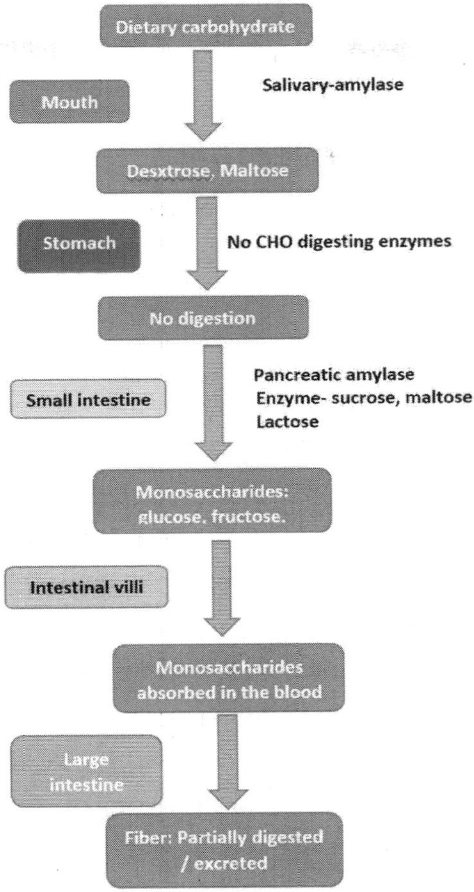

Figure 2.2. Flow chart of digestion process

2.1.5.3 *Intestine*

The main site of carbohydrate digestion is the small intestine. Upon entry of the chyme into the small intestine or the duodenum, the pancreas releases pancreatic juice through a duct. This pancreatic juice contains the enzyme, pancreatic amylase that is capable of breaking down both raw and cooked starch and converts it into smaller units. Additionally, the intestinal cells that line the villi secrete enzymes. These enzymes are sucrose, maltase and lactase. Sucrose breaks sucrose into glucose and fructose molecules. Maltase breaks the bond between the two glucose units of maltose, and lactase breaks the bond between galactose and glucose. Once carbohydrates are chemically broken down into single sugar units (monosaccharides), they are then transported to the inside of intestinal cells.

2.1.5.4 Large intestine

Carbohydrates which are not digested and absorbed by the small intestine reach the colon where they are partly broken down by intestinal bacteria. Fibre, which cannot be digested is excreted with faeces or partly digested by the intestinal bacteria.

2.1.5.5 Absorption and utilization of glucose

Once carbohydrates are broken down into their simplest forms such as glucose, fructose and galactose, they are quickly absorbed into the small intestine by small, finger-like projections, called villi.

After absorption, they are transported to the liver where galactose and fructose are converted into glucose and released into the bloodstream. Some amount of glucose remains in the blood as blood sugar and is taken up directly by the organs that need energy. In the body, glucose is mainly burnt to release energy. The extra glucose is transformed into glycogen (in a process called glycogenesis) for storage in the liver or muscles. Glycogen can be broken down to release glucose whenever needed. But only a limited amount of glucose can be stored in the body as glycogen. Once the limit of glycogen storage is exceeded, the remaining excess glucose is converted into fat and stored in the body.

2.1.6 Effects on human health

2.1.6.1 Excess intake

Excess use of carbohydrates causes problems of obesity and overweight, dental carries and type 2 diabetes mellitus.

2.1.6.2 Obesity

Weight gain occurs mainly due to consumption of refined carbohydrates or simple carbohydrates that have been processed and stripped off fibre. For example, white rice, refined flour, sweets, candies, pastries, cakes, jams, chocolates, soft drinks, etc., and most of them are also high in sugar and fats and provide satiety for a short period. These carbohydrates cause a rapid rise in glucose which stimulate the release of insulin. Insulin promotes fat storage by removing excess glucose from the blood and storing it into fat cell. When the energy intake increased expenditure, the excess is deposited as fat and over a period of time leading to overweight and obesity. Obesity is a predisposing factor for a number of health problems.

Complex carbohydrates such as whole grain cereals, pulses, beans and green vegetables are high in fibre and are important components of balanced diet which help in minimizing several health risks and also help in maintaining or promoting healthy weight loss.

2.1.6.3 *Dental carries*

Dental caries is a disease strongly related to diet. Tooth decay (destruction of tooth structure) is the disease known as caries or cavities. If sugar, milk, raisins, candy, cake, fruit juices, cereals and bread are left or remain with teeth, it can lead to tooth decay. Bacteria that normally live in the mouth change these foods into acids. The combination of bacteria, food, acid and saliva forms a substance called plaque that sticks to the teeth. Over time, the acids produced by the bacteria eat away at the tooth enamel, causing cavities.

Tooth decay can be prevented by following proper oral hygiene, including balanced diet and limiting sugary foods in the diet.

2.1.6.4 *Type 2 diabetes mellitus*

Diabetes is a condition where there is too much glucose (a type of sugar) in the blood, which causes a number of complications. In diabetes, the body cannot properly store and use glucose as fuel. Glucose comes from foods that contain carbohydrates such as bread, cereals, pasta, rice, potatoes, fruits and some vegetables. To use glucose, the body needs insulin. Insulin is made by the pancreas. When the body does not produce enough insulin, it causes an excess of blood glucose (sugar). When the glucose level of the body is too high, it becomes the chronic condition known as diabetes.

Eating in excess of calorie-dense, refined foods and beverages, such as sodas or fruit juices, which absorbs quickly, can cause blood glucose to spike. However, diet rich in raw fruits, vegetables and whole grains can significantly reduce the risk of type 2 diabetes.

2.1.7 Dietary fibre: non-available carbohydrates

Fibre is also an essential component of our diet. It is only found in foods of plant origin. It is edible but non-digestible portion of plant foods. It is also called as bulk or roughage. Fibre is available in two basic forms *soluble* and *insoluble*. Soluble fibrer dissolves in water. Examples are fruits, vegetables and oat bran. Fibre which does not dissolve in water but retains water is called insoluble. This kind of fibre is found in vegetables, whole grains, wheat bran and ragi. Fibre provides bulk in the diet, so food rich in fibre satisfies hunger without contributing excessive calories. The fibrous portion of the foods is beneficial in increasing intestinal peristalsis and consequent relief from constipation and bowel movement.

2.1.7.1 *Function*

The important functions of fibre in the body are as follows:

- Improve digestion
- Prevent constipation
- Reduce cholesterol
- Protects against colon cancer
- Lowering of blood pressure and diabetes

2.1.7.2 *Dietary requirement*

Most of the health agencies recommend that adults should consume 20–30 g of fibre daily in their diet. The dietary allowances for fibre are given in Table 2.3.

Table 2.3. Daily allowances of fibre.

Group	Particulars	Body weight (kg)	Total fibre (g/d)
Men	Adult	60	38
Women	Adult	55	25
	Expectant	55	28
	Lactating	50	28
Infants	0–6 months	5.4	ND
	6–12 months	8.4	ND
Children	1–3 years	12.9	19
	4–8years	18.0	25
Boys	10–12 years	34.3	31
Girls	10–12 years	35.0	26
Boys	14–18 years	47.6	38
Girls	14–18 years	46.6	26

2.1.7.3 *Dietary source*

The fibre content of various foods are given in Table 2.4.

Table 2.4. Fibre content of various foods.

Food sources	Fibre (g/100 g)	Food sources	Fibre (g/100 g)
Coriander seed	32.6	Pomegranate	5.1
Defatted soya flour	18.9	Cape gooseberry	4.8
Pepper dry	14.9	Drumstick	4.8
Sea buckthorn	14.0	Soya nut	4.6
Cumin seed	12.0	Peas dried	4.5
Passion fruit	9.5	Custard apple	4.0

Soya bean	9.3	Fig	4.0
Cardamom seed	9.2	Coconut fresh	3.9
Vermicelli	9.0	Barley	3.9
Rice puffed	7.6	Wheat semolina	3.9
Fenugreek seed	7.2	Black gram dal	3.8
Bael	7.0	Aonla	3.4
Guava	6.9	Grape	3.0
Chili green	6.8	Cluster bean	2.3

- Food rich in fibre are coriander seed, defatted soya flour, dry pepper, sea buckthom and cumin seed, passion fruit, soya bean, cardamom seed, vermicelli, rice puffed, fenugreek seed and bael fruit have good source of fibre.

2.1.7.4 *Effects of fibre on human health*

Deficiency

Diets of low fibre content causes constipation, which is characterized by the difficult and delayed passage of stools.

High intake

Use of large amount of fibre in regular diet irritates the intestinal mucosa and cause digestive upsets. This is the reason that when fruit pulps are given to children as source of vitamin, they are usually strained to reduce the fibre content.

Prevention/cure

Diet should contain adequate amount of fibre as recommended to meet the requirement for relief of constipation in adults.

Use of apple or grape juice which is laxative prevents constipation.

Avoid excessive or regular food which has high fibre content such as mature vegetables, whole cereals and some spices to prevent irritability of intestinal mucosa and digestive disturbances.

2.2 Water

Water is essential for life. Water is a macronutrient made of two elements hydrogen and oxygen. Water is an inorganic compound and is an essential nutrient because it is required in amounts that exceed the body's ability to produce it. All biochemical reactions occur in water. It fills the spaces in and between cells and helps to form structures of large molecules such as protein and glycogen. Water is also required for digestion, absorption, transportation, dissolving nutrients, elimination of waste products and thermo-regulation. Water is the largest constituent of the human body. The total body weight consists of 60-70% of water. The soft tissues contain 70-80% water and bones about 20%. Water is distributed in the body as intracellular water or inside the cells of the tissue and extracellular water or outside the tissue cells. Water is taken as drinking water and in food. Water is also formed in the tissue by the oxidation of hydrogen found in carbohydrates, fat and protein.

2.2.1 Functions

The important functions of water in the body are as follows:

- Water is the major component of our body, which makes about 60% total weight of adult and 75% of infant.
- Water is the medium of all body fluids: blood, saliva, digestive juices, urine, faeces, sweat or perspiration.
- Water regulates body temperature. Heat is produced in the body by the burning of carbohydrate, fat and protein. Water helps to distribute this heat throughout the body and maintain body temperature 37°C.
- Water is universal solvent. Water dissolves a variety of substances including all the products of digestion and carries them to various part of the body via blood.
- Water bathes the body cells. Water helps the body cells moist. Water present in saliva and other digestive juices helps in the passage of food, down the digestive tract. It acts as lubricant for the joints.

2.2.2 Water requirement

Water requirement for human beings is given in Table 2.5.

Table 2.5. Daily water requirement.

Group	Particulars	Body weight (kg)	Total water (L/d)*
Men	Adult	60	3.7
Women	Adult	55	2.7
	Expectant	55	3.0
	Lactating	50	3.8
Infants	0–6 months	5.4	0.7
	6–12 months	8.4	0.8
Children	1–3 years	12.9	1.3
	4–8years	25.1	1.7
Boys	9–13 years	34.3	2.4
Girls	9–13 years	35.0	2.1
Boys	14–18 years	55.4	3.3
Girls	14–18 years	52.1	2.7

* Total water includes drinking water, water-containing foods and beverages.

2.2.3 Sources of availability

2.2.3.1 Ingestion of water in the form of liquids

Intake of water as daily use of water as such and part of beverage such as fruit juices, aerated drink, tea, coffee and coconut water.

2.2.3.2 Ingestion of water in the form of solid foods

Water is present in various types of food stuffs and content varies widely. The water content of some foods are given in Table 2.6.

Table 2.6. Moisture content of food stuffs.

Food stuffs	Moisture (g/100 g)
Vegetables	
Spinach	92.1
Bottle gourd	96.1
Peas	72.1
Mushroom	88.5
Fruit	
Apple	84.6
Banana	70.1
Orange	87.6
Milk	
Cow's milk	87.5
Buffalo	81.0
Fish – Rohu	76.7
Meat	
Goat	74.2
Chicken	72.2
Cereals	
Wheat	12.8
Rice (milled)	13.7
Maize dry	14.9
Pulses	
Red gram dal	13.4
Green gram dal	10.1
Bengal gram dal	9.9

2.2.3.3 Water formed in the body from nutrient metabolism

Water is formed in the body during chemicals reaction such as in metabolism of carbohydrates, fat and protein.

2.2.3.4 Water intake and water loss

Water balance is maintained by the body when water gained by the body is equal to the water lost from the body. The intake and loss of water per day/adult is given in Table 2.7.

Table 2.7. Water intake and loss (balance) in normal human body.

Water intake	L/day	Water loss/output	L/day
Drinking water as such	1.20	Water excreted in urine	1.50
Water intake in diet/food	1.20	Water excreted in stool	0.05
Water formed during metabolism	0.30	Water loss through skin and lungs	1.15
Total intake	2.70	Total loss	2.70

Water intake is approximately equal to water loss from the body; hence, water content of the body is maintained fairly constant. Water intake and loss vary with the climatic conditions. Water requirement or water intake and water loss is generally higher in tropical climate than temperate.

2.2.3.5 Electrolytes

These are positively and negatively charged ions which are in solution in all body fluids. Cellular functions and survival require electrolytes. Total concentration of cations and anions in extracellular fluids (ECFs) and intracellular fluids (ICFs) is equal to maintain electrical neutrality. Sodium is the major cation of the ECFs and comprises over 90% of the total cations. Potassium is the major cation of the ICF. Similarly chloride (Cl^-) and bicarbonate (HCO_3^-) anions predominate in ECFs and phosphate is the principal anion of the ICFs. These four ions sodium, potassium, chloride and bicarbonate in the plasma exerts the greatest influence on water balance and acid base balance.

The balance of body water is closely associated with the balance of dissolved electrolytes. The most important of which are sodium and potassium cations. The osmotic pressure of ECF is determined by the concentration of sodium (Na^+) which accounts for over 90% of the osmolality. Similarly potassium (K^+) determines osmolality of ICFs.

2.2.4 Effects on human health

2.2.4.1 Deficiency

Water is being continuously lost from the body in various ways such as urine, sweet, expired air and faeces. If corresponding amount of water are not compensated or ingested, water deficiency occurs in the body resulting to following changes in the body.

- Decrease in volume of both ICFs and ECFs
- Rapid reduction in body weight
- Reduction in urine output
- Dehydration of cells
- Decrease in plasma and blood volume resulting to reduced cardiac output leading to circulatory failure
- Adult will be seriously ill if 5-10 L of water is lost from the body
- Death may occur if 15 L of water is lost from the body

2.2.4.2 High intake

Kidney responds to excess intake of water or increased water intake load. Normal urine flow of urine/hour rises to its peak 1.5 L/h to maintain the water balance of intake and loss. Over hydration or water intoxification (state of water excess) results due to the retention of excess water in the body which can cause nausea, vomiting, headache, weakness and convulsions.

3

Macro nutrients: Proteins and fats

3.1 Protein

Protein is a class of food nutrients which is a polymer of amino acids. It is composed of carbon, hydrogen, oxygen and nitrogen and often sulphur and phosphorus linked together by peptide bonds. Protein contains various amino acids.

3.1.1 Classification

Protein can be classified on the basis of nutritive value and chemical composition.

3.1.1.1 Classification based on nutritive value

On the basis of nutritive value, protein is classified into three groups: complete protein, partially complete protein and incomplete protein.

1. *Complete proteins*: Complete protein has high nutritive value and contains an adequate amount of all essential amino acids in the required amount and proportions to promote a normal rate of growth. These proteins are primarily of animal origins such as milk protein, egg protein, fish protein and liver protein.
2. *Partially complete proteins*: These proteins have moderate nutritive value and generally partially lacking in one or two essential amino acids, hence, promote moderate rate of growth. These proteins are supplemented with other proteins. These proteins are primarily of plant origins such as cereal and millet proteins, pulse proteins and nuts and oilseed proteins.
3. *Incomplete proteins*: Incomplete proteins have low nutritive value and deficient or completely lack in one or more essential amino acids; hence, they do not promote growth. Examples are gelatin and zein.

3.1.1.2 Classification based on chemical composition

Protein on the basis of chemical composition is classified into three groups: simple proteins, conjugated proteins and derived proteins.

1. *Simple proteins*: These proteins yield only amino acids or their derivatives on hydrolysis. These are of various types:

   - Albumins: Soluble in water, dilute salt solution and dilute acids and bases present in egg albumin, serum albumin and lactalbumin.
   - Globulins: Insoluble in water and soluble in salt solutions and found in arachin and conarchin of peanuts, myosin, etc.
   - Histones: Soluble in most common solvents found in RNA, DNA or nucleoprotein.
   - Other simple proteins are glutlins, prolamins and fibrous proteins (keratin, collagens, etc.).
2. *Conjugated proteins*: Conjugated proteins are combination of simple protein with non-protein substances which are functionally very important to the body. These are of various types:
   - Lipoproteins: Combination of proteins + lipids and found in blood plasma such as high-density lipoprotein (HDL), low-density lipoprotein (LDL), very-low-density lipoprotein (VLDL), etc.
   - Nucleoproteins: Combination of proteins + nucleic acids and found in cells of RNA and DNA, and combination of phosphoproteins (proteins + phosphoric acids) and found in milk casein.
   - Metalloproteins: Combination of proteins + metals and found in ferritin and hemosiderin.
   - Mucoproteins and glycoproteins: Combination of proteins + polysaccharides and found in gastric secretion, that is, mucin.

3. *Derived proteins*: These are proteins derived from simple or conjugated proteins by the action of heat, enzymes or chemical action. Such proteins are proteoses, peptones, peptides, meta proteins, etc.

3.1.2 Properties and functions of protein

3.1.2.1 Amino acid contents of protein

The basic building blocks of proteins are nitrogen-containing units called amino acids.

Amino acids are organic compounds containing acidic or carboxyl (COOH) and basic or amino group (NH_2) which are basic components of protein. Amino acid is required for the formation of tissue protein (during growth) enzymes, blood protein and hormones.

There are 22 or more different types of amino acids. These are vital to human life and health. Of these, 13 are synthesized in the body and nine are not synthesized. These nine amino acids have to be provided in the diet in adequate amount. These are classified as essential amino acids, semi-essential amino acids and non-essential amino acids.

1. *Essential amino acids*: Essential amino acids are those which are not synthesized in the body and these have to be provided in the diet, which include lysine, leucine, tryptophan, threonine, phenyl alanine, methionine, isoleucine, histidine and valine.
2. *Semi-essential amino acids*: Semi-essential amino acids are not synthesized in sufficient amount to meet the rapid growth of infants or pre-mature ones or intestinal metabolic function and need to be supplied in the diet. These are glycine, cystine, arginine, proline and tyrosine.
3. *Non-essential amino acids*: Non-essential acids are synthesized by the body itself and need not be provided in the diet. These are alanine, asparagine, cysteine, serine, aspartic acid, hydroxy proline, glutamic acid and glutamine.

3.1.2.2 Protein quality

Amino acid composition varies in food proteins. The quality of protein depends on types and amount of essential amino acids found in food proteins. Certain food proteins like one or more essential amino acids, for example, lysine is low in cereals high in methionine and pulses are low in methionine and high in lysine. Animal proteins contain all essential amino acids.

Protein quality can be determined by several means such as biological value, net protein utilization, protein efficiency ratio and chemical score. Biological value is a percentage of the absorbed nitrogen retained by the body, and the quality of protein is directly related to its biological value. The biological value increases with the increase in the percentage of nitrogen retained which are absorbed. Proteins of high biological value are egg protein (96), milk (90), fish (80), meat (74), rice (73) and whole wheat (65).

3.1.2.3 Functions of protein

1. *Bodybuilding and repair of tissues*: Protein is a building block of the body, as it contains amino acids that are needed for building new body tissues, maintenance and replacement of worn-out issues. Body uses protein to build and maintain muscles, bone, hair, skin, eyes, blood and organs. They are required throughout life for growth and maintenance.

2. *Maintain body structure and composition*: Structural proteins are fibrous, stingy and provide support. For example, keratin is a type of protein found in hair, nails and skin which helps to give structures strength. Collagen, found in various connective tissues, provides support for the ligaments and tendons.
3. *Helps in the formation of antibodies to fight infection*: Protein is used to build white blood cells and antibodies which prevent infection and disease and thus, participate in the body's immune system.
4. *Forms enzymes and hormones to regulate body*: Proteins also regulate body processes. All enzymes are proteins and are essential catalysts in digestion and metabolic processes in the tissue. Hormones secreted by various glands are protein in nature. Hormones are chemical messengers; they regulate and coordinate body processes and activities. Examples are insulin, thyroxine, growth hormones, etc.
5. *Act as a carrier*: Protein acts as a carrier for the transportation of certain molecules. For example, haemoglobin is a protein that transports oxygen throughout the body. Protein as lipoprotein transports triglycerides, cholesterol, phospholipids and fat soluble vitamins across the cell wall.
6. *Provides energy*: Protein also contributes to body's energy need. If the diet does not furnish enough calories from carbohydrates and fats, proteins are broken down to give energy. One-gram protein yields 4-kcal energy.
7. *Act as a Storage:* It stores nutrients. Casein stores protein in milk, supplies amino acids for baby mammals. Ferritin store iron in the spleen and liver.

3.1.3 Dietary requirements

The protein requirements depend on age and physiological state. Requirements of dietary protein for Indians are given in Table 3.1.

Table 3.1. Daily allowances of protein.

Group	Particulars	Body weight (kg)	Protein (g/d)
Men	Sedentary work		60
	Moderate work	60	
	Hard work		

Women	Sedentary work		
	Moderate work	55	55
	Hard work		
	Expectants		78
	Lactating		
	0–6 months	–	74
	6–12 months		68
Infants	0–6 months	5.4	1.16 g/kg/d
	6–12 months	8.4	1.69 g/kg/d
Children	1–3 years	12.9	16.7
	4–6 years	18.0	20.1
	7–9 years	25.1	29.5
Boys	10–12 years	34.3	39.9
Girls	10–12 years	35.0	40.4
Boys	13–15 years	47.6	54.3
Girls	13–15 years	46.6	51.9
Boys	16–18 years	55.4	61.5
Girls	16–18 years	52.1	55.5

3.1.4 Dietary sources

Protein contents of various foods sources are given in Table 3.2.

Table 3.2. Protein contents of various foods.

Food sources	Protein content (g/100g)	Food sources	Protein content (g/100 g)
Plant sources		*Plant sources*	
Soya bean	43.2	Pistachio nut	19.8
Ground nut	25.3	Dry peas	19.7
Field bean dry	24.9	Gingelly seed	18.3
Green gram dal	24.5	Bengal gram whole	17.1
Cow pea	24.1	Walnut	15.6
Black gram dal	24.0	Oat meal	13.6
Green gram whole	24.0	Wheat flour	12.1
Rajma	22.9	Bajra	11.6
Red gram dal	22.3	Maze dry	11.1
Cashew nut	21.2	Jawar	10.4
Almond	20.8	Rice para boiling	8.5

Bengal gram dal	20.8	Ragi	7.3
Mustard	20.0		
Animal sources		*Animal sources*	
Shrimp (small dry)	68.1	Prawn	19.1
Poultry meat	25.0	Pork muscle	18.7
Beef muscle	22.6	Rohu fish	16.6
Goat meat	21.4	Egg	13.3
Goat liver	20.0		

Among plant-based foods soya bean, ground nut, pulses and dry fruits are rich source of protein. Dry shrimps and various flesh foods such as poultry, goat and beef are good source of protein among animal-based foods.

3.1.5 Digestion and absorption of protein

Dietary protein chiefly consists of small and large chain of amino acids. Digestion of proteins involves the breakdown of amino acid chains in the stomach and in small intestine into their constituent amino acids (Fig. 3.1).

Protein digestion does not begin in the mouth as the saliva contains no proteolytic enzyme which can breakdown protein. Protein digestion mainly occurs in the stomach with the action of an enzyme called pepsin. Pepsin is a protein-digesting enzyme, present in gastric juice of the stomach which breaks the bonds that hold the protein molecule together, called peptide bonds and changes the large protein into short chain of amino acids called polypeptides. Since food remains in the stomach for a limited time, pepsin cannot complete the digestion of proteins. Partially broken down protein or polypeptides from stomach enter into the small intestine where further digestion of protein takes place. In the small intestine, there are several proteolytic enzymes called proteases. The proteases involved in digestion are trypsin, chymotrypsin and carboxypeptidase secreted from pancreatic juice also called pancreatic enzymes. They act on the polypeptides and convert them to even smaller amino acid chains or peptides. Further breakdown of peptides is aided by another proteolytic enzyme called peptidases which convert them into single amino acids.

The amino acids are absorbed in the small intestines, carried by the blood to the liver. Here amino acids are used for building blood proteins or some are retained in the liver to build proteins for its own maintenance and repair and rest of them enter the blood circulation as amino acids. The amino acids are thereby distributed to all the body tissues, where they are taken up by the cells to repair and reform the protein structures wherever needed.

Only protein of good quality is utilized by the body for synthesis of its own protein. Protein which contains all essential amino acids are of good quality as in animal protein, for example, egg, milk, meat, etc. Protein which lacks one or more essential amino acids are of poor quality as in plant-based protein like wheat and pulses.

Thus, the amino acids present in good quality proteins can be utilized optimally for body protein synthesis while the proteins of poor quality are broken down and converted into energy for immediate use.

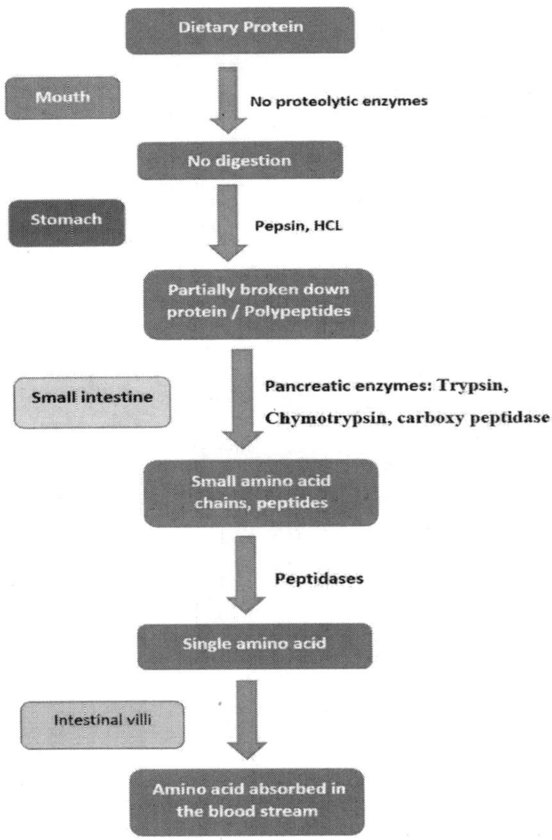

Figure 3.1. Flow chart of digestion of protein.

3.1.6 Effects on human health

3.1.6.1 Protein energy malnutrition

Protein energy malnutrition (PEM) is a range of pathological conditions arising from the deficiency of protein and energy and is commonly associated with infection. In developed countries, PEM deficiency is not a serious problem. However, in developing countries, it is common among young children of age group 1-6 years because their requirement is high due to rapid growth and development. In all forms of PEM, growth failure or low body weight is common

Severe forms of PEM are kwashiorkor, marasmus and marasmic kwashiorkor.

3.1.6.2 Kwashiorkor

Kwashiorkor is a severe form of malnutrition, caused by a deficiency in dietary protein characterized by oedema and very low body weight for age. It is more common among children of age group between 1 and 3 years and is often precipitated by series of infections. This disease occurs when the children who are mostly weaned from the breast althrough their life suddenly switched to a dilute diet high in carbohydrates especially sugar and little protein because of the arrival of a younger sibling.

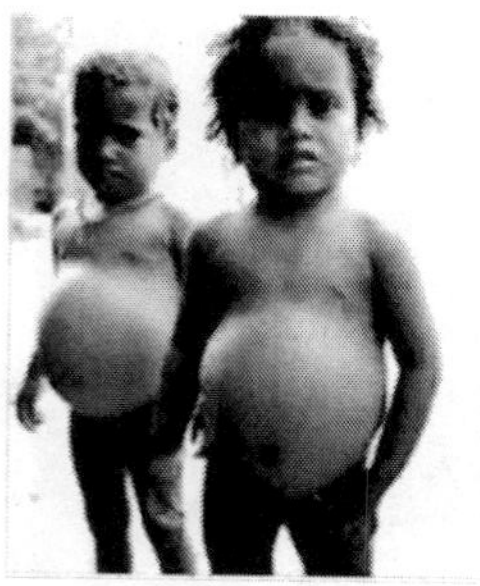

Figure 3.2. Kwashiorkor.

Other signs include a distended abdomen, an enlarged liver with fatty infiltrates, thinning hair, loss of teeth, skin de-pigmentation, dermatitis, irritability and anorexia (Fig. 3.2).

3.1.6.3 Marasmus

Marasmus is an acute form of PEM, more common in infants and very young children. It is characterized by very low body weight and severe wasting of fat and muscle which the body breaks down to make energy.

3.1.6.4 Marasmic kwashiorkor

Deficiency of protein in the diet of children causes this condition. This has characteristic symptoms of both kwashiorkor and marasmus.

Dietary guidelines for prevention are as follows:

- The diet should be rich in protein and calories and other dietary essentials.
- Diet may consist of skimmed milk powder, sugar, banana and cooked cereals. Fat may also be included after a week.
- The daily protein intake 3-5 g/kg body weight and calorie intake should be 140-150 kcal/kg body weight.
- Treatment for any infection (bacterial or parasitic) present.

3.2 Fats and oils (lipids)

Fat and oils are esters of glycerol and fatty acids. They contain carbon, hydrogen and oxygen but the proportion of oxygen present is much smaller than carbohydrates. Fats and oils are more concentrated source of energy than carbohydrates. Each gram of oil or fat supplies 9 kcal of energy. Oils and fats are obtained from plants and animals. Fats and oils are made up of glycerol and fatty acid. A molecule of fat or oil has three fatty acids and a molecule of glycerol called *triglycerides*. Fats and oils are composed of many triglycerides molecule. Both are triglycerides but fats are solid at room temperature (20°C or 68°F), have a relatively high melting point and have a higher proportion of saturated fatty acids, for example, ghee and butter. However, oils are liquid at room temperature (20°C), have a lower melting point and have more unsaturated fat, for example, sunflower, soya bean and sesame oil.

3.2.1 Classification of lipids

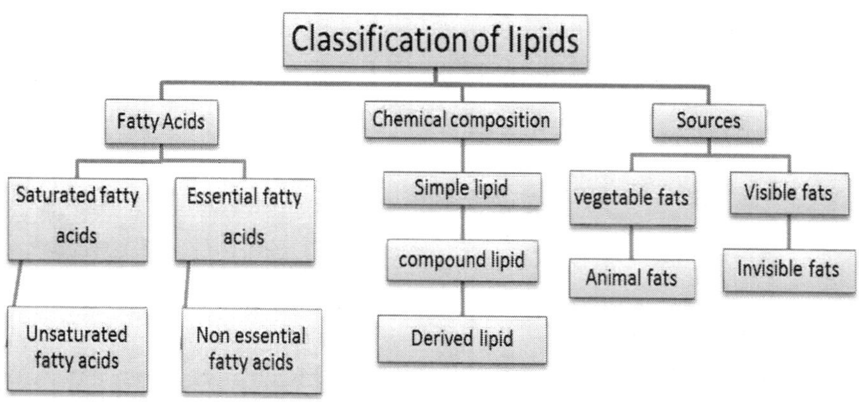

Figure 3.3. Classification of lipids

Lipids can be classified on the basis of chemical composition and fatty acids (Fig. 3.3).

3.2.1.1 Classification based on chemical composition

Lipids based on chemical composition can be classified into three groups: simple lipids, compound lipids and derived lipids.

1. *Simple lipids*: Simple lipids are fatty acid esters of glycerol called triglycerides and they are the major fats present in food like ghee and oil.
2. *Compound lipids*: Compound lipids are simple lipids which combine with proteins (lipoprotein), carbohydrates (glycerol), phosphates (phospholipids), etc.
3. *Derived lipids*: Fats obtained after hydrolysis and digestion are called derived fats like glycerol, fatty acids, cholesterol, etc.

3.2.1.2 Classification based on fatty acids

The major constituents of all fats and oil are fatty acids and glycerol. Fatty acids are mainly composed of long chains of carbon atoms linked to hydrogen atoms.

The number of carbon atoms in fatty acids decides the chain length. On the basis of length of the carbon chain, fatty acids are classified into three groups: (a) *short chain fatty acids* with fewer than six carbon atoms, (b) *medium chain* with 6-12 carbons and (c) *long chains* with 13-21 carbons.

Fatty acids are also classified according to their saturation and essentiality. They are classified as saturated, unsaturated and essential and non-essential fatty acids. These acids occur naturally in foods.

Saturated fatty acids

Saturated fatty acids are fats that contain no double bonds between the carbon atoms, so it is saturated with hydrogen. In other words, saturated fatty acids carry the maximum possible number of hydrogen atoms and have no point of unsaturation. They are mostly found in food of animal origin like meat, eggs and dairy. For example, stearic acid found in animal fats and butyric acid in butter. It is also found in few plant sources. Rich source of saturated fats are coconut, palm oil, mahua oil and butter fat.

Unsaturated fatty acids

Unsaturated fatty acids have one or more double bonds between carbon atoms, and hence, are not saturated with hydrogen atoms and called unsaturated fat. Unsaturated fatty acid lacks some hydrogen atoms and has one or more point of unsaturation. This is divided into two groups: monounsaturated and polyunsaturated.

Monounsaturated acids are fatty acids which have one double bond in the fatty acid chain with all of the remainder carbon atoms being single bonded or contain one point of unsaturation such as palmitoleic found in olive oil, fish oil and beef fat, oleic acid in olive oil and erucic in rapeseed oil. Other plant sources of monounsaturated fatty acid are mustard, groundnut, palm oil and gingelly oil.

Polyunsaturated fatty acids are fatty acids that contain more than one double bond or have two or more point of unsaturation. For example, linoleic present in soya bean, corn, safflower and cottonseed oil, linolenic in mahua, soya bean, rapeseed and mustard oil, arachidonic in fat, liver, meat and eicosapentaenoic in fish oil.

Essential fatty acids

Essential fatty acids are required by the human body but it is not synthesized in the body. Therefore, it must be obtained from foods. They are linoleic, linolenic and arachidonic. These are used by the body to make prostaglandins (hormone-like compounds) which reduce blood clotting rate and clot blocking the coronary arteries. Essential fatty acids play a role in immunity. Low availability of essential fatty acids leads to affect growth, mental and physical capacities.

Fats obtained from the vegetable sources are known as vegetable fat, for example, fat found in groundnuts, soya bean, coconuts, palm oil, etc. Vegetable oils except coconut and palm oils are a rich source of essential fatty acids or unsaturated fats.

Hydrogenation of vegetable oil converts unsaturated fatty acids into saturated fatty acids and partial hydrogenation converts it into trans fats as well and eliminates most essential fatty acid content. It converts liquid vegetable oils into solid or semi-solid fats which increase the shelf life and they are the predominant fat used as shortening in most commercially backed food.

Fats obtained from animal sources like milk, butter, meat, ghee, egg, etc., are known as animal fat.

3.2.1.3 Invisible and visible fats

Invisible fats

Invisible fat is present naturally in many foods, such as nuts, seeds, oil-bearing plants, meat, poultry, fish, dairy products and eggs.

Visible fats

Visible fats are fats prepared from natural food products. Generally, oil-bearing plants store their fat as triglycerols. Sunflower and soya bean store oil in seed endosperm, avocado in flesh mesocarp, palm in mesocarp (palm oil) and in endosperm (palm kernel oil).

3.2.2 Properties and functions of fat

3.2.2.1 Properties

The physical properties of fat are greasy to touch, insoluble in water but soluble in organic solvent and have less specific gravity than water. Fats containing saturated fatty acids are solid at room temperature and fats containing unsaturated fatty acids are liquid at room temperature and fats have definite melting point.

The chemical properties of fat are acrolein formation which has unpleasant smell, hydrogenation, saponification (hydrolysis of fat by alkali) and rancidity that is a chemical change resulting unpleasant smell and taste in storage due to exposure to moisture, heat and air.

The important characteristics of fats are saponification number and iodine number. Saponification is defined as the number of milligrams of potassium hydroxide required to saponify 1 g of fat. It indicates molecular weight such as butter has saponification number of 210-230 and coconut oil 253-262. Saponification number decreases with the increase in molecular weight. Iodine value is the number of grams of iodine absorbed by 100 g of fat. This measures the unsaturated fatty acids found in fats and oils. Higher the iodine number, the higher is the degree of unsaturation.

3.2.2.2 Functions of fat

1. *Source of energy*: Fat is a concentrated source of energy. One gram of fat provides 9 kcal energy which is more than the double the amount of calories from carbohydrates and proteins.
2. *Transporting fat-soluble vitamin*: Fat-soluble vitamins like A, D, E and K are absorbed and synthesized in the body only in the presence of fat. Without fat in the diet, these vitamins would not be able to function. This would result in severe problems with eyesight, skin, nail formation, blood clotting, kidney function, bone growth, repair, etc.
3. *Fats provide essential fatty acids*: Essential fatty acids which are not synthesized in the body; hence, it must be obtained from food. The essential fatty acids are linoleic, linolenic acid and arachidonic acids. They are structural components of all tissues and are important for controlling inflammation, blood clotting and brain development.
4. *Energy store*: Only a small amount of energy is used for body's energy need. The excess calories consumed, which are not required for immediate use, are stored for future use in special fat cells called adipose tissues. Deposited fats in adipose tissues serve as a reserve source of energy during starvation, cold and physiological damage.

5. *Insulation and padding*: Layers of fat stored under the skin also known as subcutaneous fat, act as an insulator and keep the body warm. Many of the vital organs, especially the kidneys, heart and intestines are cushioned by fat that helps protect them from injury and hold them in position.
6. *Provides satiety value*: Fats take more time to digest; therefore, they provide satiety value.
7. *Improves palatability of the diet*: Fats provide taste, flavour and variety to food.
8. *Act as a lubricant*: Fats provide lubrication to skin and digestive organs like stomach, intestine, etc.

3.2.3 Dietary requirements

The recommended dietary allowance for fats and oil is given in Table 3.3.

Table 3.3. Daily allowances of fats and oil.

Group	Particulars	Body weight (kg)	Visible fat (g/d)
Men	Sedentary work		25
	Moderate work	60	30
	Hard work		40
Women	Sedentary work		20
	Moderate work		25
	Hard work	55	30
	Expectants		30
	Lactating		
	0–6 months	50	30
	6–12 months	50	30
Infants	0–6 months	5.4	–
	6–12 months	8.4	19
Children	1–3 years	12.9	27
	4–6 years	18.0	25
	7–9 years	25.1	30
Boys	10–12 years	34.3	35
Girls	10–12 years	35.0	35
Boys	13–15 years	47.6	45
Girls	13–15 years	46.6	40
Boys	16–17 years	55.4	50
Girls	16–17 years	52.1	35

Fat and oils are very rich in butter, ghee, vanaspati, red palm oil, dry coconut, walnut oil, almond oil and pistachio nut. Coconut fresh, ground nut, cashew nut, mustard, gingelly, soya bean, sunflower and egg yolk are also the good source of fats and oils.

Fats of the animal sources (fish, liver oil, butter and ghee) are rich in vitamin A and vegetable fats contain vitamin E.

3.2.4 Dietary sources

The fat and oil content of various foods are given in Table 3.4.

Table 3.4. Fat and oil content of plant- and animal-based food.

Fat and oil sources	Oil and fat (g/100 g)
Plant-based sources	
Red palm oil	100
Vanaspati	100
Walnut	64.5
Coconut dry	62.3
Almond	58.9
Pistachio nut	53.5
Mahua kernel	48.5
Cashew nut	46.9
Gingelly seed	43.3
Coconut fresh	41.6
Ground nut	40.1
Sun flower	40.0
Mustard seed	39.7
Soya bean	19.5
Avocado	16.0
Animal-based sources	
Ghee	100
Butter	86.0
Egg yolk	32.5
Khoa	31.2
Whole milk powder	26.7
Cheese	25.1
Mutton	13.3

3.2.5 Digestion and absorption of fat

Fat in the human diet is mostly in the form of *triacylglycerol*, which consists of three fatty acids linked to glycerol. In the processes of digestion, fat is broken down to its constituent components fatty acid and glycerol (Fig. 3.4).

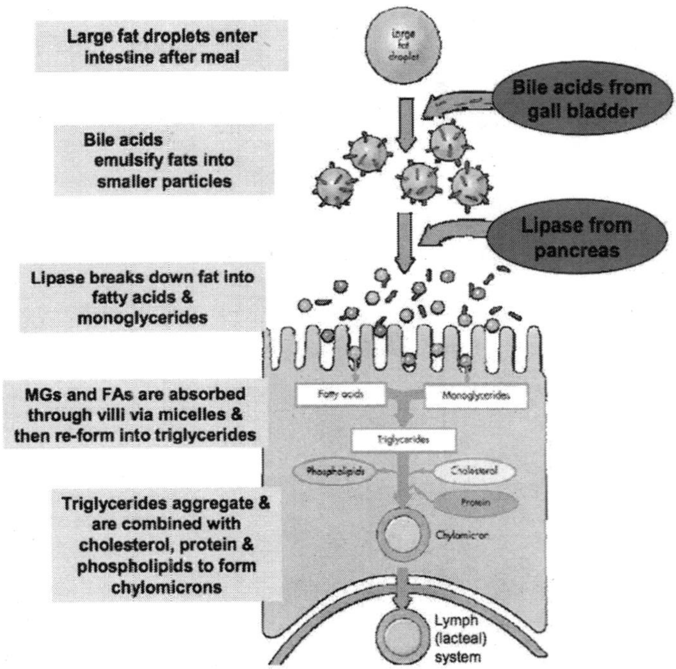

Figure 3.4. Flow chart of digestion and absorption of fat

Fat digestion occurs mostly in the small intestine. The major digestive enzyme in this process is *gastric lipase* present in gastric juice and *pancreatic lipase* poured into the small intestine from the pancreas. The fats in the ingested foods are insoluble in water and clump together to form large fat droplets. For enzyme action, fats need to be dispersed or mixed in water since pancreatic lipase is a water-soluble enzyme. A secretion produced by the liver and stored in the gallbladder called bile mixes with large fat droplet and break them into small droplets. These fat droplets are then dispersed in the liquid digestive juice and are easily acted upon by enzymes. Since bile is not present in the stomach, the action of gastric lipase is not very significant. This is the reason fats are chiefly digested in the small intestine where pancreatic lipase breaks them into glycerol (monoglycerides) and fatty acids aided by the action of bile.

The end products of fat digestion are glycerol and fatty acids that are present in the intestine move into the intestinal cells. The fatty acids cannot enter intestinal cells as such because of low solubility in water. Bile salts play an important role in fat absorption by dispersing the fatty acids into small tiny water-soluble units called micelles which can easily move into the intestinal cells.

After they pass through the small intestine, fatty acids are converted to triglycerides, which combine with cholesterol, phospholipids and protein to form a structure called a chylomicron. The protein coating of the chylomicron makes it water-soluble so it can travel through the lymph vessels to the heart and eventually the blood stream. Blood then carries them either to the adipose tissues where they are stored as concentrated sources of energy or to cells where they are broken down to provide energy.

3.2.6 Effects on human health

Fatty acid in the diet has different effects on human health.

1. *Deficiency*: Deficiency causes dryness of the skin and malnutrition.
2. *Dryness of skin*: Prolonged deficiency of fat in the diet may cause dryness of the skin.
3. *Malnutrition*: Much of the malnutrition particularly in children is due to low intake of fat. The expert group of FAO/WHO recommended that 30% of our total caloric requirement must be met by oil and fats and ratio of saturated and polyunsaturated fatty acid should be 1:1.
4. *High intake*: High intake causes risk of cardiovascular disease, risk of obesity and diabetes, risk of cancer and artherosclerosis.
5. *Risk of cardiovascular disease*: Excess intake of saturated fatty acids and cholesterol in the diet increases the level of serum lipids and LDL cholesterol that causes the risk of cardiovascular disease.
6. *Risk of obesity and diabetes*: Besides cardiovascular disease, high fat intake particularly the saturated fatty acids is also a risk factor in obesity and diabetes.
7. *Risk of cancer*: High intake of fat particularly saturated fatty acids associated with the occurrence of cancer at several sites particularly the breast, prostate and large bowel.
8. *Atherosclerosis*: The blood of normal human beings contains 150-250 mg/100 mL cholesterol. When the blood cholesterol exceeds over 250 mg/100 mL, the incidence of atherosclerosis is high.

Dietary guidelines are as follows:

- Intake of those foods or dietary sources which raise bad cholesterol and increases the risk for heart attack or stroke should be curtailed. These bad fats are present in many foods and are called saturated fat and trans fat. Sources of saturated fat include butter, shortening, red meat, cheese and whole milk. Trans fat is found in some margarine, snack foods and fast foods.

- Limit saturated fat intake by cutting down on eating red meat and whole milk and dairy product. Add beans, legumes, fish or poultry to your diet in the place of the red meat.
- Trans fats can be avoided by lowering or altogether cutting out the processed foods. Include whole grain products and healthy snack alternatives such as nuts and fruits instead of packaged cookies, crackers and snacks.
- Fats rich in essential fatty acid have been found to reduce blood cholesterol level. Polyunsaturated fatty acid, linoleic and linolenic lower the serum cholesterol and serum triglycerides; these healthy fats are found in fish, nuts and vegetable oils.

4

Micro nutrients: Vitamins

The 'vita' part of the word 'vitamin' means 'life'. Vitamins are the organic substances occurring in natural foods either as such or as utilizable precursors which are required in minute quantity for normal growth, maintenance and reproduction. Plants are able to synthesize vitamins whereas animals depend on plants for their supply of vitamins. Vitamins defer from hormones which are supplied with the diet, whereas hormones are produced by glands in the body. Vitamins are usually found within the cell in minute amount and mostly function as co-factors in enzymatic reaction. Vitamins are vital and essential for life and health. They regulate metabolism, help in growth and protect against diseases.

Vitamins belong to several chemical groups. They are classified according to their solubility. Some of the vitamins are soluble in fat while others are soluble in water; hence, they are classified into two categories: fat soluble and water soluble.

4.1 Fat-soluble vitamins

The fat-soluble vitamins generally occur together in the fats and oils of food. The characteristics of fat-soluble vitamins are soluble or dissolve in fat, require bile for absorption, stored in tissues and can be toxic in excess. Fat-soluble vitamins are A, D, E and K.

4.1.1 Vitamin A and carotene

Vitamin A is certainly one of the most versatile vitamin with diverse function. Vitamin A (retinol) is found only in foods of animal origin. Carotene is found in foods of plant origin. It is a precursor of vitamin A and called provitamin A. Among the various carotenoids present in plants, β-carotene is the most important and is the most widely distributed carotenoid among colourful fruits and vegetables. Most of the yellow and orange colour of vegetables and fruits is due to this carotenoid pigment. Green leafy vegetables also contain β-carotene but the yellow and the orange colour of the carotenoid pigments is masked due to the presence of another pigment called chlorophyll which is green in colour.

The body converts these plant pigments into vitamin A. Conversion of β-carotene into vitamin A takes place in the intestinal walls and only half of the β-carotene absorbed is converted to retinol. About 4 μg of β-carotene is equal to 1 μg of vitamin A. Thus people who consume less animal foods need to consume enough plant foods such as green leafy vegetables and orange-yellow fruits to meet vitamin A needs.

Vitamin A is stable to heat (100°C) for a short time in the absence of oxygen but destroyed rapidly by oxidation. It is slowly destroyed in the presence of light.

4.1.1.1 Functions of vitamin A

1. *Maintains normal vision*: Vitamins A occurs in the retina of the eyes. The retina has two kinds of cells, that is, rods and cones. Both rods and cones are sensitive to changes in light. Rods are sensitive to dim light and cones respond to bright light. Rods contain a retinol pigment called rhodopsin needed for vision in the dim light.
2. *Maintain the integrity of the epithelial tissue*: Vitamin A helps in keeping skin and tissue (in the mouth, stomach, intestines, respiratory, genital and urinary system) healthy; hence, protecting against infection and several diseases.
3. *Supporting new cell growth*: It is stimulus for new cell growth and cell division. It has an important role in reproduction, embryonic development and organ formation.
4. *Essential for bone formation*: Vitamin A is essential for growth of skeleton. Bones do not grow to their full length and the overall growth of the body is affected with the deficiency of vitamin A. It increases the release of calcium and phosphate in the bones which is necessity for skeletal growth. Retinoic acid is known to play a hormone-like function in control of growth and development of tissue in musculo skeletal system.
5. *Helps in maintaining healthy immune system*: It is anti-infective. Many of the epithelial tissues are important barrier to infection. Vitamin A helps to maintain the lymphocyte pool. Vitamin A also functions in T-cell-mediated response. The immune response such as immunoglobulin production is affected by retinoids.
6. *Protection against night blindness*: Vitamin A helps eyes to see in the dark by adjusting to the lower level of light.
7. *Protection against diseases*: β-Carotene is a powerful antioxidant that helps the immune system and many chronic diseases. It protects against some epithelial cancers and bronchinal cancers.

4.1.1.2 *Dietary requirement*

Recommended dietary allowances (RDAs) for vitamin A by ICMR are given in Table 4.1.

Table 4.1 Daily allowances of vitamin A.

Group	Particulars	Vitamin A (μg/d)	
		Retinol	β-Carotene
Men	Sedentary work	600	2400
	Moderate work	600	2400
	Hard work	600	2400
Women	Sedentary work	600	2400
	Moderate work	600	2400
	Hard work	600	2400
	Expectant	800	3200
	Lactating	950	3800
Infants	0–6 months	350	1400
	6–12 months	350	1400
Children	1–3 years	400	1600
	4–6 years	400	1600
	7–9 years	600	2400
Boys	10–12 years	600	2400
Girls	10–12 years	600	2400
Boys	13–15years	600	2400
Girls	13–15 years	600	2400
Boys	16–17 years	600	2400
Girls	16–17 years	600	2400

4.1.1.3 *Dietary sources*

The carotene content and its equivalent to vitamin A content of plant- and animal-based foods are given in Table 4.2.

Table 4.2 Carotene/vitamin A content of various foods.*

Plant-based food sources	Carotene (μg/100 g)	Equivalent vitamin A (μg/100 g)	Plant-based food sources	Carotene (μg/100 g)	Equivalent vitamin A (μg/100 g)
Red palm oil	29,000	7250	Chili green	2430	607.5
Amaranth	20,160	5040	Fenugreek leaves	2340	685.0

Sea buckthorn	12,839	3209.7	Persimmon	2268	567.0
Colocasia leaves	10,278	2569.5	Sweet potato	2200	550.0
Spinach	9440	2360	Pumpkin	2100	525.0
Coriander leaves	6918	1729.5	Papaya	2020	505.0
Radish leaves	5295	1323.7	Carrot	1890	472.5
Cape gooseberry	5000	1250	Bathua leaves	1740	435.0
Mango	4800	1200	Raspberry	1248	312.0
Ginger fresh	3027	756.7	Cabbage	1200	300.0
Tomato	3010	752.5	Barbados cherry	1000	250.0
Mustard leaves	2622	655.5	Jackfruit	992	248.0
Carambola	700	175.0	Phalsa	750	187.5

Animal-based food	Vitamin A (retinol µg/100 g)	Animal-based food	Vitamin A (retinol µg/100 g)
Cod liver oil	10,000	Butter	960
Fish liver oil	6000	Ghee	650
Shark liver oil	9000	Egg yolk	600
Liver (sheep)	6690	Egg whole (hen)	420
Liver (goat)	6000	Buffalo milk	60
Whole milk powder	1400	Cow milk	50

* 4 µg carotene = 1 µg vitamin A.

Vitamin A is found almost exclusively in animal products, such as organ meats, liver and cod fish liver oils, egg yolk and whole milk and dairy products such as butter, ghee, etc. Provitamin A carotenoids are found in green leafy vegetables (e.g., spinach, amaranth, colocassia, fenugreek, bathua, pumpkins, sweet potatoes and carrots). Carotenoids are also found in citrus fruits, mangoes, papaya, etc. Red palm oil produced in several countries worldwide is especially rich in provitamin.

4.1.1.4 Absorption

Vitamin A is mostly absorbed in the intestine and passes along with fat through the lymphatic system into the bloodstream. Approximately 90% of the total absorbed vitamin is stored in the liver and the remaining 10% is distributed in other organs and glands like the kidneys, lungs and adrenal glands. Being a fat-soluble vitamin, the presence of bile and fats greatly aids in vitamin A absorption.

4.1.1.5 *Effects on human health*

1. *Deficiency*: Deficiency of vitamin A in the diet causes following disorders:

    - Night blindness: Inability to see and read in dim light
    - Frequent respiratory infection: Reduced resistance to infection
    - Xerophthalmia: Dryness of the conjunctiva of the eyes
    - Bitot's spot: Greyish patches on the white of the eyes
    - Keratomalacia: Opacity of the cornea (Fig. 4.1)
    - Phrynoderma: Failure of growth in children or skin becomes rough and dry with papules
    - Faulty bone modelling

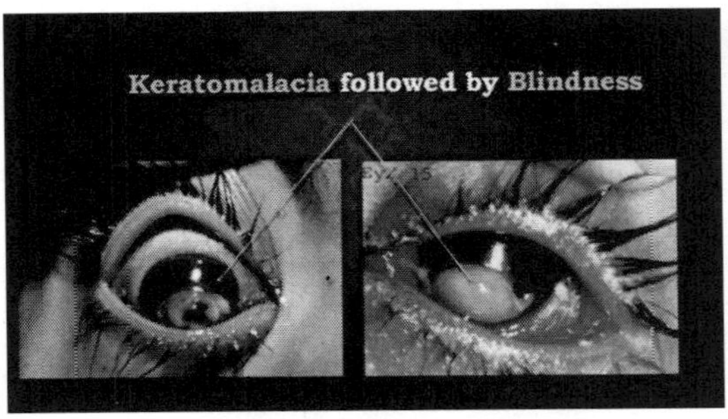

Figure 4.1 Keratomalacia.

2. *High intake of vitamin A*: Vitamin A is fat soluble and stored in the liver. Routine consumption of large amounts of vitamin A over a period of time can result in toxicity but it would be difficult to reach this level consuming food alone. Some multivitamin supplements contain high doses of vitamin A, which could lead to toxicity. β-Carotene from fruits and vegetables are considered safe because it is not converted efficiently into vitamin A to cause toxicity. Children are particularly more vulnerable to toxicity because they need less vitamin A and generally on supplements. Toxicity is characterized by following symptoms:

    - Headache
    - Dry itching of skin
    - Anorexia
    - Swelling over the bones

3. *Prevention/cure*:
    - Diet should contain an adequate level of vitamin A to meet the requirement.
    - Administration of 10,000 μg of fat-soluble vitamin A orally daily for a period of 10 days.

4.1.2 Vitamin D (calciferol)

Vitamin D is unique and different from other fat-soluble vitamins. Body can synthesize it from 7-dehydro cholesterol in the skin of the body by exposure to ultraviolet B radiation from sunlight for a short time over a period of a month; therefore, it is also called as sunshine vitamin. The easiest way to get the vitamin D is through enough exposure to sunlight and do not need to depend only on dietary sources.

Vitamin D is also naturally present in fewfoods of animal origin. It is fat-soluble vitamin and insoluble in water. It is fairly stable to heat. Bile is essential for effective absorption of fats and therefore, of vitamin D.

4.1.2.1 Functions

The functions of vitamin D in human body are as follows:

- It increases the absorption of calcium and phosphorus and regulates their concentration in the blood.
- It helps directly in building strong and healthy bones and teeth.
- Vitamin D regulates cell differentiation and growth.
- Support the health of the immune system.

4.1.2.2 Dietary requirement

The AI for vitamin D recommended by National Academy of Science (USA) is given in Table 4.3.

Table 4.3 Daily allowances of vitamin D.*

Group	Particulars	Vitamin D	
		μg	IU
Men	Adult	15	600
Women	Adult	15	600
Women	Expectant	15	600
Women	Lactating	15	600
Geriatric	Age above 70 years	20	800
Infants	0-6 months	10	400
	6-12 months	10	400

Children	1-3 years	15	600
	4-8 years	15	600
Boys	9-13 years	15	600
Girls	9-13 years	15	600
Boys	14-18 years	15	600
Girls	14-18 years	15	600

* 1 μg of vitamin D = 40 IU.

Tolerable upper intake level (UL) is 4000 IU or 100 μg/d for people ages 9 and over. The UL for infants is 1000-1500 IU/d, for children ages 1–8 years is 2500-3000 IU/day.

The amount of sun needed will also depend on skin colour, age, the time of the day, season and geographic location.

4.1.2.3 *Dietary sources*

Vitamin D is present in foods of animal origin. The vitamin D content of animal-based foods is given in Table 4.4.

Table 4.4 Vitamin D content of animal-based foods.

Animal-based sources	Vitamin D content	
	μg/100 g	IU
Fish cod liver oil	475.0	19,000
Fish cod liver oil BP	200.0	8000
Shark liver oil	65.0	2600
Fatty fish oil	17.0	680
Egg yolk	4.0	160
Egg hen whole	1.5	60
Butter	1.0	40
Ghee	0.85	34
Whole milk powder	0.5	20
Fresh milk	0.1	4.0

The fish liver oils are the richest sources. Foods of animal origin like eggs, liver and butter contain the vitamin D in significant amounts. However, most of the commonly used foods of plant origin do not contain vitamin D.

4.1.2.4 *Absorption*

The ingested vitamin D is absorbed along with fats from the small intestine. After absorption, the vitamin is then taken to the liver. Some of it is stored there and the remaining is distributed by the blood to various body tissues.

4.1.2.5 Effects on human health

1. *Deficiency*: Deficiency of vitamin D causes rickets in children and osteomalacia in adults.

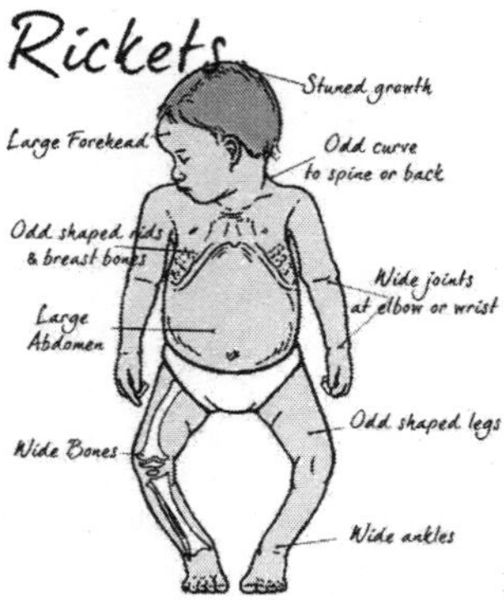

Figure 4.2 Rickets

Rickets in children: The disease is characterized by the following symptoms (Fig. 4.2):

- Rickety rosary
- Bone deformities, that is, pigeon breast, knock knees and bow legs

Osteomalacia in adults: The disorder occurs commonly in pregnant women. It is characterized by the following symptoms:

- Bone deformities (spine bending and leg bowing) occur due to the body weight in pelvis, legs and ribs
- Difficulty in the delivery of baby due to deformities of pelvis

2. *Excess or toxicity*: Being a fat-soluble vitamin, it is stored in the liver, too much vitamin D can be toxic and could lead to confusion, problems with heart rhythm and kidney stone. An overdose is more likely due to dietary supplements of vitamin D, not food. High doses of vitamin D supplements coupled with large amounts of fortified foods may cause accumulations in the liver and produce signs of poisoning. Excessive sun exposure also does not cause vitamin D toxicity because body limits its own vitamin D production. The symptoms of vitamin D toxicity are poor appetite, constipation, weakness, nausea and weight loss.

3. *Prevention/cure*:
   - Diet should contain adequate level of vitamin D (400 IU) to meet the requirement
   - Administration of about 1000-3000 IU vitamin D orally for about 4 weeks followed by 800 IU daily for 6 months
   - Avoid high dose of vitamin D supplement with fortified food to prevent toxicity

4.1.3 Vitamin E

Vitamin E consists of a group of tocopherol. The α-tocopherols are most active form. Vitamin E is widely distributed in plant foods. It is destroyed by high heat. Vitamin E is also present in animal foods. Vitamin E is insoluble in water and soluble in fats and fat solvent. Being fat-soluble vitamin, absorption of vitamin E also requires the presence of fat and bile.

4.1.3.1 Functions

The functions of vitamin E are as follows:

- Prevents oxidation of β-carotene
- Protecting resistance to diseases such as heart, diabetes and cancer
- Essential for reproduction
- Protecting red blood cells from haemolysis by oxidizing agent
- Acts as an antioxidant and protect polyunsaturated fatty acids in membrane cells and tissues
- Protecting liver injury caused by poisoning

4.1.3.2 Dietary requirements

The AI for vitamin E recommended by National Academy of Science (USA) is given in Table 4.5.

Table 4.5 Daily allowances of vitamin E.*

Group	Particulars	Vitamin E (mg)
Men	Adult	15
Women	Adult	15
Women	Expectant	15
Women	Lactation	19
Infants	0–6 months	4
	7–12 months	5

Children	1–3 years	6
	4–8 years	7
Boys	9–13 years	11
Girls	9–13 years	11
Boys	14–18 years	15
Girls	14–18 years	15

* The tolerable UL for teens aged 14-18 is 800 mg/d. For adults, 19 years and above is 1000 mg of α-tocopherol/d.

4.1.3.3 Dietary sources

Vitamin E content of various foods is given in Table 4.6.

Table 4.6 Vitamin E content of various foods.

Food sources	Vitamin E (mg/100 g)	Food sources	Vitamin E (mg/100 g)
Plant source			
Wheat germ oil	255	Hazelnuts	15.03
Soya bean oil	118	Peanuts	8.33
Sunflower seed oil	91	Avocados	2.07
Cotton seed oil	81	Spinach	2.03
Safflower seed	80	Kiwi	1.46
Sunflower seed oil	70	Asparagus	1.13
Ground nut oil	22	Blackberries	1.17
Coconut oil	8.3	Broccoli	0.78
Sunflower seed kernels dried	35.7	Poppy seeds	1.77
Almonds	25.63	Flax seeds	0.31
Animal sources			
Butter	2.4	Mackerel fish	1.52
Egg yolk	2.58	Liver, chicken	0.70
Herring fish	1.07	Lard	2.7

Vegetable oils like wheat germ, soya bean, cotton seed and safflower and sunflower are rich sources of vitamin E. Other good sources are nuts and oil seeds. Dark green vegetables and fruits are fair sources. Foods of animal origin are low in vitamin E. However, foods like egg yolk, butter and liver contain some amount of vitamin E.

4.1.3.4 Absorption

Absorption of vitamin E requires the presence of fat and bile. After absorption from upper part of small intestine, vitamin E as part of chylomicrons is carried to the liver through the bloodstream and is distributed to various body tissues. Mostly all body tissues have small amount of vitamin E but mainly stored in muscles and adipose tissue.

4.1.3.5 Effects on human health

1. *Deficiency*: Deficiency of vitamin E is very rare. Vitamin E deficiency usually occurs in premature, very low birth weight of infants and people with poor fat absorption or have other chronic health problems. Since vegetable oils are good sources of vitamin E, people generally meet their vitamin E requirement easily but people who restrict total dietary fat may not get enough vitamin E. In such cases, nervous system and immune response could get affected.
2. *Excess of vitamin E*: Vitamin E obtained from food usually does not pose a risk for toxicity. Supplemental vitamin E is not recommended due to lack of evidence supporting any added health benefits. Mega doses of supplemental vitamin E may pose a hazard to people taking blood-thinning medications, increased risk of bleeding and impaired vitamin K functions.
3. *Prevention/cure*:
   - Do not restrict total fat or oil in the diet that causes deficiency of vitamin E
   - Avoid mega dose of supplement of vitamin E to prevent hazards or toxicity

4.1.4 Vitamin K

Vitamin K is also known as the clotting or antibleeding or anti-haemorrhagic vitamin because blood would not clot without it. Vitamin K is a group of naphthoquinones with long branched hydrocarbon side chain. Plant based foods are rich in vitamin K. Vitamin K is soluble in fat and stable to heat (100°C) for a short period. Vitamin K is also produced by the bacteria, present in the lower intestinal tract. Approximately half of the vitamin K needed is made in the intestinal tract and the other half is obtained from animal and plant foods.

4.1.4.1 Functions

The functions of vitamin K are as follows:

1. Required for synthesis of procoagulant factors or blood coagulation.
2. Increases the level of prothrombin.
3. Helps to produce proteins for blood, bones and kidneys.

4.1.4.2 Dietary requirements

The AI of vitamin K recommended by Food and Nutrition Board is given in the Table 4.7.

Table 4.7 Daily allowances of vitamin K.*

Group	Particulars	Vitamin K (mg)
Men	Adult	120
Women	Adult	90
Women	Expectant	90
Women	Lactating	90
Infants	Birth-6 months	2
	7–12 months	2.5
Children	1–3 years	30
	4–8 years	55
	9–13 years	60
Boys	9–13 years	60
Girls	9–13 years	60
Boys	14–18 years	75
Girls	14–18 years	75

* No tolerable UL is established.

4.1.4.3 Dietary sources

Vitamin K content of various foods is given in Table 4.8.

Table 4.8 Vitamin K content of various foods.

Food sources	**Vitamin K (μg/100 g)**	**Food sources**	**Vitamin K (μg/100 g)**
Plant sources			
Parsley	1640	Olive oil	60.2
Swiss chard	830	Pine nuts	53.9
Kale	704.8	Cabbage	76
Spinach	482.9	Soya bean	37

Watercress	250	Peas green	24.8
Lettuce, green leaf	126.3	Blueberries	19.3
Broccoli	101.6	Carrot	16.9
Soya bean oil	183.9	Cauliflower	15.5
Canola oil	71.3	Raspberry	7.8
Animal source			
Fish	5		
Liver, beef	3		
Egg yolk	0.7		

The rich sources of vitamin K are green leafy vegetables such as parsley, Swiss chard, kale and spinach. Oil and nuts are the also good sources of vitamin K. Animal sources, such as fish, liver and eggs, contain little amounts vitamin K.

4.1.4.4 Absorption

Vitamin K is fat soluble, hence, absorption requires bile. After absorption from upper part of the small intestine, the vitamin is distributed to various body tissue. It is stored in very small amount in the body. The concentration is not high in any specific tissues.

4.1.4.5 Effects on human health

1. *Deficiency*: Deficiency occurs either due to poor intake or poor intestinal absorption. Prolonged use of antibiotics also induces deficiency because it destroys intestinal bacteria that produce vitamin K. Poor intake of vitamin K in expectant causes
   - uncontrolled bleeding (Fig. 4.3),
   - haemorrhagic disease in infants,
   - low level of prothrombin in infants and
   - osteoporosis.
2. *Excess of vitamin K*: No tolerable UL has been established for vitamin K. No adverse effects has been observed but large doses are not recommended. People taking blood-thinning drugs or anticoagulants should moderate their intake of foods with vitamin K because excess vitamin K can make blood clot faster.
3. *Prevention/cure*:
   - The diet should contain an adequate amount of vitamin K by rich dietary sources to meet the requirements.
   - Administration of vitamin K by injection in infants.
   - Do not take excess supplement to avoid blood clotting.

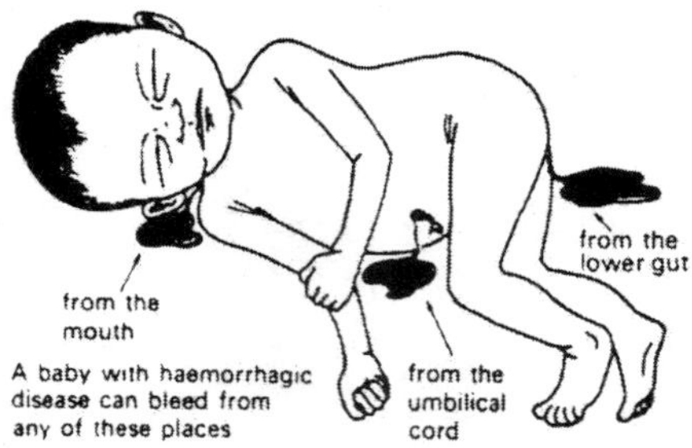

Figure 4.3 Haemorrhagic disease in infants due to deficiency of Vitamin K

4.2 Water-soluble vitamins

The characteristic of water-soluble vitamins are soluble or dissolved in water, easily absorbed and excreted, not stored extensively in tissues and seldom reach toxic level. The water-soluble vitamins are B complex, vitamin C and vitamin P.

4.2.1 Vitamin B complex

This is large group of B vitamins. These are vitamin B_1, B_2, B_3, B_5, B_6, B_9, B_{12}, biotin and choline which play an important role in nutrition.

4.2.1.1 Thiamine (vitamin B_1)

Thiamine is widely distributed in plant and animal foods. It is soluble in water and slightly soluble in alcohol. It is stable in acid medium. It is commonly found in most of the plant and animal foods. Generally thiamine needs will be met if a person eats balanced diet to meet energy needs, except in the case of chronic alcoholics who may not consume enough or their body may not convert thiamine to a bioactive form. It is utilized to perform several important functions.

Functions

1. It acts as a coenzyme and plays an important role in the metabolism of carbohydrate, fat and proteins.
2. Essential for maintenance of good appetite and normal digestion.
3. Required for normal functioning of nerve tissue.

Dietary requirements

The RDA for thiamine (ICMR) is given in Table 4.9.

Table 4.9 Daily allowances of thiamine.*

Group	Particulars	Thiamine mg/d
Men	Sedentary work	1.2
	Moderate work	1.4
	Hard work	1.7
Women	Sedentary work	1.0
	Moderate work	1.1
	Hard work	1.4
Women	Expectants	+0.2
Women	Lactating	
	0–6 months	+0.3
	6–12 months	+0.2
Infants	0–6 months	0.2
	6–12 months	0.3
Children	1–3 years	0.5
	4–6 years	0.7
	7–9 years	0.8
Boys	10–12 years	1.1
Girls	13–15 years	1.0
Boys	16–18 years	1.4
Girls	10–12 years	1.2
Boys	13–15 years	1.5
Girls	16–18 years	1.0

* No adverse effects has been associated with excess of thiamine. No upper level has been determined.

Dietary sources

Thiamine contents of various food stuffs are given in Table 4.10.

Table 4.10 Thiamine content of various foods.

Food sources	Thiamine (mg/100 g)	Food sources	Thiamine (mg/100 g)
Plant-based food			
Jackfruit	3.0	Cashew nut	0.63
Rice bran	2.7	Cabbage	0.60
Wheat germ	2.5	Capsicum	0.55
Banana	1.5	Dry field bean	0.52

Gingelly seed	1.0	Cowpea	0.51
Oatmeal	0.98	Wheat flour whole	0.49
Ground nut	0.90	Bengal gram dal	0.48
Amaranth	0.83	Green gram dal	0.47
Litchi	0.80	Skimmed milk powder	0.45
Soya bean	0.73	Ragi	0.42
Pistachio nut	0.67	Almond	0.40
Animal-based food			
Pork, chop lean	0.98	Meat and fish	0.14
Liver	0.40	Milk	0.05
Egg yolk	0.17		

Foods rich in thiamine content are wheat germ, rice bran and oatmeal in cereals, gingelly seed and groundnut in oil seeds, jackfruit, banana in fruits, and amaranth in vegetable. Good source of thiamine are dry field beans, cowpea (pulses), cashew nut, pistachio nut, cabbage, capsicum and litchi. Animal-based foods such as milk, meat and liver are fair sources of thiamine except meat of pork which is exceptionally rich in thiamine.

The processing of cereals and pulses can significantly, alter their thiamine content. Sprouting and fermentation can increase their content markedly. Prolonged cooking can destroy thiamine, it leaches into the water when foods are boiled or blanched. Cooking methods such as steaming or microwave heating which requires little or no water can conserve thiamine as well as other water-soluble vitamins.

Absorption

After ingestion, thiamine is absorbed and enters the bloodstream. Excess thiamine or the amount in excess of the body needs is excreted in the urine.

Effects on human health

Deficiency of thiamine in the diet causes a disease known as beriberi. The disease occurs both in infants and in adults.

1. *Infantile beriberi*: This disease occurs in infants and characterized by the symptoms restlessness, loss of appetite, palpitation, breathlessness and mortality may occur in case of severe deficiency and delayed treatment.
2. *Beriberi disease in adults*: This occurs in adults and characterized by the symptoms loss in appetite, enlargement of heart, paralysis of limb, oedema in legs, nervous trouble, irritability, fall in body temperature, muscle wasting and loss of skin sensitivity (Fig. 4.4).

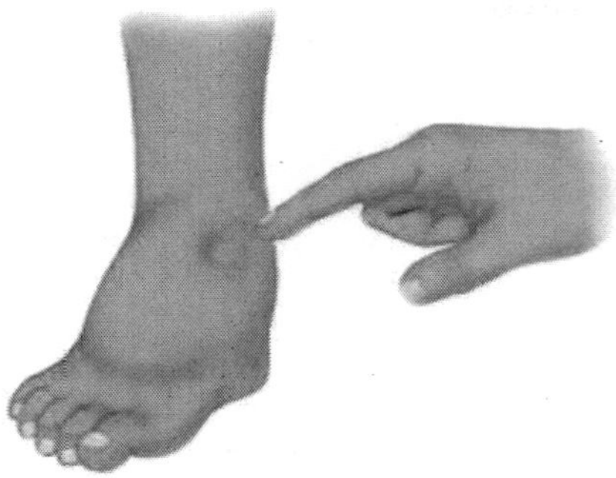

Figure 4.4 Oedema in leg.

3. *Prevention/cure*:
   - Include thiamine rich food in the diet like whole cereals and whole wheat flour or enriched cereals with thiamine, as sufficient thiamine can be obtained from them.
   - Regular intake of oatmeal, seeds, nuts, beans, eggs and meats would be helpful in meeting the requirement.
   - Infantile beriberi can be prevented or controlled by administering 5 mg of thiamine intramuscularly for a week followed by 5 mg oral for a month.
   - In case of adult beriberi administer 25 mg of thiamine intramuscularly for a week followed by 10 mg oral for a month or two.

4.2.1.2 Riboflavin (vitamin B2)

It is water-soluble vitamin, stable in acid medium but destroyed in alkaline medium. It is widely distributed in plant and animal foods. An average mixed diet including milk, green leafy vegetables, whole cereals and pulses (especially when sprouted) can take care of the riboflavin needs of vegetarians. Non-vegetarians can also obtain riboflavin from animal foods.

Functions

Play role in metabolism of carbohydrates, protein and fat. It forms part of two important coenzymes: flavin mononucleotide (FMN) and flavin adenine dinucleotide (FAD) which helps to release energy from the end products of digestion of carbohydrates, fats and proteins.

- Helps in cell respiration essential for growth
- Provides antioxidant protection
- Helps in maintaining smooth skin and eye health

Dietary requirements

The RDAs for riboflavin are given in Table 4.11.

Table 4.11 Daily allowances of riboflavin.*

Group	Particulars	Riboflavin (mg/d)
Men	Sedentary work	1.4
	Moderate work	1.6
	Hard work	2.1
Women	Sedentary work	1.1
	Moderate work	1.3
	Hard work	1.7
Women	Expectants	+0.3
Women	Lactating	
	0–6 months	+0.4
	6–12 months	+0.3
Infants	0–6 months	0.3
	6–12 months	0.4
Children	1–3 years	0.6
	4–6 years	0.8
	7–9 years	1.0
Boys	10–12 years	1.3
Girls	13–15 years	1.2
Boys	16–18 years	1.6
Girls	10–12 years	1.4
Boys	13–15 years	1.8
Girls	16–18 years	1.2

* No adverse effects has been associated with excess of riboflavin. No upper level has been determined.

Dietary source

Riboflavin content of various foods is given in Table 4.12.

Table 4.12 Riboflavin content of foods.

Food sources	Riboflavin (mg/100 g)	Food sources	Riboflavin (mg/100 g)
Plant-based food			
Wood apple (bael)	3.0	Soya bean	0.39
Cashew nut	1.9	Gingelly	0.34
Pineapple	1.2	Fenogreek leaves	0.31
Litchi	1.0	Green gram whole	0.27

Pomegranate	1.0	Calocasia leaves	0.26
Almond	0.57	Papaya	0.25
Rice bran	0.48	Bajra	0.25
Reddish leaves	0.47	Mushroom shitake	0.217
Walnut	0.40	Green gram dal	0.21
Garlic	0.40	Black gram dal	0.20
Chili green	0.39	Cowpea	0.20
Animal-based food			
Liver, raw (beef)	2.75	Egg	0.29
Liver (sheep)	1.7	Milk	0.4
Meat	0.20	Fish	0.20
Egg powder	1.6	Whole milk powder	1.4

Among plant-based foods, wood apple, pineapple, litchi, pomegranate fruits and leafy vegetables and milk, liver, kidney and eggs in animal-based foods are good sources of riboflavin. Wholegrain cereals, legumes, pulses and nuts contain fair amounts.

Refining causes significant loss of the vitamin. However, sprouting and fermentation of wholegrain cereals and pulses can markedly increase their riboflavin content. Cooking does not destroy riboflavin, as it is stable to heat. Ultraviolet rays and irradiation destroy riboflavin. Because of this, most milk is packed in opaque plastic or cardboard containers not in clear glasses.

Absorption

The ingested riboflavin is absorbed from upper part of the small intestine into the bloodstream and is taken to various body tissues to perform specific function. Excess of riboflavin is excreted in the urine.

Effects on human health

1. *Deficiency*: Deficiency of riboflavin in the diet causes following disorders (Fig. 4.5):
   - Swelling and fissuring of the lips (cheilosis)
   - Ulceration and cracking of the angles of the mouth (angular stomatitisis)
   - Oily, scaly skin rashes on the scrotum, vulva or area between the nose and lip
   - Inflammation of the tongue
   - Red, itchy eyes that are sensitive to light

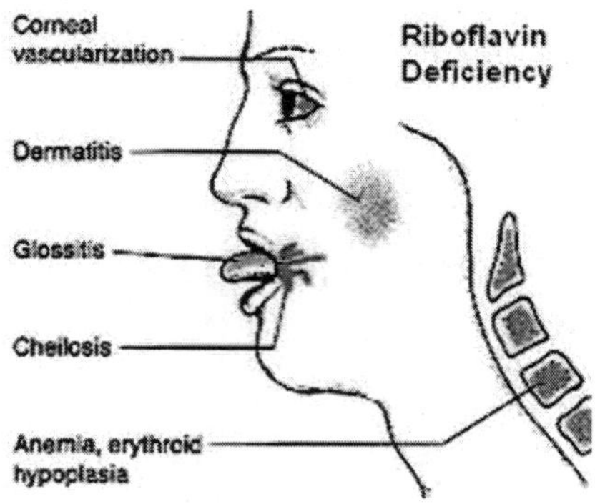

Figure 4.5 Symptoms of riboflavin deficiency.

2. *Prevention/cure*:
   - The diets commonly consumed should have adequate amount of riboflavin to meet the requirements. Include dairy products, and dark green vegetables, fruits, nuts, grains and legumes (beans and peas), that contribute riboflavin to the diet.
   - Administering 5 mg riboflavin orally for a month in children. In case of adult, administration of 10 mg riboflavin for a month is recommended.

4.2.1.3 Niacin (vitamin B3)

This is also known as nicotinic acid and nicotinamide. It is found in both animal and plant foods. It is water soluble and stable to heat. Among B vitamins, niacin is unique because it can also be formed in the body from an amino acid called tryptophan. Milk is a good example of a food rich in tryptophan but not in niacin. The tryptophan present in milk protein can be converted to niacin in the body; hence, milk provides appreciable amounts of niacin. About 60 mg of tryptophan can produce 1 g of niacin.

Functions

Niacin has following function in the body:

1. Niacin forms a part of two important co-enzyme namely nicotinamide adenine dinucleotide (NAD) and nicotinamide adenine dinucleotide phosphate (NADP) which helps to release energy from the end-products of digestion of carbohydrates, fats and proteins and hence essential for their metabolism.
2. Essential for normal functioning of nervous system, skin and intestinal tract.

Dietary requirement

The RDA of niacin is given in Table 4.13.

Table 4.13 Daily allowance of niacin.*

Group	Particulars	Niacin (mg/d)
Men	Sedentary work	16
	Moderate work	18
	Hard work	21
Women	Sedentary work	12
	Moderate work	14
	Hard work	16
	Expectant	+2
Lactating	0–6 months	+4
	6–12 months	+3
Infants	0–6 months	710 µg/kg
	6–12 months	680 µg/kg
Children	1–3 years	8
	4–8 years	11
	7–9 years	13
Boys	10–12 years	15
Girls	10–12 years	13
Boys	13–15 years	16
Girls	13–15 years	14
Boys	16–18 years	17
Girls	16–18 years	14

* The tolerable upper level is 35 mg daily for adults and 30 mg daily for teens aged 14 to 18.

Dietary sources

The niacin content of both plant- and animal-based foods is given in Table 4.14.

Table 4.14 Niacin content of various foods.

Food sources	Niacin (mg/100 g)	Food sources	Niacin (mg/100 g)
Plant-based food			
Rice bran	29.8	Rice puffed	4.1
Ground nut	19.9	Rice parboiled	4.0
Garden cress seed	14.3	Mustard	4.0
Almond	4.4	Mushroom, shiitake	3.877
Gingelly seed	4.4	White millet (jowar)	3.3
Wheat flour whole	4.3	Red gram dal and Bengal gram whole	2.9

Animal-based food			
Liver (sheep)	17.6	Prawn	4.8
Mutton	6.8	Pam fret white fish	2.6
Beef muscle	6.4	Cat fish	2.5

Foods high in protein are also rich sources of niacin such as liver, meat, fish and poultry, groundnuts and oil seeds. Among vegetables, mushroom is the richest source. Cereals, legumes and pulses are also good sources of niacin.

Niacin in natural foods tends to be relatively stable and less vulnerable during food processing and storage as compared to other water-soluble vitamins. Being heat resistant, it can withstand fairly reasonable cooking time. Main loss occurs from leaching into the cooking water. Microwaving, steaming or quick boil which keeps the time of submersion in water to a minimum would help to reduce nutrient loss during cooking. Niacin can be eaten preformed or can be made in the body from tryptophan one of the amino acid.

Effects on human health

1. *Deficiency*: Deficiency of niacin in the diet causes Pellagra disease (Fig. 4.6). The disease is characterized by symptoms soreness of mouth and tongue, dermatitis in hands, feet and neck, diarrhoea and mental disturbance (delirium).

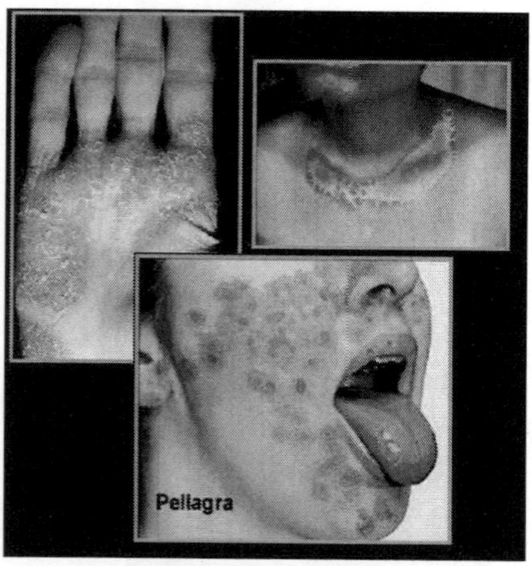

Figure 4.6 Pellagra disease.

2. *Excess or toxicity*: High doses of niacin can be toxic. Niacin overdose is unlikely from eating niacin-rich foods and causes no harm but taking supplements or drugs in large amount can be harmful. Most common effect of niacin overdose is niacin flush. It dilates blood vessels

and creates a sensation of warmth. Other effects are rashes, itching and gastrointestinal disturbances, such as nausea and vomiting. Niacin is available over the counter as a supplement as well as with a prescription as a cholesterol-lowering agent. Doses higher than the RDA except under doctor's prescription may lead to adverse effect; hence, upper limit for niacin is established. The upper tolerable level is 35 mg daily for adults and 30 mg daily for teens aged 14 to 18.

3. *Prevention/cure*:
   - Use foods in the diet from various important sources which are rich or good source of niacin.
   - Administration of nicotinamide (50 mg) twice daily, intramuscularly for a week followed by 100 mg twice a day orally for about 2 weeks.
   - Do not use excess supplement or more than upper limit of niacin to prevent toxicity.

4.2.1.4 Pantothenic acid (vitamin B5)

Pantothenic acid exists in two forms, that is, free form and in a combination of adenine, β-mercapto-ethylamine, ribose and phosphoric acid is known as coenzyme A. Coenzyme A is essential to many biochemical reactions that sustain life. It is highly soluble in water, stable to heat in neutral solution and rapidly lost in acid and alkaline medium. It is widely distributed in foods of plant and animal origin and normal diet provides sufficient amount of vitamin B_5; hence, dietary deficiency is very rare.

Functions

Pantothenic acid has following functions:

- Essential for oxidation of pyruvic acid
- In the form of coenzyme A, participate in carbohydrate and fat metabolism.

Dietary requirement

A little information is available on the requirements of pantothenic acid in humans; hence, Food and Nutrition Board, IMNA (USA) set an AI based on observed dietary intakes in healthy population groups. It reflects the amount needed to replace daily losses. Pantothenic acid requirement is given in Table 4.15.

Table 4.15 Pantothenic acid requirement.*

Groups	Particulars	Pantothenic acid (mg/d)
Men	Adult	5.0
Women	Adult	5.0
	Expectant	6.0

Lactation	Lactating	7.0
Infants	0–6 months	1.7
	6–12 months	1.8
Children	1–3 years	2
	4–8 years	3
Boys	9–13 years	4
Girls	9–13 years	4
Boys	14–18 years	5
Girls	14–18 years	5

* An AI has been set for Pantothenic acid. No tolerable UL has been set.

Dietary sources

The pantothenic acid contents of both plant- and animal-based foods are given in Table 4.16.

Table 4.16 Pantothenic content of various foods.

Food sources	Pantothenic acid (mg/100 g)	Food sources	Pantothenic acid (mg/100 g)
Plant-based food			
Rice polishing	3.3	Rice parboil	1.4
Green gram	2.5	Wheat whole	1.4
Wheat germ	2.2	Cowpea	1.2
Split pea	2.2	Cauliflower	1.0
Peanut roasted	2.1	Apricot	1.0
Soya bean	1.7	Walnut	0.97
Oats	1.5	Sweet potato	0.93
Lentil	1.5	Green peas	0.82
Avocado	1.5	Whole wheat	0.79
Animal-based food			
Beef liver	9.3	Chicken meat	0.80
Lamb liver	7.2	Fish	0.6
Pork liver	7.2	Milk	0.4
Egg	1.5	Meat	0.3

Beef and lamb are the richest sources of pantothenic acid. Cereals, grains, lentils and vegetables are good sources.

Pantothenic acid is stable to heat in slightly acid to neutral conditions, but its stability decreases in alkaline environment. Pantothenic acid is quite stable during cooking when foods are cooked at a neutral pH. Some pantothenic acid lost into cooking water when boiling. Losses are also substantial during food preservation such as freezing, canning and refining process.

Effects on human health

1. *Deficiency*: Deficiency of pantothenic acid causes following disorders:
   - Burning of feet syndrome (Fig. 4.7)
   - Diabetic problem
   - Kidney disorder
   - Nausea and vomiting

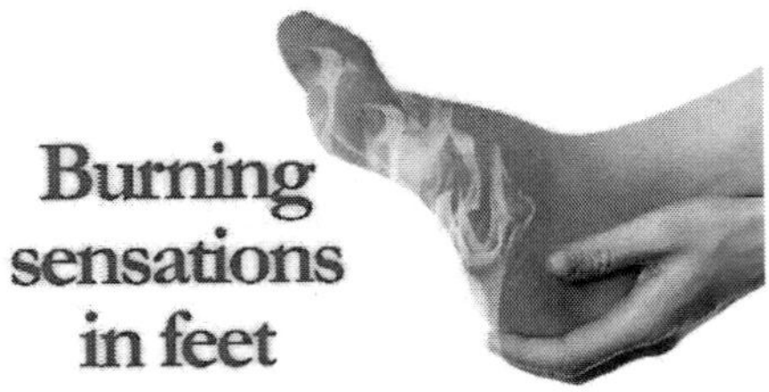

Figure 4.7 Symptom of pantothenic acid deficiency.

2. *Prevention/cure:*
   - The diets commonly consumed should have adequate amounts of pantothenic acid to meet requirements
   - Administration of 20-40 mg CA-pantothenate intramuscularly.

4.2.1.5 Pyridoxine (vitamin B_6)

Pyridoxine contains pyridine and related compounds pyridoxal, pyridoxine and pyridoxamine. Pyridoxine is slowly destroyed in neutral alkaline solution in exposed light and partial destruction in an autoclave at 120°C.

Functions

- Essential for maintaining nerves
- Pyridoxal phosphate acts as coenzyme in amino acid metabolism

Dietary requirements

The RDA for pyridoxine (ICMR) is given in Table 4.17.

Table 4.17 Daily allowances of pyridoxine.

Group	Particulars	Pyridoxine (mg/d)
Men	Sedentary work	2.0
	Moderate work	2.0
	Hard work	2.0

Women	Sedentary work	2.0
	Moderate work	2.0
	Hard work	2.0
	Expectant	2.5
Lactating	0-6 months	2.5
	6-12 months	2.5
Infants	0-6 months	0.1
	6-12 months	0.4
Children	1-3 years	0.9
	4-8 years	0.9
	7-9 years	1.6
Boys	10-12 years	1.6
Girls	10-12 years	1.6
Boys	13-15 years	2.0
Girls	13-15 years	2.0
Boys	16-18 years	2.0
Girls	16-18 years	2.0

Dietary sources

Pyridoxine content of various foods is given in Table 4.18.

Table 4.18 Pyridoxine content of various foods.

Food sources	Pyridoxine (mg/100 g)	Animal sources	Pyridoxine (mg/100 g)
Plant-based food			
Wheat bran	1.2	Banana	0.4
Wheat germ	1.1	Lime	0.4
Rice polishing	0.7	Leafy vegetables	0.3
Nuts and oil seeds	0.5	Grapes	0.08
Legumes	0.4	Milled cereals	0.07
Whole cereals	0.4	Apricot	0.06
Animal-based food			
Egg whole	0.7	Milk powder whole	0.5
Liver (sheep, beef, pork)	0.6	Meat	0.3
Milk skimmed	0.6	Milk fresh	0.09

Animal sources such as egg, meat, liver and milk are rich in vitamin B_6. Cereals, vegetables and fruits are good sources of vitamin B_6.

Pyridoxine is susceptible to light-induced degradation and exposure to water can cause leaching and consequent losses. However, vitamin B_6 is fairly stable during storage.

Alcohol causes destruction and losses of vitamin B_6. Several medications act as a B_6 antagonist such as anti-tuberculosis drugs, anti-parkinsonians, non-steroidal anti-inflammatory drugs may interfere with vitamin B_6 metabolism and induce its deficiency.

Effects on human health

1. *Deficiency*: Deficiency of pyridoxine in the diet causes following disorders:
   - Development of skin lesions around mouth, eyes and nose in adults (Fig. 4.8)
   - In infants, development of convulsions and nervous irritability

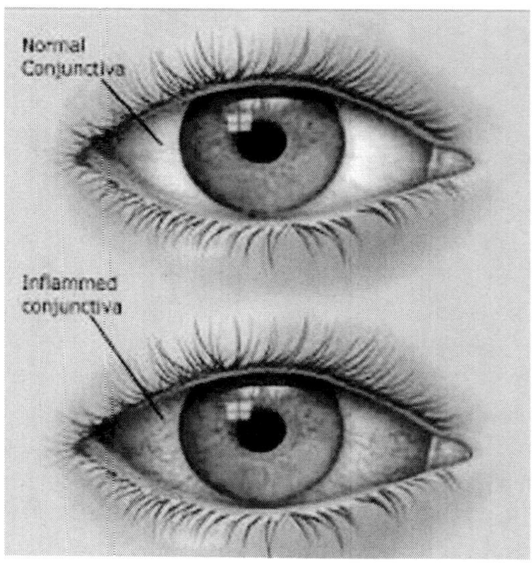

Figure 4.8 Inflammed conjunctiva due to pyridoxine deficiency.

2. *Excess or toxicity*: Pyridoxine toxicity from natural food sources is rarely seen but taking vitamin B_6 supplements in high amounts can cause nerve damage.
3. *Prevention/cure*:
   - The diets commonly consumed should have adequate amounts of pyridoxine to meet requirements.
   - Administration of pyridoxine in adult and infants cures the disorders caused by pyridoxine deficiency.
   - Avoid taking supplement in high dose to prevent toxicity.

4.2.1.6 Folic acid (vitamin B_9)

This is also known as *Folate*. The word folate is derived from the Latin Folium, a leaf, a pretty good clue to its high concentration in green leafy vegetables (Fig. 4.9). Folic acid is water soluble. Water-soluble vitamins dissolve in water. Leftover amounts of the vitamin leave the body through the urine. Body does not store folic acid and need a continuous supply of it. After absorption, folic acid is taken to various body tissues through the bloodstream for specific functions.

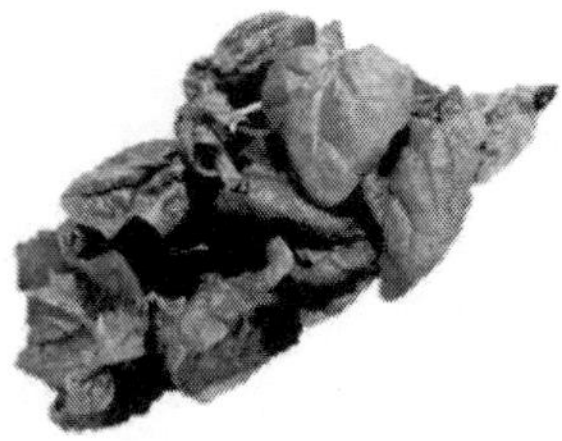

Figure 4.9 Green leafs: rich source of folic acid.

Functions

- Stimulates the formation of red blood cells.
- Folic acid is crucial for proper brain function and plays an important role in mental and emotional health.
- It plays a vital role in the production of DNA and RNA, the body's genetic material, and is especially important when cells and tissues are growing rapidly, such as in infancy, adolescence and pregnancy. It also helps in preventing change to DNA that may lead to cancer.
- Folic acid also works with vitamin B_{12} to form haemoglobin in red blood cells, help iron to work properly in the body and prevent anaemia.
- Folic acid intake during pregnancy reduces the risk of neural tube defects and some other specific kinds of birth defects in newborn.
- Reduces blood homocysteine levels that help to reduce the risk of cardiovascular diseases.

Dietary requirements

The RDAs for folic acid (ICMR) is given in Table 4.19.

Table 4.19 Daily allowances of folic acid.

Group	Particulars	Folic acid (μg/d)
Men	Sedentary work	200
	Moderate work	200
	Hard work	200

Women	Sedentary work	200
	Moderate work	200
	Hard work	200
	Expectant	500
Lactating	0–6 months	300
	6–12 months	300
Infants	0–6 months	25
	6–12 months	25
Children	1–3 years	80
	4–8 years	100
	7–9 years	120
Boys	10–12 years	140
Girls	10–12 years	140
Boys	13–15 years	150
Girls	13–15 years	150
Boys	16–18 years	200
Girls	16–18 years	200

Dietary sources

Folic acid content of both plant- and animal-based foods is given in Table 4.20.

Table 4.20 Folic acid content of various foods.

Food sources	Folic acid (μg/100 g)	Food sources	Folic acid (μg/100 g)
Plant-based food			
Cowpea	69.0	Kiwi	20.0
Strawberry	60.0	Red gram	19.0
Gingelly seed	51.0	Groundnut	16.0
Spinach	51.0	Colocasia	16.0
Cluster bean	50.0	French bean	15.5
French bean	45.0	Coconut dry	15.3
Amaranths	41.0	Bajra	14.7
Bengal gram whole	34.0	Lentil	14.5
Bengal gram dal	32.0	Wheat whole	14.2
Oatmeal	32.0	Jowar	14.0
Okra	25.0	Maze dry	14.0
Green gram dal	24.5	Tomato ripe	14.0

Black gram dal	24.0	Cabbage	13.3
Curry leaves	23.5	Cucumber	12.6
Bengal gram roasted	22.0	Wheat flour	12.1
Mango	20.0	Coconut fresh	11.7
Animal-based food			
Egg (duck)	80.0	Shrimp fresh	15.7
Egg (hen)	70.0	Mrigal fish	9.7
Liver (sheep)	65.6	Cow milk	5.6
Liver (goat)	61.2	Buffalo milk	3.3

Lentils are good source but they require prolonged cooking. It should be soaked overnight, and preferably sprouted prior to cooking. The prolonged cooking is likely to destroy the folic acid. Fresh, raw fruits and vegetables often contain more folate than cooked one. Overcooking or heat destroy vitamin in the food.

Folate losses during harvesting, storage, distribution and cooking can be considerable. Likewise, folate derived from animal products is subject to loss during cooking. Some staples, such as white rice and unfortified corn, are low in folate.

Effects on human health

1. *Deficiency*: Deficiency of folic acid causes macrocytic anaemia (Fig. 4.10), birth defects, cancer, heart disease and nervous system. Folate deficiency is a common cause of megaloblastic anaemia because body stores of folate are more easily depleted and even a minor degree of dietary lack or malabsorption can precipitate deficiency. Folate metabolism may be adversely affected by the ingestion of alcohol.

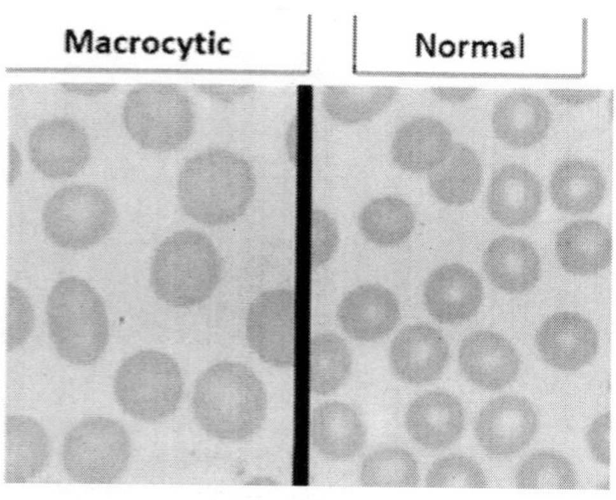

Figure 4.10 Macrocytic anaemia.

Macrocytic anaemia in infants and children: Macrocytic anaemia occurs among malnourished children. It is characterized by low haemoglobin content (5-8 g/100 mL blood) and RBC count 2.5-3 million/mm³.

Macrocytic anaemia in adults: This disease commonly occurs in pregnant and lactating women. Most often the combined result of deficient dietary intake increase demands. The haemoglobin content may vary from 6-9% and RBC counts 2-3 million/mm³.

2. *Prevention/cure*:
    - Include rich sources of folic acid such as green leafy vegetables, organ meat, citrus fruits, legumes and fortiefied cereals in diet.
    - In case of children, oral administration of 1-2 mg folic acid daily. Iron salts, that is, 6 mg iron/kg body weight and 100 µg of vitamin B_{12} intramuscularly once in a week.
    - In case of adults, administration of 5 mg folic acid orally and 500 µg vitamin B_{12} intramuscularly is needed for the cure. Foods in the diet should have a high content of folic acid.

4.2.1.7 Vitamin B_{12}

Vitamin B_{12} has 4–5% cobalt. This is sparingly soluble in water and stable to heat at 100°C. Vitamin B_{12}, derived from a substance called cobalamin, is mainly found in meats and other animal products. Plant foods do not contain the vitamin. Vitamin B_{12} is readily absorbed in the last part of the small intestine (ileum); however, its absorption depends in the presence of intrinsic factor, a substance that is secreted by the lining of the stomach and is vital for the absorption of vitamin B_{12} in the intestines. Intrinsic factor attaches itself to vitamin B_{12}, so it can be absorbed from the food. Without intrinsic factor, vitamin B_{12} moves through the intestine and is excreted in stool. Bacteria present in the intestine can also produce vitamin B_{12}. But this cannot be absorbed without the intrinsic factor which is found only in the stomach. The vitamin B_{12} produced by the bacteria is hence excreted from the body through faeces.

Because of its predominantly animal source, strict vegetarians develop B_{12} deficiency over a period of many years, unless they take special measures or supplements to avoid it.

Functions

- Stimulates the formation of red blood cells with folate
- It is necessary for the proper functioning of the digestive tract, nervous system and the bone marrow
- Cures the neurological symptoms of pernicious anaemia
- Helps body to use fatty acids and some amino acids
- It plays a vital role in cell division and growth

Dietary requirements

The RDA for vitamin B_{12} by ICMR is given in Table 4.21.

Table 4.21 Dietary allowances of vitamin B_{12}.

Group	Particulars	Vitamin B_{12} (μg/d)
Men	Adult	1.0
Women	Adult	1.0
Women	Expectants	1.2
Women	Lactating	1.5
Infants	0–6 months	0.2
	6–12 months	0.2
Children	1–3 years	0.2
Children	4–6years	0.2
	7–9 years	1.0
Boys	10–12 years	0.2
Girls	10–12 years	1.0
Boys	13–15 years	0.2
Girls	13–15 years	1.0
Boys	16–17 years	0.2
Girls	16–17 years	1.0

Dietary sources

Vitamin B_{12} is found only in foods of animal origin. Vitamin B_{12} content of animal-based foods is given in Table 4.22.

Table 4.22 Vitamin B_{12} content of animal-based food.

Animal sources	Vitamin B_{12} (μg/100 g)
Liver (sheep)	133
Liver (goat)	122
Liver (pig)	59
Meat (sheep)	30
Fish	23
Meat (goat)	11
Egg (hens)	11
Egg (ducks)	9
Herring fish	10

Mackerel fish	8.7
Skimmed milk powder	3.2
Whole milk powder	2.4
Milk fresh (cows)	0.5
Milk fresh (buffalo)	0.4
Milk fresh (goat)	0.1

The rich dietary sources are meat and its products, good sources are poultry and fish and, to a lesser extent, milk. Fruit, vegetables, cereals and cereal products are devoid of vitamin B_{12}.

Effects on human health

Deficiency of this vitamin causes pernicious or macrocytic anaemia (Fig. 4.11). The characteristic symptoms of the disease are as follows:

- Low level of haemoglobin (8-9%) and RBC count (1.5-2.5 million/ mm^3)
- Soreness and inflammation of tongue
- Tingling and numbness of fingers and toes
- Degenerative signs of spiral cord

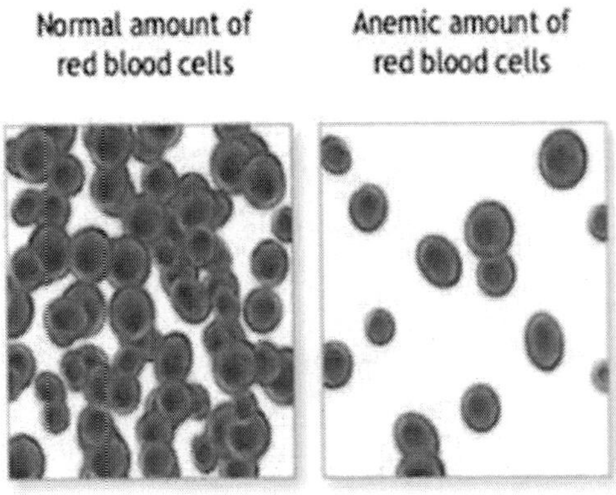

Figure 4.11 Macrocytic anaemia.

Prevention/cure:

- Diet should contain an adequate level of vitamin B_{12} to meet the RDAs.
- Administration of 1000 µg of vitamin B_{12} two times in the first week by injection. Subsequently a dose of 250 µg/week for 2 months and same dose for few months.

4.2.1.8 Biotin (vitamin H)

Biotin is also called vitamin H. It is freely soluble in hot water and sparingly in cold water and alcohol. It is stable to heat at 120°C. Biotin is widespread in foods so eating a healthy diet protects against deficiency. It is also synthesized by intestinal bacteria but does not produce in significant amount.

Functions

- Helps in producing energy
- Act as a coenzyme and plays an important role in metabolism of protein, fat and carbohydrates from food
- Regulate hormone synthesis
- Maintain the skin and nervous system

Dietary requirements

The AI for biotin recommended by Food and Nutrition Board IMNA (USA) is given in Table 4.23.

Table 4.23 Daily allowances of biotin.*

Group	Particulars	Biotin (μg/d)
Men	Adult	30
Women	Adult	30
Women	Expectants	30
Women	Lactating	35
Infants	0-6 months	5
Infant	6-12 months	6
Children	1-3 years	8
Children	4-8 years	12
Boys	9-13 years	20
Girls	9-13 years	20
Boys	14-18 years	25
Girls	14-18 years	25

* The biotin does not have the upper level because no adverse effect from high/excess biotin has been reported.

Dietary source

Biotin is found in foods of both plant and animal origin. The biotin content of various foods is given in Table 4.24.

Table 4.24 Biotin content of various foods.

Food sources	Biotin (μg/100 g)	Food sources	Biotin (μg/100 g)
Plant-based food			
Soya bean	61.0	Cauliflower	17.0

Rice polishing	57.0	Wheat whole	16.0
Walnut	37.0	Lentil	13.2
Peanut	34.0	Rice paraboil	10.0
Barley	31.0	Peas green	9.4
Oats	24.0	Green gram	7.5
Corn	21.0	Spinach	6.9
Cowpea	21.0	Rice white	5.0
Split pea	18.4	Banana	4.4
Almond	18.0	Sweet potato	4.3
		Cabbage	2.4
Animal sources			
Lamb liver	127.0	Salmon fish	15.0
Pork liver	100	Chicken meat	11.2
Beef liver	96.0	Mutton	6.5
Eggs	21.0	Fresh cow milk	5.5

The rich sources of biotin are liver of lamb, pork and beef. Soya bean polished rice walnut, peanut, barley and oats are the good source of biotin. Corn cowpea, cauliflower, whole wheat and fish are the fair source of biotin.

Effects on human health

Deficiency in human beings causes following disorders:

Dermatitis on the hand, neck, arms and legs (Fig. 4.12)
Depression and muscle pain
Hyperesthesia
Occasional nausea and increase in serum cholesterol

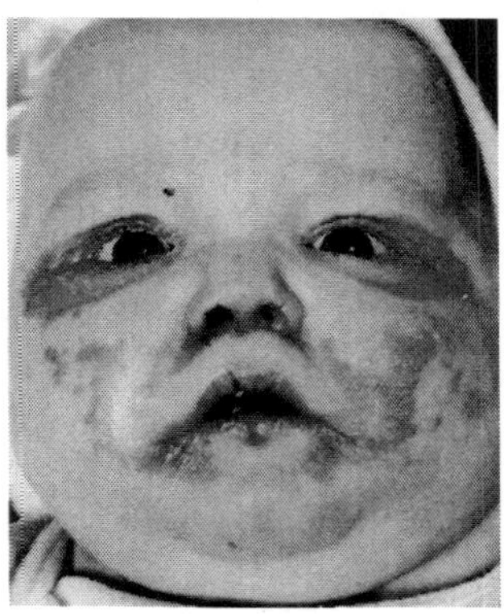

Figure 4.12 Dermatitis.

Prevention/cure:

- Diet should contain an adequate level of biotin to meet the requirement.
- Injection of biotin 75-300 μg brings rapid cure within a week.

4.2.1.9 Choline

Choline is an essential water-soluble nutrient that is usually grouped in as part of the B vitamin complex. It is a nitrogen-containing compound found in foods and made in the body from the amino acid methionine. It is an integral part of phospholipids and neurotransmitter which are found in nervous tissue and essential for life processes. It is highly soluble in water and alcohol.

Functions

- It is a component of lecithin, which is critical to normal liver metabolism
- Prevents fat accumulation in the liver
- It plays an important role in the synthesis of phospholipids which are key structural components of the human cell membrane
- It is a precursor for neurotransmitter acetylcholine which is vital to nerve and muscle function
- It plays important roles in brain and memory development in the foetus

Dietary requirement

The AI for cholin recommended by Food and Nutrition Board IMNA (USA) is given in Table 4.25.

Table 4.25 Daily allowances of choline.*

Group	Particulars	Choline (μg/d)
Men	Adult	550
Women	Adult	425
Women	Expectant	450
Women	Lactating	550
Infants	0-6 months	125
Infants	6-12 months	150
Children	1-3 years	200
Children	4-8 years	250
Boys	9-13 years	375
Girls	9-13 years	375
Boys	14-18 years	550
Girls	14-18 years	400

* Tolerable UL for adults is 3.5 g/d. Teens aged 14-18 years: 3 g/d.

Dietary sources

Choline content of various foods is given in Table 4.26.

Table 4.26 Choline content of various foods.

Food sources	Choline (mg/100 g)	Food sources	Choline (mg/100 g)
Plant-based food			
Wheat germ	406	Rice parboiled	98
Soya bean	340	Wheat whole	94
Cowpea	257	Peas green	75
Lintel	223	Beef muscle	68
Green gram	209	Corn yellow	61
Split pea	201	Rice whole	59
Peanut roasted	162	Wheat flour	52
Oats	156	Potato	29
Rice polishing	102	Cabbage	23
		Spinach	22
Animal-based foods			
Liver pork	552	Pork ham	122
Liver (beef)	510	Salmon fish, pink	97
Liver (lamb)	508	Lamb muscle	84
Egg large	147	Pork beacon	80
		Beef muscle	68

Animal food sources such as liver of pork, beef and lamb and plant sources such as wheat germ, soya bean, cowpea and lentil are the rich source of choline.

Effects on human health

Choline deficiency is not likely to occur in human beings.

4.2.2 Ascorbic acid (vitamin C)

Vitamin C is also known as ascorbic acid. It oxidized rapidly when exposed to air. Oxidation is faster at higher temperature during food cooking which means vitamin gets lost at higher temperature; hence, it is also termed as the 'fresh food vitamin' because fresh fruits and vegetables are its major sources. Organs and glands like the spleen, bone marrow, liver, pancreas, kidney and the retina of the eye have a high concentration of ascorbic acid.

Functions

1. *Wound healing*: Vitamin C plays an important role in the formation of special protein called collagen. Formation of collagen at the site of wound helps in healing and use to form skin, cartilage, tendons, ligament and blood vessel.
2. *Release of hormones*: Ascorbic acid plays an important role in the release of two hormones, epinephrine and norepinephrine, which help the body to deal with stressful situations like day to day tensions, stresses of infections and injury.
3. *Absorption of iron*: Iron is essential component of red blood cells. Ascorbic acid helps absorption of iron from plant sources by reducing the ferric iron to ferrous iron.
4. *Protection of certain substances from destruction*: Ascorbic acid protects certain substances such as vitamin A and unsaturated fatty acids from being destroyed.
5. *Acts an antioxidant*: Ascorbic acid is also an antioxidant, protect cells from damage by free radicals and protect from infection by stimulating the antibody. It also boosts immunity.
6. *Maintain healthy gums and healing fractures*: Ascorbic acid keeps our gums healthy and heals bone fractures by forming connective tissues.

Dietary requirements

The RDAs for ascorbic acid by ICMR are given in Table 4.27.

Table 4.27 Daily allowances of ascorbic acid.

Group	Particulars	Ascorbic acid (mg/d)
Men	Sedentary work	40
	Moderate work	40
	Hard work	40
Women	Sedentary work	40
	Moderate work	40
	Hard work	40
	Expectant	60
Lactating	0–6 months	80
	6–12 months	80
Infants	0–6 months	25
	6–12 months	25
Children	1–3 years	40
	4–8 years	40

	7–9 years	40
Boys	10–12 years	40
Girls	10–12 years	40
Boys	13–15 years	40
Girls	13–15 years	40
Boys	16–17 years	40
Girls	16–17 years	40

Dietary sources

The ascorbic acid content of various plant-based foods is given in Table 4.28.

Table 4.28 Ascorbic acid content of plant-based foods.

Plant-based food	Ascorbic acid (mg/100 g)	Plant-based food	Ascorbic acid (mg/100 g)
Barbados cherry	4500	Strawberry	60
Sea buckthorn	1600	Litchi	60
Amla	700	Papaya	57
Guava	300	Cauliflower	56
Kiwi	300	Carambola	50
Ber	150	Spinach	48
Capsicum	137	Jamun	46
Coriander leaves	135	Turnip	43
Cabbage	124	Cape goose berry	43
Drumstick	120	Custard apple	40
Chili green	111	Tomato ripe	32
Amaranth	99	Pointed gourd	29
Bitter gourd	88	Musk melon	26
Pineapple	70	French bean	24
Citrus fruits	65	Sweet potato	24

Fresh foods such as cherry, sea buckthorn, aonla, guava and kiwi are rich source of vitamin C. Ber, citrus fruits, litchi and fresh vegetables such as capsicum, coriander leaves, cabbage, drum stick and green chilies are also good source of vitamin C. Cereals and pulses as such are poor in vitamin C but when sprouted and fermented become good sources. Animal foods like fish, meat, milk, poultry and eggs contain little or no ascorbic acid.

Absorption

Ascorbic acid is readily absorbed from the digestic tract and distributed to various body tissues. Organ and glands like spleen, bone marrow, liver, pancreas, kidney and retina of the eyes have high concentration of ascorbic acid.

Effects of on human health

1. *Deficiency*: Deficiency of ascorbic acid causes scurvy disease in adults and infants.

   Scurvy in adults: The characteristic symptoms of scurvy in adults are as follows (Figs. 4.13 and 4.14):

   - Bleeding of gums
   - Loose teeth
   - Swollen tendered joints
   - General weakness
   - Haemorrhages under the skin and in tissues

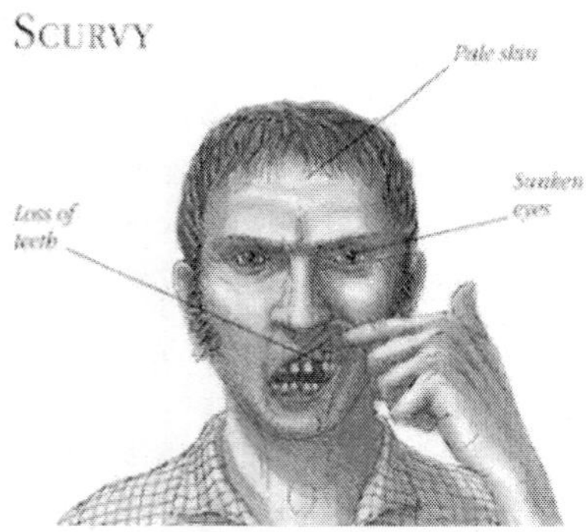

Figure 4.13 Scurvy.

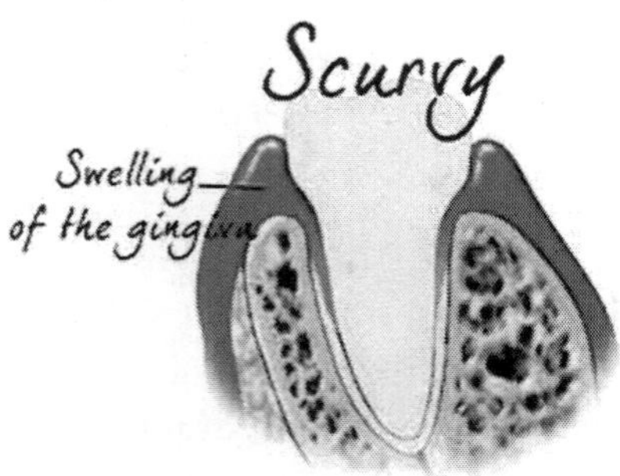

Figure 4.14 Scurvy tooth.

Scurvy in infants: Scurvy in infants is known as infantile scurvy. The characteristic symptoms of infantile scurvy are as follows:

- Defective bone growth
- Loss of appetite
- Listlessness
- Swollen gums
- Swelling at the ends of long bone
- Haemorrhages

2. *Prevention/cure*:
    - Diet should contain adequate level of vitamin C to meet the requirements.
    - In adult, administration of 100 mg ascorbic acid intramuscularly for a week followed by oral administration of 500 mg daily for a month.
    - In infants, administration of 50 mg of ascorbic acid intramuscularly twice a day for a week followed by oral administration of 100 mg daily for a month.

4.2.3 Vitamin P (bioflavonoid)

Bioflavonoids are mostly found in fruits and vegetables. Various glycosides having 'P' activity have been isolated from foods and vegetables called flavonoids. The important bioflavonoid occurring in nature are citrine (citrus juice, lemon peel) has peredin (sweet orange), naringin (grapefruit), tangerine (loose skin orange), catechin (apple, grape), epicatechin (dates), queretin (mango, apple, strawberry, onion) and rutin and kaemferol (onion, snap beans, lettuce, broccoli).

Functions

- Capillary protection
- Control allergies
- Control cancer initiation and heart disease
- Reduces cholesterol

Dietary requirement

Requirement of bioflavonoid in the diet is not known. Regular consumption of fresh fruits and vegetables has an adequate amount to meet the requirement.

Dietary sources

Vitamin P activity (bioflavonoid) of some fruits and vegetables is given in Table 4.29.

Table 4.29 Vitamin P content of plant-based food.

Plant-based food	Vitamin P content (units)*
Lemon peel	500
Orange juice and peel	490

Lemon juice	450
Rose hips syrup	300
Spinach	130
Lettuce	100
Walnut	100
Tomato	70
Water cress	70
Apple	60
Blackberry	60
Cherry	60
Cabbage	60
Plum	50
Pea	40
Parsnip	40
Carrot	40
Cauliflower	40
Potato	35
Beetroot	15

*1 unit = activity of 1mg of citrine.

Effects on human health

Bioflavonoid deficiency causes following disorders in human beings:

- Capillary resistance decreases which leads petechial bleeding and pain across the shoulders and legs
- Fatigue and lassitude

Prevention/cure:

- Diet should contain adequate level of vitamin P to meet the requirements.
- A dose of 200 mg orally four times a day have been found effective to cure decreased capillary resistance.

5
Minerals

Minerals are inorganic substances present in food and play an important role in nutrition. Body needs variety of minerals for a variety of function and maintaining proper health.

Minerals play various roles in human system, such as:

- Component of skeleton or constituents of bones and teeth
- Constituent of body cells of soft tissue
- Regulators of the body neutrality
- Constituents of vitamin, hormone, and enzymes for specific functions

The minerals required by the human body are classified into two groups macro minerals and micro minerals, which are given in Table 5.1.

Table 5.1 Minerals required in human nutrition.

Macro minerals	Micro minerals
Calcium	Iron
Phosphorus	Zinc
Magnesium	Copper
Sodium	Iodine
Potassium	Manganese
Chloride	Fluorine
Sulphur	Chromium
	Cobalt
	Molybdenum
	Selenium

5.1 Macro minerals

Macro minerals are major minerals and required in excess of 100 mg/d in diet. In other words, minerals present at level more than 0.05% in human body are called as macro minerals. These are calcium, phosphorus, magnesium, sodium, potassium, chloride and sulphur. Each macro minerals play some special roles which are described in the following sections.

5.1.1 Calcium

Calcium content is the highest in the body as compared to other minerals. The adult human body contains about 1–1.5 kg calcium which is deposited in the bone during the growth of body. Calcium is found maximum (99%) in skeleton (bone and teeth). Normal serum level is 9–11 mg/100 mL. The functions of calcium in body are:

- Gives strength and firmness to the bodies
- Necessary for the bone and teeth formation
- Necessary for the clotting of bloods
- Necessary for the movement of muscles
- Necessary for the heart and muscle contraction
- Regulates the permeability of capillary walls and excitability of nerve fibres
- Nerve transmission and membrane excitability
- Cell division
- Activates number of enzymes

5.1.1.1 Dietary requirements

Recommended dietary allowances for calcium (ICMR) are given in Table 5.2.

Table 5.2 Daily allowances of calcium.

Group	Particulars	Calcium (mg/d)
Men	Sedentary work	600
	Moderate work	600
	Hard work	600
Women	Sedentary work	600
	Moderate work	600
	Hard work	600
	Expectant	1200
Lactating	0–6 months	1200
	6–12 months	1200
Infants	0–6 months	500
	6–12 months	500
Children	1–3 years	600
	4–8 years	600
	7–9 years	600
Boys	10–12 years	800

Girls	10–12 years	800
Boys	13–15 years	800
Girls	13–15 years	800
Boys	16–17 years	800
Girls	16–17 years	800

5.1.1.2 Dietary sources

The calcium contents of various foods from both plant- and animal-based sources are given in Table 5.3.

Table 5.3 Calcium content of various foods.

Food sources	Calcium (mg/100 g)	Food sources	Calcium (mg/100 g)
Plant-based foods			
Gingelly seed	1450	Almond	230
Curry leaves	810	Buffalo milk	210
Mustard seed	490	Bengal gram dal	202
Colocasia leaves	460	Fig	200
Drumstick leaves	440	Tamarind	170
Coconut dry	400	Black gram dal	154
Amaranth	397	Coriander leaves	144
Fenugreek leaves	395	Phalsa	130
Mustard seed	490	Custard bean	130
Colocasia leaves	460	Green gram whole	124
Drumstick leaves	440	Walnut	100
Coconut dry	400	Lime	90
Amaranth	397	Bael	90
Fenugreek leaves	395	Carrot	80
Chironji	300	Spinach	73
Rajma	260	Litchi	70
Soya bean	240	Okra	66
Animal-based foods			
Shrimp dried	4384	Chela fish fresh	590
Chela fish dried	2950	Katla fish	530
Skimmed milk powder	1370	Prawn	320
Khoa (cow)	960	Buffalo milk	210

Whole milk powder	950	Mutton	150
Cheese	700	Curd	149
Rohu fish	650	Cow milk	120
Khoa buffalo	650	Egg	60

Plant-based foods rich in calcium content are gingelly seed (sesame seed), curry leaves, mustard, colocasia leaves, drumstick leaves, dry coconut, ragi, amaranth, fenugreek leaves and chironji. Other fruits of plant origin have good to fair sources.

Animal-based foods rich in calcium content are dried shrimp, dried chela fish, skimmed milk powder, cow milk khoa, whole milk powder, cheese, rohu fish, buffalo milk khoa, fresh chela, fish katla fish and prawn.

5.1.1.3 Absorption

Absorption chiefly occurs in duodenum or from upper part of the intestine. Only a small proportion of the calcium (20–30%) in the diet gets absorbed. The rest is excreted in the faeces. Part of the absorbed calcium is also excreted in the urine. The absorbed calcium is used to perform various functions.

Factors influencing calcium absorption are body need such as during deficiency or rapid growth and nutrients in the diet such as vitamin D through its active form calciferol. Protein, gastric acidity, sugar such as lactose promote calcium uptake by intestinal cells.

Factors which hinder or decreased calcium absorption are oxalates (green vegetables), phytates (cereals) and fatty acids which form insoluble salts with calcium.

5.1.1.4 Effects on human health

1. *Deficiency*: Deficiency of calcium in the diet causes following disorders in human body:
    - Rickets (In children bones) or defective calcification of bones. Vitamin D level is decreased in the body
    - Osteoporosis (In adults) demineralization of bones, thus loss of bone mass which results in increased incidence of fractures
    - Decay of teeth
    - Stunted growth, pigeon chest and irritability in children
2. *Prevention/cure*:
    - Diet should contain adequate amount of calcium (1000–1500 mg) along with 400–800 IU vitamin D to meet the requirements of deficiency.

5.1.2 Phosphorus

Phosphorus is the second most abundant mineral in the body. Phosphorus is found in the body in the form of inorganic phosphorus such as calcium phosphate in bone and teeth, sodium and potassium phosphates in fluids and soft tissues, and organic compounds containing phosphorus such as phospholipids, nucleic acid, nucleoprotein, creatine phosphate, adenosine triphosphate (ATP), adenosine diphosphate, hexose phosphate and glycerol phosphate. The adult human body contains 400–700 g phosphorus as phosphates. The large amount (80%) is found in bone and teeth and remaining in other tissues. The inorganic phosphate content of blood serum in normal adult ranges from 3 to 4 mg/100 mL and in children 4–6 mg/100 mL.

5.1.2.1 Functions

- Formation of bone and teeth
- Formation of phospholipids: integral part of cell structures or membranes
- Assists in energy metabolism
- Constituents of nucleic acid, nucleoprotein and certain coenzymes
- Acid-base regulation for maintaining pH of the body fluids

5.1.2.2 Dietary requirement

The retention of phosphorus in the body depends on the calcium content of the body and quantity of phosphorus ingested. The calcium and phosphorus ratio of diet consumed in various countries vary from 1:1.5 to 1:3. The optimal calcium:phosphorus ratio for infants and children is 1:1, that is, phosphorus requirement is equal to that of calcium. In adult this ratio of calcium and phosphorus is 1:2. Excess of phosphorus lowers calcium absorption. Phosphorus requirement of person consuming cereal-based diet will be higher than those consuming milk, meat, fish and dried nuts.

Dietary intake for phosphorus recommended by Food and Nutrition Board IMNA (USA) is given in Table 5.4.

Table 5.4 Dietary intake for phosphorus.

Group	Particulars	Phosphorus (mg/d)
Men	Adult	700
Women	Adult	700
Women	Expectant	700
Women	Lactating	700
Infants	0–6 months	100

Infants	6–12 months	275
Children	1–3 years	460
Children	4–8 years	500
Boys	9–13 years	1250
Girls	9–13 years	1250
Boys	14–18 years	1250
Girls	14–18 years	1250

5.1.2.3 Dietary sources

The phosphorus content of plant- and animal-based sources is given in Table 5.5.

Table 5.5 Phosphorus content of various foods.

Food sources	Phosphorus (mg/100 g)	Food sources	Phosphorus (mg/100 g)
Plant-based foods			
Rice brown	1410	Ragi	283
Chironji	580	Rice paraboil	280
Carrot	530	Jwar	222
Almond	490	Rice milled	160
Cashew nut	450	Colocasia	140
Oat meal	380	Peas green	139
Walnut	380	Tamarind	110
Wheat flour whole	355	Drumstick	110
Maze dry	348	Amaranth	83
Litchi	310	Ber	80
Bajra	296		
Animal sources			
Shrimp	1160	Liver goat	279
Skimmed milk powder	1000	Prawn	278
Whole milk powder	730	Egg	220
Cheese	520	Goat meat	193
Khoa	420	Rohu fish	175
Liver sheep	380	Milk buffalo	130
Pomphret fish	290	Milk cow	90

Plant-based foods rich in phosphorus are rice brown, oat meal, whole wheat flour, maize dry, bajra, carrot, almond, cashew nut, walnut and litchi. Other plant-based foods have good to fair source.

The animal-based foods rich in phosphorus are fishes (shrimp, pomfret, prawn and rohu fish), goat, liver, skimmed milk, whole milk powder, cheese and khoa. Egg, goat meat and cow milk have fair sources. Animal protein is the excellent source of phosphorus.

5.1.2.4 Absorption

Absorption of phosphorus is also takes place from upper part of the small intestine. Considerable amount of phosphorus in cereals and pulses and nuts is found in a bound form which is not absorbed. The body absorbs only the free form. The absorbed phosphorus is used in the body for various functions.

5.1.2.5 Effects on human health

The deficiency of phosphorus causes bad bones and teeth and body weakness. The diet shall contain adequate amount of phosphorus from food sources to meet the requirement. However, under normal circumstances, deficiencies of phosphorus are unknown.

5.1.3 Magnesium

The adult human body contains about 25 g of magnesium. About 50% of this quantity is found in bones and remaining in other tissues. The magnesium content of blood serum is 2–3 mg/100 mL and whole blood 1.6 mg/100 mL.

5.1.3.1 Functions

- Required for metabolism of calcium and phosphorus
- Essential to the function of several enzyme system as cofactor
- Maintains electrical potential in nerves and membranes
- It is an important constituent of bone and teeth
- Magnesium along with calcium, sodium and potassium controls neuro muscular irritability

5.1.3.2 Dietary requirements

The recommended dietary allowances for magnesium by ICMR are given in Table 5.6.

Table 5.6 Daily allowances of magnesium.

Group	Particulars	Magnesium (mg/d)
Men	Sedentary work	340
	Moderate work	340
	Hard work	340

Women	Sedentary work	310
	Moderate work	310
	Hard work	310
	Expectant	310
Lactating	0–6 months	310
	6–12 months	310
Infants	0–6 months	30
	6–12 months	45
Children	1–3 years	50
	4–8 years	70
	7–9 years	100
Boys	10–12 years	120
Girls	10–12 years	160
Boys	13–15 years	165
Girls	13–15 years	210
Boys	16–17 years	195
Girls	16–17 years	235

5.1.3.3 Dietary sources

The magnesium content of various foods is given in Table 5.7.

Table 5.7 Magnesium content of various foods.

Food sources	Magnesium (mg/100 g)	Food sources	Magnesium (mg/100 g)
Plant-based food			
Cocoa	420	Bajra	125
Almond	267	Dry peas	124
Tea	254	Banana	108
Coffee	235	Masur dal (lentil)	94
Cowpea	230	Tamarind	92
Black gram dal	185	Spinach	84
Groundnut	181	Tapioca	66
Green gram whole	171	Coriander leaves	64
Bengal gram whole	168	Apricot	63
Maize	144	Dates	59
Wheat whole	139	Wheat flour	55
Green gram dal	139	Celery	52

Red gram dal	133	Coconut fresh	52
Barley	127	Rice polished	48
		Okra	43
Animal sources			
Whole milk powder	112	Skimmed milk powder	111

Plant-based foods rich in magnesium are cocoa, tea, coffee, almond and cowpea. Other food such as black gram dal, whole green gram, whole Bengal gram, groundnut, green gram dal and maize have also good source of magnesium.

Animal-based foods such as whole milk and skimmed milk powder are fair source of magnesium.

5.1.3.4 Absorption

Magnesium is absorbed by the small intestine. Absorption is somewhat similar to that of calcium. Factor affecting the absorption is the body need that is when body's demand increases the absorption increases. Absorption of magnesium is inhibited by inhibitors such as phytates and oxlates. Excretion of magnesium of the body is regulated by kidneys.

5.1.3.5 Effects on human health

1. *Deficiency*: Deficiency of magnesium in human body causes following disorders:
   - Osteoporosis
   - Nervous breakdown
   - Depression
   - Muscular weakness
2. *Prevention/cure*:
   - Diet should contain adequate amount of magnesium to meet the requirements.
   - Administration of 100 mg magnesium chloride parenterally cures the deficiency symptoms.

5.1.4 Sodium

Sodium is the major cation of the extracellular fluids. Sodium attracts water. It is found in the body in association with chloride, bicarbonate, phosphate, lactate and proteinate anions. The adult human body contains about 100 g sodium ions which are distributed in plasma, tissue fluids and lymph. Normal sodium serum level is 135–145 mEq/L.

5.1.4.1 Functions

The functions of sodium ion in the human body are:

- Chief intracellular ions of the body and regulate acid-base balance of the body
- Regulates osmotic pressure of plasma or cell fluid
- Originating and maintaining heartbeat
- Maintains the muscular and nerve irritability
- Involved in cell permeability membrane
- Helps in active transport of glucose, galactose and amino acid across the intestinal mucosa

5.1.4.2 Dietary requirements

Dietary intake for sodium recommended by Food and Nutrition Board IMNA (USA) is given in Table 5.8.

Table 5.8 Daily allowances of sodium chloride.

Group	Particulars	Sodium chloride (g/d)
Men	Adult	15
Women	Adult	15
Women	Expectants	15
Women	Lactating	15
Infants	0–6 months	0.12
	6–12 months	0.37
Children	1–3 years	1.0
	4–8 years	1.2
Boys	9–13 years	15
Girls	9–13 years	15
Boys	14–18 years	15
Girls	14–18 years	15

5.1.4.3 Dietary sources

The sodium content of various foods is given in Table 5.9.

Table 5.9 Sodium content of plant- and animal-based foods.

Food sources	Sodium (mg/100 g)	Food sources	Sodium (mg/100 g)
Plant-based foods			
Cowpea	95	Red gram dal	66
Celery	91	Beat root	66

Spinach	89	Sesame seed	60
Field bean	89	Green gram whole	57
Black gram whole	80	Okra	54
Black gram dal	75	Green gram dal	49
Coffee	74	Carrot	47
Bengal gram dal	72	Tea	44
Bengal gram whole	71	Radish	41
Raisin	67	Cashew nut	41
		Jackfruit	41
Animal-based sources			
Skimmed milk powder	450	Liver	83
Whole milk powder	410	Rohu fish	69
Milk condensed	140	Mutton	63
Egg whole	129	Chicken meat	58

Plant-based foods have lower content of sodium than animal-based foods. Sodium content of animal-based food varies from 58 to 450 mg/100 g. Skimmed milk and whole milk powder, condensed milk and whole egg are richer in sodium than liver, rohu fish, mutton and chicken meat.

5.1.4.4 Absorption

Sodium is absorbed by the digestive tract. The excessive amount of sodium is lost from the body through urine, sweat and faeces. Diarrhoea also causes excessive loss. Intake of fluids and salt are taken to makeup the loss during such period. The major regulation of the sodium in the body is done by the kidney.

5.1.4.5 Effects on human health

1. *Deficiency*: Deficiency of sodium causes following disorders in the body:
    - Weakness
    - Nausea
    - Dehydration
    - Muscle cramps
    - Vomiting
    - Constant thirst
    - Abdominal cramps
2. *High intake*: Consumption of high amount of sodium or salt causes:
    - Increased blood pressure in hypertension
    - Oedema in protein deficiency

3. *Prevention/cure*: Loss of excessive sodium chloride from the body (10–12 g/d) due to excessive sweating causes muscular cramps or heat cramps (painful contraction of skeleton muscle). This can be prevented by using 0.3–0.5% sodium chloride to drinking water. Diet should contain foods of adequate amount of sodium to meet the requirements. However, diet rarely lacks sodium.

Patient suffering from high blood pressure should have low sodium diet. Concentration between salt and blood pressure in salt-sensitive person is direct. The more salt you eat, the higher is the blood pressure.

5.1.5 Chloride

Chloride is the major anion in the extracellular space. On an average, 5–10 g of sodium corresponding to 10–20 g sodium chloride ingested/d in average diet. The normal serum level is 95–110 mEq/L.

5.1.5.1 Functions

The functions of chloride in the body are:

- Essential for the formation of stomach's hydrochloric acid by the gastric mucosa to digest proteins
- Essential for activation of enzyme amylase
- Essential for water balance as a part of sodium chloride
- Involved in chloride shift
- Regulates osmotic pressure and acid-base balance

5.1.5.2 Dietary requirement

Dietary intake for chloride recommended by Food and Nutrition Board IMNA (USA) is given in Table 5.10.

Table 5.10 Daily allowances of chloride.

Group	Particulars	Chloride (g/d)
Men	Adult	2.3
Women	Adult	2.3
Women	Expectants	2.3
Women	Lactating	2.3
Infants	0–6 months	0.18
	6–12 months	0.57
Children	1–3 years	1.5
	4–8 years	1.9

Boys	9–13 years	23
Girls	9–13 years	23
Boys	14–18 years	23
Girls	14–18 years	23

5.1.5.3 Dietary sources

The important sources of chloride are common salt, wholegrains, leafy vegetables, milk and egg.

5.1.5.4 Absorption

Chloride is absorbed from upper part of the intestine. Excretion of excess chloride is through urine and to some extent by the sweat and faeces.

5.1.5.5 Effects on human health

Low salt diet results persistent vomiting, renal, tubular damage, excessive, sweating and Addison's disease.

Excessive consumption of sodium chloride causes increased blood pressure in hypertension patient and oedema in protein deficiency.

Prevention/cure:

- Diet should contain adequate amount of sodium chloride to meet the requirement.
- Patient suffering from hypertension should be prescribed for low salt diet.

5.1.6 Potassium

Potassium is the principal intracellular cation. It is found almost entirely about 98% in cells of various tissues and muscles. A little quantity is also found in extracellular fluids. The human adult body contains about 250 g potassium. The concentration in serum is 4.5 mEq/L.

5.1.6.1 Functions

The functions of potassium in human body are:

- Regulates intracellular osmotic pressure and pH equilibria of cell contents
- Increases the relaxation of heart muscles
- Required for transmission of nerve in pulses
- Assists nuclear activity and protein synthesis

5.1.6.2 Dietary requirements

The dietary intake for potassium recommended by Food and Nutrition Board IMNA (USA) is given in Table 5.11.

Table 5.11 Daily allowances of potassium.

Group	Particulars	Potassium (g/d)
Men	Adult	4.7
Women	Adult	4.7
Women	Expectants	4.7
Women	Lactating	5.1
Infants	0–6 months	0.4
	6–12 months	0.7
Children	1–3 years	3.0
	4–8 years	3.8
Boys	9–13 years	4.5
Girls	9–13 years	4.5
Boys	14–18 years	4.7
Girls	14–18 years	4.7

5.1.6.3 Dietary sources

The potassium content of various foods is given in Table 5.12.

Table 5.12 Potassium content of various foods.

Food sources	Potassium (mg/100 g)	Food sources	Potassium (mg/100 g)
Plant-based food			
Tea	2160	Bajra	402
Coffee	2020	Field bean	386
Cocoa	1522	Bengal gram dal	386
Dried apricot	1200	Onion	385
Dry plum	1100	Bitter gourd	382
Peas dry	956	Sweet potato	373
Almond	856	Tomato	360
Sesame seeds	725	Wheat whole	349
Coconut dry	700	Peas green	346
Groundnut roasted	700	Coconut fresh	336
Dried fig	680	Lettuce	329

Black gram dal	643	Radish	325
Green gram dal	643	Cowpea	323
Raisin (dried grapes)	629	Bengal gram whole	322
Tamarind	628	Beat root	300
Green gram whole	583	Kiwi	312
Spinach	570	Celery	293
Date	537	Maize	290
Black gram whole	523	Cauliflower	285
Red gram dal	482	French bean	282
Carrot	482	Cabbage	277
Colocasia	464	Pumpkin	259
Drumstick	463	Potato	249
Coriander leaves	453	Grape	249
Yam	422	Brinjal	229
Lentil	402	Aonla	201
		Grape fruit	200
Animal-based foods			
Skimmed milk powder	1210	Chicken	322
Whole milk powder	1100	Mutton	244
Milk malted dry	720	Rohu fish	225
		Milk fresh	130

Plant-based foods rich in potassium are tea, coffee, cocoa in beverages, dried apricot, dry plum, almond, dried coconut, dried fig, dried grape, tamarind, date in fruits, dry peas, spinach, carrot, colocasia, drumstick, coriander leaves, yam in vegetables, sesame seeds, roasted groundnut lentil in oil seeds, black gram dal, green gram dal, whole green gram, whole black gram, red gram dal in pulses and bajra in cereals.

Animal-based foods rich in potassium are skimmed milk and whole milk powder and dry malted milk. Chicken, mutton and rohu fish have fair source of potassium.

5.1.6.4 Absorption

Potassium is absorbed by the upper part of intestine. The absorbed potassium is used for various functions in the body. Excess potassium is excreted in the urine and faeces.

5.1.6.5 Effects on human health

1. *Deficiency*: Diuretics can deplete the potassium. Dehydration also leads to potassium loss from cells. Deficiency causes following disorders in the body:
   - Weakness
   - Muscular paralysis
   - Hypertension or blood pressure
2. *High intake*: High intake of potassium causes muscular weakness similar to that of potassium deficiency. Excessive potassium in the stomach triggers the vomiting.
3. *Prevention/cure*:
   - Potassium occurs in various foods abundantly and deficiency rarely occurs in human body; hence, potassium supplement is not required.
   - Avoid intravenous administration for excess of potassium in the body.
   - Use diet which is adequate in potassium.

5.1.7 Sulphur

Sulphur is also considered major mineral although it occurs only as part of other compounds such as protein. The body receives sulphur through proteins as sulphur-containing amino acids such as methionine and cysteine. Skin, hair and nails contain some of the body's more rigid protein which have high sulphur content. Sulphur is constituents of protein, glycosaminoglycans, bile acids and compounds like insulin and glutathione. Sulphur is excreted by the kidneys in urine in the form of inorganic, organic and ethereal sulphate.

5.1.7.1 Dietary requirements

There is no recommended dietary intake for sulphur and deficiency is unknown.

5.1.7.2 Dietary sources

The sources of sulphur are cereals, pulses, legumes, cauliflower, eggs and plant and animal protein.

5.2 Micro minerals

Micro minerals are trace elements and required in amounts less than 10 mg/d in diet. In other words, the minerals present at levels less than 0.05% in the human body are called micro minerals. The important micro minerals are iron, copper, iodine, zinc, manganese, cobalt, fluorine, chromium, cobalt, molybdenum and selenium.

5.2.1 Iron

The iron content of the adult human body is estimated about 4.5 g. The greater part of the iron is found in haemoglobin. The iron in the body exists in complex forms bound to protein. Iron exists in two forms: ferrous and ferric. Iron is absorbed from intestine in the form of ferrous salts. Ferrous salts have been found more effective in haemoglobin formation than ferric salts. About 70% of the iron is present in red blood cells (RBCs) called haemoglobin and in muscle cells called myoglobin and some are stored in the body organs such as the liver, spleen, kidney and bone marrow.

Ascorbic acid enhances the absorption of iron, whereas oxalic acid and excess of calcium and phosphorus interferes or lowers the absorption.

5.2.1.1 Functions

The functions of iron in human body are as follows.

1. *Oxygen transport*: Iron is a major component of haemoglobin present in the blood. Iron is present in the haem part of haemoglobin. It represents about two-thirds of the body's iron. Haemoglobin is necessary for transport of oxygen from lungs to various parts of the body.
2. *Helps in muscle contraction*: Iron is an essential component of myoglobin. Myoglobin is the protein (bound to iron) present in muscle tissues that help in the transport and short-term storage of oxygen in muscle cells. This oxygen is used for muscle contraction and for other immediate needs of the muscle cells.
3. *Energy metabolism*: Iron is needed for energy production. It helps with the conversion of nutrients into ATP, which is the form of energy, the body uses to carry out its functions.
4. *Brain development*: Iron is also a component of neurotransmitters and plays an important role in brain development and function, especially cognitive abilities, and mood
5. *DNA synthesis*: Iron is needed for making a genetic material called DNA.
6. *Antioxidant activity*: It acts as antioxidants and protects tissues from free radicals. Free radicals are a contributing factor for aging and cardiovascular diseases.

5.2.1.2 Dietary requirement

Recommended dietary allowances for iron by ICMR are given in Table 5.13.

Table 5.13 Daily allowances of iron.

Group	Particulars	Iron (mg/d)
Men	Sedentary work	17
	Moderate work	17
	Hard work	17
Women	Sedentary work	21
	Moderate work	21
	Hard work	21
	Expectant	35
Lactating	0–6 months	21
	6–12 months	21
Infants	0–6 months	46 μg/kg
	6–12 months	5
Children	1–3 years	9
	4–8 years	13
	7–9 years	16
Boys	10–12 years	21
Girls	10–12 years	27
Boys	13–15 years	32
Girls	13–15 years	27
Boys	16–17 years	28
Girls	16–17 years	26

5.2.1.3 Dietary source

The iron content of plant- and animal-based foods is given in Table 5.14.

Table 5.14 Iron content of foods.

Food sources	Iron (mg/100 g)	Food sources	Iron (mg/100 g)
Plant-based food			
Cauliflower	40.0	Bengal gram roasted	9.5
Karonda	39.0	Gingelly seed	9.3
Jamun	39.0	Carrot leaves	8.8
Rice bran	35.0	Cowpea	8.6
Cumin seed	31.0	Bajra	8.0
Amaranth	25.5	Watermelon	7.9
Rice flakes	20.0	Coconut dry	7.8
Tamarind	18.0	Pistachio nut	7.7

Coriander leaves	18.0	Peas dry	7.0
Fenugreek leaves	16.5	Rice puffed	6.6
Mustard leaves	16.3	Cashew nut	5.8
Beetroot green	16.2	Drumstick	5.3
Mint	15.6	Almond	5.1
Loquat	12.0	Phalsa	5.0
Spinach	10.9	Aonla	4.5
Soya bean	10.4	Custard apple	4.3
Colocasia leaves	10.0	Jaggery	2.6
Animal-based foods			
Chela fish	10.0	Khoa	5.8
Liver sheep	6.3	Prawn	5.3

Plant-based foods rich in iron are fruits (karonda, jamum, tamarind, loquat), vegetables [cauliflower, amaranth, coriander leaves, fenugreek leaves, mustard leaves, beetroot green, colocasia leaves, spinach, soya bean, herb (mint), spice (cumin seed)] and cereals (rice bran, rice flakes, Bengal gram, roasted). Foods which have also good source of iron are gingelly seeds, carrot leaves, cowpea and bajra.

Among animal-based foods, liver is an excellent source. Other organ meats like kidney and spleen also contain substantial amounts of iron.

5.2.1.4 Absorption

Absorption of iron from food takes place in duodenum and the small intestine. Only about 10% of the iron is absorbed in normal adult. However, this value increases markedly with iron deficiency. Iron once enters the body is absorbed by the upper part of the intestine. The extant of absorption of iron in plant and animal-based foods is different. Iron absorption from animal-based food is higher than plant-based foods. Plant-based foods such as cereals and green vegetables have inhibitors that hinder the absorption. Protein and vitamin C present in the food promote the absorption of iron. Iron after absorption is transported by the blood to body cells for various functions. Amount of iron to some extant is transferred to the liver spleen, kidney and bone marrow. The loss is through bile or sloughing of gastrointestinal epithelium.

The extent of iron absorption from different food stuffs depends on the type of iron. There are two types of iron present in the food, heme and non-heme irons. Heme iron is an easily absorbed form of iron found in animal foods because it comes from haemoglobin and myoglobin contained in the flesh of the animal.

Non-heme iron is a less easily absorbed form of iron found in plant foods. The absorption of non-heme iron is strongly influenced by enhancers and inhibitors present in the same meal.

Substances that can reduce the amount of non-heme iron absorption are called as inhibitors and substance that can increase its absorption is called enhancers.

5.2.1.5 *Inhibitors of non-heme iron*

1. *Polyphenols or phenolic compounds*: The phenolic compounds are released from food or beverages during digestion, and can combine with iron in the intestine making it unavailable for absorption. Phenolic acid present in herbal teas, black teas, coffee and cocoa can inhibit iron absorption. The effect can be reduced by the presence of vitamin C.
2. *Phytic acid*: Phytic acid is present in legumes, dried beans and peas, seeds, nuts, wholegrains - especially in the bran or outer hull. Even low levels of phytate (about 5% in cereal whole flours) have a strong inhibitory effect on iron bioavailability. Fermentation and refining of grain can reduce phytic acid content.
3. *Oxalate*: It occurs naturally in many common plants, especially in dark leafy green vegetables such as spinach, chard, beet greens and kale. They inhibit the body's iron absorption by combining with iron to form a insoluble compound called iron oxide.
4. *Calcium*: High intakes of calcium can inhibit iron absorption if both are present in the same meal. Separating foods high in calcium from those high in iron during meals and snacks may prevent some of this calcium-induced inhibition.

5.2.1.6 *Enhancers of non-heme iron absorption*

1. *Vitamin C*: Pairing sources of non-heme iron with foods containing vitamin C, or ascorbic acid, boosts iron absorption. The ascorbic acid forms a complex with iron and chemically modifies iron into a form that body can easily absorb, it reduces iron from ferric to ferrous forms, which increases its absorption. Vitamin C rich foods are guava, aonla, oranges ,lemon, pineapple, broccoli, tomatoes, fortified fruit juices, etc.
2. *Citric acid*: Citric acid and lactic acid from foods (fermentation) as well as HCl from the stomach can enhance iron absorption.
3. *Animal food*: The inclusion of animal foods in the diet greatly enhances non-heme iron absorption.

5.2.1.7 Effects on human health

1. *Deficiency*: Iron deficiency results either from poor dietary intake of iron, the inability to absorb iron from the digestive tract, or from excessive loss, such as in heavy menstrual bleeding. Because the majority of iron goes into the production of RBCs, iron deficiency results in anaemia. Iron deficiency anaemia causes microcytic anaemia, in which the body produces fewer and smaller RBCs, which decreases their capacity to transport oxygen.

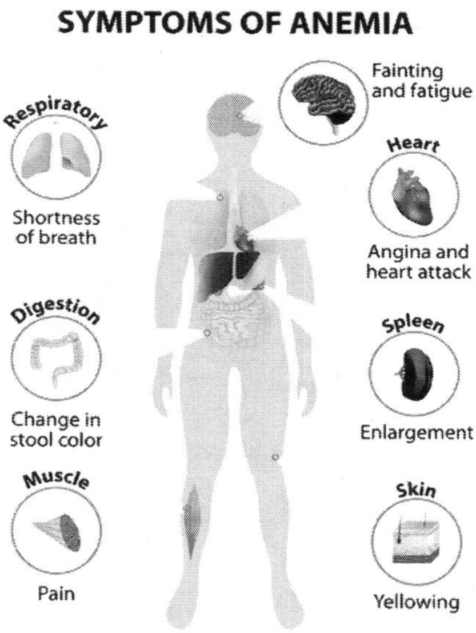

Figure 5.1 Symptoms of anaemia.

1. *Anaemia*: Anaemia is prevalent in infants, children, adolescent girls, expectant and lactating mother (Fig. 5.1). The characteristic symptoms of this disease are:
   - Low level of haemoglobin
   - The normal level of haemoglobin ranges between 13 and 15 g/100 mL of blood in human beings. The range commonly falls between 5 and 9 g/100 mL in anaemic cases. As a result, the oxygen-carrying power of the blood is diminished.
   - Lassitude, fatigue, exertion and giddiness in women.
   - Retarded growth, poor appetite, dullness or inactive and pallor of the skin in infants and children.
2. *Excess intake of iron*: Excessive iron intake caused by dietary iron overload, excessive oral or parenteral iron supplementation and blood transfusion can be highly toxic.

Genetic factors can also influence iron retention, with diseases such as haemochromatosis characterized by excessive iron absorption that leads to life-threatening organ damage.

3. *Prevention/cure*:
    - Diet should contain an adequate amount of iron to meet the requirement for preventing iron deficiency.
    - Infant should receive a mixture containing 0.2 g ferrous ammonium citrate sweetened with sugar three times a day.
    - Anaemic children should be given 0.4–0.9 g of ferrous ammonium citrate in the form of a mixture.
    - Anaemic women should be given ferrous sulphate tablets of 0.2 g three times a day. The treatment should continue till the haemoglobin level raised or restored to a normal level.
    - Avoid excess supplement of iron to prevent toxicity.

5.2.2 Zinc

Zinc is found in small amount in all tissues of human body. The adult human body may contain 1.4–2.3 g zinc. The amount of zinc is found slightly higher in bones/teeth, pancreas than other tissues. Whole blood and blood serum contain 0.7 and 0.1 mg/100 mL, respectively.

5.2.2.1 Functions

The important functions of zinc are:

- It is an essential component/cofactor for more than 300 enzymes involved in synthesis and metabolism of carbohydrates, lipids, proteins, nucleic acids and other micronutrients.
- Essential for cell division and is needed for normal growth and development.
- Zinc is also needed for the senses of smell and taste.
- It is involved in DNA synthesis and the process of genetic expression.
- It helps to maintain optimum immune function, boosts immunity and helps in wound healing.
- Zinc is needed to balance most hormones, including insulin, the main hormone involved in the regulation of blood sugar.
- Zinc stabilizes the molecular structure of cellular components and membranes and contributes in this way to the maintenance of cell and organ integrity.

5.2.2.2 Dietary requirements

The recommended dietary allowances for zinc by ICMR are given in Table 5.15.

Table 5.15 Daily allowances of zinc.

Group	Particulars	Zinc (mg/d)
Men	Sedentary work	12
	Moderate work	12
	Hard work	12
Women	Sedentary work	10
	Moderate work	10
	Hard work	10
	Expectant	12
Lactating	0–6 months	12
	6–12 months	12
Infants	0–6 months	–
	6–12 months	–
Children	1–3 years	5
	4–8 years	7
	7–9 years	8
Boys	10–12 years	9
Girls	10–12 years	9
Boys	13–15 years	11
Girls	13–15 years	11
Boys	16–17 years	12
Girls	16–17 years	12

5.2.2.3 Dietary sources

The zinc content of plant- and animal-based foods is given in Table 5.16.

Table 5.16 Zinc content of various foods.

Food sources	Zinc (mg/100 g)	Food sources	Zinc (mg/100 g)
Plant-based foods			
Yeast	7.91	Soya bean	3.6
Cashew nuts	5.78	Paushṭik atta	2.9
Soya bean	4.89	Kidney beans	2.79
Almonds	4.46	Chick peas	2.76
Lentils	3.7	Defatted soya flour	2.7
Animal-based foods			
Crustaceans, crab	5.95	Turkey	1.78
Beef	4.55	Chicken	1.31

Goat	4.0	Fish salmon	0.64
Pork	1.74		

High-protein foods contain high amounts of zinc. Beef, pork and goat contain more zinc than fish. Other foods which are rich source of zinc are yeast, nuts, wholegrains, soya bean and lentils.

Fruits and vegetables are not good sources, because the zinc in plant protein is not as available for use by the body as the zinc from animal proteins. Therefore, low-protein diets and vegetarian diets tend to be low in zinc.

5.2.2.4 Absorption

Dietary zinc absorbed (about 20–30%) in small intestine. Absorbed zinc is transported to blood plasma mostly by albumin and α-2-macroglobulin. Excretion of zinc is through urine, bile and pancreas.

Phytates in wholegrain, cereals, nuts, legumes and some other foods inhibit zinc absorption and so affect the bioavailability of zinc from plant foods. Absorption of zinc from animal sources are high because of the absence of substances that inhibit zinc absorption, in fact animal protein enhance zinc absorption. Fermentation and refining of grain can reduce phytic acid content. Refining of wholegrains not only remove phytic acid but also the other essential nutrient.

5.2.2.5 Effects on human health

1. *Deficiency*: Zinc deficiency due to dietary inadequacy is unlikely in healthy individuals. Zinc deficiency is more likely to occur due to medical conditions which causes zinc malabsorption or increased zinc loss, such as severe burns or prolonged diarrhoea, etc. Deficiency of zinc in the diet causes following disorders:
   - Frequent infections
   - Impaired wound healing
   - Impaired sense of taste and smell
   - Retardation of growth
   - Dwarfism or delayed genital maturation in children
2. *Excess intake*: The tolerable upper intake level (UI) for zinc is 35 mg/d for teens aged 14–18 years. For adults 40 mg/d. High doses of zinc or zinc supplements can cause:
   - Decreased immunity
   - Interfere with the absorption of copper, leading to copper deficiency
   - Nausea, headache, lethargyness, irritability, stomach irritation and vomiting

3. *Prevention/cure*:

- Diets having adequate amount of zinc do not cause zinc deficiency in human beings
- Avoid high dose of zinc supplement to prevent toxicity

5.2.3 Copper

Copper is an essential trace mineral present in all body tissues. The adult human body contains 100–150 mg of copper. Copper found in blood is in the form of copper-protein complex in RBC as hemocuprein and in plasma as ceruloplasmin.

5.2.3.1 Functions

The functions of copper in human beings are:

- Copper is a constituent of several enzymes that act as catalyst in number of body functions
- Helps in energy production
- Keeps our brain and nervous system healthy
- Helps to form collagen, a key part of bones and connective tissue
- Act as an antioxidant, reducing free radicals that can damage cells and DNA
- Helps in formation of pigment melanin, required for the pigmentation of hair and skin
- Important for the production of haemoglobin and RBCs, as well as for the proper utilization of iron and oxygen within the blood

5.2.3.2 Dietary requirements

The adequate intake for copper recommended by the Food and Nutrition Board, IMNA (USA) is given in Table 5.17.

Table 5.17 Daily allowances of copper.

Group	Particulars	Copper (μg/d)
Men	Adult	900
Women	Adult	900
Women	Expectants	1000
Women	Lactating	1300
Infants	0–6 months	200
	6–12 months	250
Children	1–3 years	340
	4–8 years	440
Boys	9–13 year	700

Girls	9–13 year	700
Boys	14–18 years	890
Girls	14–18 years	890

5.2.3.3 Dietary sources

The copper content of various foods is given in Table 5.18.

Table 5.18 Copper content of various foods.

Food sources	Copper (mg/100 g)	Food sources	Copper (mg/100 g)
Plant-based food			
Sesame seeds	4.082	Coffee	0.82
Cashew nuts	2.195	Bengal gram whole	0.76
Sunflower seeds	1.8	Cowpea	0.75
Soya bean	1.658	Black gram dal	0.72
Tea	1.59	Rice polished	0.72
Walnuts, black dried	1.36	Lentil	0.66
Red gram dal	1.25	Drumstick	0.60
Green gram dal	1.13	Bajra	0.55
Bengal gram dal	0.98	Coriander leaves	0.225
Green gram whole	0.97	Wheat flour	0.49
Cocoa	0.92	Pears	0.08
Peas dried	0.85	Pineapple	0.11
Animal-based food			
Beef liver	9.75	Mollusks oyster	1.576

Plant-based foods rich in copper content are sesame seeds, cashew nut, sunflower seeds, soya bean and tea. Pulses are also good source of copper. Animal-based organ meats such as liver and fish (Mollusks oyster) are rich source of copper.

5.2.3.4 Effects on human health

1. *Deficiency*: Copper deficiency occurs in infants fed only on milk diet. The deficiency causes:
   - Anaemia
   - Osteoporosis
   - Lowered resistance to infections
   - Impaired brain function
   - Impaired growth

2. *Excess intake*: Copper toxicity is unlikely due to excess of dietary intake in healthy individual. Copper toxicity generally can result from ingesting or absorbing excess copper, for example, from ingesting an acidic food or beverage that has prolonged contact with a copper container. In large amounts, copper is poisonous and can result in:
   - Nausea, vomiting and diarrhoea
   - Kidney damage, liver damage, coma

3. *Prevention/cure*:
   - Foods containing adequate amount of copper should be used to prevent disorders.
   - Infants suffering from anaemia should be given copper salt with iron.
   - Avoid excess amount or supplement to prevent copper toxicity.

5.2.4 Iodine

The adult body of human being contains 15–20 mg of iodine. The maximum concentration of this mineral approx. 70–80% is found in the thyroid gland which is located in the neck region. Iodine is a constituent of thyroxin which is active principle component of thyroid glands.

5.2.4.1 Functions

The thyroid glands play a role in:

- Metabolism of energy
- Body growth
- Foetal and infant development

5.2.4.2 Dietary requirements

The adequate intake for iodine recommended by Food and Nutrition Board, IMNA (USA) is given in Table 5.19.

Table 5.19 Daily allowances of iodine.

Group	Particulars	Iodine (μg/d)
Men	Adult	150
Women	Adult	150
Women	Expectants	220
Women	Lactating	290
Infants	0–6 months	110
	6–12 months	130
Children	1–3 years	90
	4–8 years	90

Boys	9–13 year	120
Girls	9–13 year	120
Boys	14–18 years	150
Girls	14–18 years	150

5.2.4.3 *Food sources*

The common foods contain small amount of iodine. The amount varies in food with iodine content of the soil. Crops such as vegetables grown in coastal areas where iodine content of the soil is high have substantial amounts of iodine. However, in hilly region the iodine content of both the soil and water is low hence the crops grown in such areas contain less iodine.

The iodine content of animal foods like eggs, dairy products and meat depends on the iodine content of the food that is part of the animal's diet. Sea foods like fish and shell fish are the best sources of iodine. Crude common salt prepared from sea water and iodized salt are among the good source of iodine.

5.2.4.4 *Effects on human health*

1. *Deficiency*: Iodine deficiency is rare in areas where iodine is added to table salt. Deficiency of iodine in the diet causes following disorders:

Hypothyroid: It causes lower than normal heart rate, a chronic feeling of being cold, constipation, unexplained weight gain, dry skin, hair loss or coarse dry hair, weakness, muscle aches, depression and fatigue.

Goitre disease: The disease is characterized by enlargement of thyroid glands. The normal weight of thyroid gland in adult is about 25 g. This increases 200-500 g or more in goitre. The disease generally occurs in people of hilly or mountainous region (Fig. 5.2).

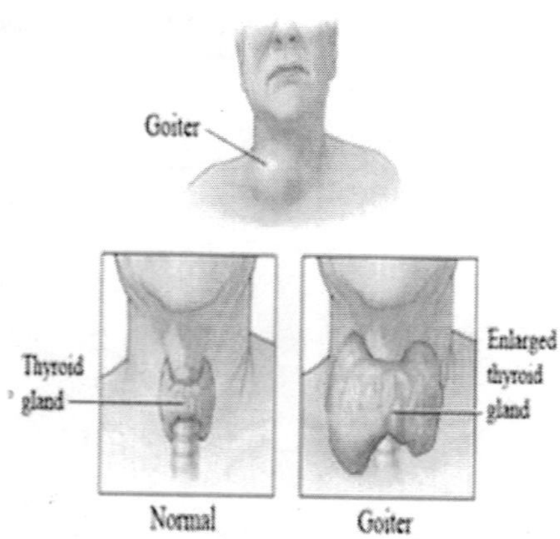

Figure 5.2 Goitre.

Cretinism in children: Children of mothers with severe iodine deficiency during pregnancy can cause cretinism. Cretinism is a syndrome characterized by permanent brain damage, mental retardation, deaf mutism, spasticity and short stature.

Excess intake: Excess consumption of iodine is uncommon. It usually results from taking iodine supplements or people who live near the sea, consume too much iodine or drink water that is high in iodine and can results in:

Hyperthyroidism: An excessively high metabolic rate. People with this condition have rapid heart rates and often palpitations, excessive sweating, weight loss and experience muscle weakness.

2. *Prevention/cure*: The disease can be prevented by the regular use of iodized salt. This can be prepared by mixing 1 g of sodium iodate in 100 kg of common salt. Thyroid can become normal if the treatment with iodized salt is started early otherwise enlargement of the glands persist in delayed treatment.
   - Avoid the consumption or use of large quantity of those foods which contain goiterogenic substances such as cabbage, cauliflower, broccoli, brussels sprouts, turnips, kale, rutabaga, spinach, mustard, soya bean-related foods and peanuts. These foods should be eaten in cooked form and not raw because cooking inactivates the goitrogenic compound to some extent.
   - These goitrogens or substances react with iodine present in food and make iodine unavailable.
   - Avoid to take iodine supplement to prevent hyperthyroidism.

5.2.5 Manganese

The adult normal human body contains 12–20 mg manganese which is distributed throughout the body such as bone, kidney, liver, pancreas and other tissues. The blood content of human body is low about 2–3 μg/100 mL. Manganese present in the diet is absorbed only 3–4%.

5.2.5.1 Functions

The manganese plays an important role in:

- Required for the metabolism of carbohydrate, amino acid and fat
- Growth and reproduction
- Functioning central nervous system
- Skeleton/bone development
- Plays a role in wound healing by helping in the formation of collagen
- Manganese is a component of the antioxidant enzyme superoxide dismutase, which helps in fighting free radicals.

5.2.5.2 Dietary requirement

The adequate intake for manganese recommended by the Food and Nutrition Board, IMNA (USA) is given in Table 5.20.

Table 5.20 Daily allowances of manganese.*

Group	Particulars	Manganese (mg/d)
Male	Adult	2.3
Female	Adult	1.8
Women	Expectant	2.0
Women	Lactation	2.6
Infants	0–6 months	0.003
	6–12 months	0.6
Children	1–3 years	1.2
	4–8 years	1.5
Boys	9–13 years	1.9
Girls	9–13 years	1.6
Boys	14–18 years	2.2
Girls	14–18 years	1.6

* The tolerable UL for manganese is 9 mg/day for teens aged 14–18 years. For adult 11 mg/d.

5.2.5.3 Dietary sources

Manganese is found in several foods including mussels, nuts, seeds, tea, wholegrains and leafy green vegetables. Absorption of manganese can be adversely affected by other minerals such as calcium, phosphorus and soy protein. Even though vegetarian sources are high in manganese but its absorption from vegetarian food is not good because certain substances in food greatly inhibit its absorption. High phytate content, present in nuts, seeds, legumes and wholegrains and oxalic acid present in green leafy vegetable reduces manganese absorption. Although tea is rich in manganese, but tannin present in it reduces its absorption. Animal foods are not very good source of manganese but bioavailability from animal food is better.

The manganese content of plant- and animal-based foods is given in Table 5.21.

Table 5.21 Manganese content of foods.

Food sources	Manganese (mg/100 g)	Food sources	Manganese (mg/100 g)
Plant-based food			
Hazelnuts	5.6	Peanuts	1.93

Tofu, dried or frozen	3.86	Lima beans	1.67
Brown rice, long grain	2.85	Pineapple	0.93
Flax seeds	2.48	Spinach	0.90
Almonds	2.18	Tea, black brewed	0.20
Whole wheat bread	2.1		
Animal-based food			
Mussels cooked	6.8	Chicken liver	0.26

5.2.5.4 Effects on human health

1. *Deficiency*: Deficiency of manganese in human beings is not known. This is normally supplied by average diet.

Toxicity symptoms have been reported in mine workers due to dust containing manganese ores. The symptoms are tremors of hand, blurred speech and spastic gait.

5.2.6 Fluorine

Fluorine is found in little amount in bones and teeth. The fluorine requirement of the body is 1–2 ppm which is met by drinking water containing 1–2 ppm.

5.2.6.1 Functions

The functions of fluorine are:

- Required for proper formation of bone and teeth.
- Crystalline mineral of bones and teeth form fluorapatite which increases hardness of bone and teeth.
- Provide protection against dental caries and acid attack.

5.2.6.2 Dietary requirement

The adequate intake for fluorine recommended by the Food and Nutrition Board, IMNA (USA) is given in Table 5.22.

Table 5.22 Daily allowances of fluorine.*

Group	Particulars	Fluoride (mg/d)
Male	Adult	4.0
Female	Adult	3.0
Women	Expectant	3.0
Women	Lactation	3.0
Infants	0–6 months	0.01
Infants	6–12 months	0.5

Children	1–3 years	0.7
Children	4–8 years	1.0
Boys	9–13 years	2.0
Girls	9–13 years	2.0
Boys	14–18 years	3.0
Girls	14–18 years	3.0

* The tolerable UI for fluoride is 10 mg/d for ages above 9 years.

5.2.6.3 Dietary sources

Drinking water is the main source. Tea and some sea fish also have small amount of fluoride.

5.2.6.4 Absorption

Fluoride is readily absorbed in the stomach and small intestine. It is distributed entirely to bone and teeth. Generally 50% of daily intake is excreted through urine.

5.2.6.5 Effects on human health

1. *Deficiency*: Fluorine deficiency occurs high in those area where drinking water contains fluorine less than 0.5 ppm. The deficiency causes dental caries in children and adult and osteoporosis.
2. *Toxicity*: Excess of fluorine in human beings causes toxic effects which are as follows:

   Mottled enamel or dental fluorosis: Mottled enamel occurs when drinking water contains excessive amount of fluorine (3–5 ppm). Enamel of teeth loses its lustre and becomes rough. White patches with yellow or brown staining appear irregularly over teeth surface.
   Skeletal fluorosis: Skeletal fluorosis occurs when drinking water contains fluorine over 10 ppm. This is characterized by increased bone density and hyper calcification of bone of the spine, limbs and pelvis. Ligament of the spine also becomes calcified. Such persons are crippled, difficult bending and squatting.
3. *Prevention/cure*:
   - Drinking water containing 1-2 ppm can prevent dental caries.
   - Removal of excess fluorine from water supplies by treatment with suitable fluorine absorbents such as activated carbon can prevent toxic fluorosis.

5.2.7 Chromium

The chromium content of adult human body is estimated about 6 mg. Generally adult tissue contains 0.02–0.04 ppm and blood contains in traces 0.009–0.055 ppm. This is also present in skin, hair, brain and body fats.

5.2.7.1 *Functions*

Functions of chromium are as follows:

- Chromium is considered as cofactors for insulin.
- Essential for activating enzymes involved in carbohydrate, fat and protein digestion and metabolism.

5.2.7.2 *Dietary requirement*

The adequate intake for chromium recommended by the Food and Nutrition Board, IMNA (USA) is given in Table 5.23.

Table 5.23 Daily allowances of chromium.*

Group	Particulars	Chromium (μg/d)
Male	Adult	35
Female	Adult	25
Women	Expectant	30
Women	Lactation	45
Infants	0–6 months	0.2
Infants	6–12 months	5.5
Children	1–3 years	11
Children	4–8 years	15
Boys	9–13 years	25
Girls	9–13 years	21
Boys	14–18 years	35
Girls	14–18 years	24

* No tolerable UI for chromium is established.

5.2.7.3 *Dietary sources*

Chromium is widely distributed in the food. It is present in vegetables, fruits, cereal grains, legumes, nuts/seeds, brewers yeast, sea food, organ meats such as liver and dairy products. Chromium present in food is in very small amounts less than 2 μg.

5.2.7.4 *Effects on human health*

Deficiency of chromium causes following disorders.

- Impaired growth
- Disturbs metabolism of protein, glucose and lipids

Prevention/cure:
Chromium is required in traces. The average diet appears to be sufficient to meet the requirements of chromium.

5.2.8 Cobalt

Cobalt is found in traces in all tissues of human body. Liver and kidney have high concentration of cobalt. Vitamin B_{12} has most of the cobalt. The deficiency of cobalt in human beings is not observed. The traces of cobalt found in foods meet the requirement of human beings.

5.2.8.1 Functions

- Biological activity of vitamin B_{12}
- Taking part in enzymatic action and thyroid functions

5.2.8.2 Dietary requirement

Deficiency of cobalt is not common among human beings; hence, dietary allowance per day is not established.

5.2.8.3 Dietary sources

Cereals, beans and peas among plant-based foods and organ meats such as liver and kidney in animal-based foods.

5.2.8.4 Effects on human health

1. *Deficiency*: Cobalt deficiency is accompanied by all the signs and symptoms of vitamin B_{12} deficiency. The most important is anaemia.
2. *Toxicity*: Administration of cobalt in excess amount is toxic and causes polycythaemia (increased number of RBC in blood).
3. *Prevention/cure*:
   - Cobalt is not synthesized in the body hence, dietary source is vitamin B_{12}.
   - Avoid administration of large amount of cobalt to prevent toxicity.

5.2.9 Molybdenum

Molybdenum is required in only trace amounts in the body.

5.2.9.1 *Functions*

The functions of molybdenum are:

- It acts as a catalyst for enzymes and to help facilitate the breakdown of sulphur-containing amino acids in the body.
- It helps to metabolize toxins and leftover by-products of digestion.

5.2.9.2 *Dietary requirement*

The adequate intake for molybdenum recommended by the Food and Nutrition Board, IMNA (USA) is given in Table 5.24.

Table 5.24 Daily allowances of molybdenum.*

Group	Particulars	Molybdenum (μg/d)
Male	Adult	45
Female	Adult	45
Women	Expectant	50
Women	Lactation	50
Infants	0–6 months	2
Infants	6–12 months	3
Children	1–3 years	17
Children	4–8 years	22
Boys	9–13 years	34
Girls	9–13 years	34
Boys	14–18 years	43
Girls	14–18 years	43

* The tolerable upper intake level (UI) for molybdenum is 1100 mg for children aged 9–13 years, 1700 mg/d for teens aged 14–18 years. For adults 2000 mg/d.

5.2.9.3 *Dietary sources*

Molybdenum is primarily found in foods that are consumed on a regular basis. A few foods that are extremely molybdenum-rich include legumes, leafy vegetables, wholegrain cereal meats, cheese and milk.

5.2.9.4 *Absorption*

Molybdenum is readily absorbed by the intestine and is excreted in urine and bile.

5.2.9.5 *Effects on human health*

- The human body requires very little molybdenum to receive the benefits that it provides. This means that molybdenum deficiencies are extremely rare. However, its deficiency causes xanthimuria with low plasma and urinary uric acid concentration.
- The most commonly documented form of excess molybdenum appearing in the human system occurs with individuals that work in factories where supplements are processed. In these cases, the most frequent complaints associated with excess amounts of molybdenum include nose and throat irritation accompanied by possible coughing.

Prevention/cure:

- Diet rich in molybdenum meet the requirements.
- Avoid to take supplement for preventing toxicity.

5.2.10 Selenium

Selenium is found in the body as selenium analogues of sulphur-containing amino acids such as seleno cysteine and seleno methionine.

5.2.10.1 *Functions*

- Prevents membrane lipid peroxidation along with vitamin E
- Acts as a prosthetic group of enzyme glutathione peroxidase
- Prevents hepatic necrosis and muscular dystrophy
- Reduces the requirement of vitamin E
- Provide protection against carciogenic chemicals

5.2.10.2 *Dietary requirement*

Dietary intake for selenium recommended by Food and Nutrition Board, IMNA (USA) is given in Table 5.25.

Table 5.25 Daily allowances of selenium.

Group	Particulars	Selenium (μg/d)
Male	Adult	55
Female	Adult	55
Women	Expectant	60
Women	Lactation	70
Infants	0–6 months	15
Infants	6–12 months	20

Children	1–3 years	20
Children	4–8 years	30
Boys	9–13 years	40
Girls	9–13 years	40
Boys	14–18 years	55
Girls	14–18 years	55

5.2.10.3 Dietary source

Foods which are good source of selenium are cereals, sea foods and organ meat such as liver and kidney.

5.2.10.4 Effects on human health

1. *Deficiency*: Deficiency causes following disorders:
    - Liver necrosis
    - Pancreas degeneration
    - Infertility
    - Muscular dystrophy
    - Cardio myopathy
2. *Toxicity*: Excess intake of selenium causes selenosis which leads to dermatitis, diarrhoea, weight loss and emotional disturbances.
3. *Prevention/cure*:
    - Deficiency can be avoided by using adequate amount of foods rich in selenium.
    - Toxicity can be avoided by avoiding large amount of selenium administration.

6

Nutritive value of plant-based foods

Plant-based foods are cereals, pulses, fruits, vegetables, spices and herbs, nuts and oil seeds, fats and oils, sweetening agents and beverages. The nutritive values of these foods are discussed in this chapter.

6.1 Cereals

The term cereal includes plants that produce grains. The grains themselves and food products made from these grains. Cereals largely used in India are wheat, rice, jwar, maize, bajra, barley and finger millet (ragi). Rice wheat and barley are classified as fine cereals. Bajra, ragi, maize, oat and jwar are the coarse cereals and referred as millets. Cereals and millets form stable food of the diet. Cereals are consumed in large quantity by a vast majority of the population in the world. Cereals are rich source of carbohydrate and form main source of energy in Indian diet. It is fairly rich in protein, B vitamins and some minerals. Cereals are poor in carotene content and have no vitamin C. The nutritive values of cereals are as follows.

6.1.1 Macro nutrients

The moisture protein, fat, fibre, carbohydrate and energy values are given in Table 6.1.

Table 6.1. Nutritive value of cereals, macro nutrients/100 g.

Cereals	Moisture (%)	Protein (%)	Fat (%)	Fibre (%)	Carbohydrate (%)	Energy (kcal)
Whole wheat/flour	12.8	12.1	1.7	2.2	69.4	341
Wheat flour refined	13.3	11.0	0.9	0.3	73.9	348
Wheat bread white	42.0	7.0	0.7	0.2	52.0	238
Wheat bread brown	40.8	8.0	1.1	0.8	49.0	238
Wheat semolina	13.4	11.1	0.8	0.3	74.4	349
Rice brown	10.9	7.5	1.0	0.9	77.1	346
Rice polished white	11.0	7.1	0.4	0.1	80.9	346
Hand pounded	12.2	8.5	0.6	0.9	78.1	349
Para boiled rice	13.6	7.0	0.8	0.1	78.0	345

Rice flakes	12.6	6.6	1.2	0.3	77.5	347
Rice puffed	14.7	7.5	0.1	7.6	74.0	327
Barley	12.5	11.5	1.3	3.9	69.3	335
Bajra	12.4	11.6	5.0	1.2	67.9	361
Jwar	12.0	10.4	1.9	1.6	72.6	349
Maize dry	14.9	11.3	3.6	2.8	66.8	342
Oatmeal	10.7	13.6	7.6	3.5	62.8	374
Ragi	13.1	7.4	1.3	3.7	72.9	328

6.1.1.1 Moisture

The moisture content of cereals varies from 10% to 14%. Brown rice and oat have lower amount of moisture. Breads of wheat have 40–42% moisture.

6.1.1.2 Protein

Protein content of cereals varies from 7% to 13.6%. Embryo scutellum and aleurone layer have higher concentration of protein than endosperm, pericarp and testa. The protein content of wheat, barley, bajra, jwar and maize is higher than the rice but protein quality of rice is better than other cereals. The types of protein present in cereals are gliadins (prolamines), glutelins, albumins and globulins. Gliadins and glutelins are gluten proteins which are important in baking bread, chapaties and other products due to its unique elasticity and flow properties. Cereals provide more than 50% of the protein requirements as they are consumed in greater quantities.

6.1.1.3 Fat

Cereals are low in fat content. Most of the cereals have less than 2% fat except oatmeal, bajra and dry maize which have comparatively higher content. Fat present in cereals meet about 50% of essential fatty acids requirements.

6.1.1.4 Fibre

The constituents of fibre are cellulose, hemicellulose and pentosans. These are concentrated in bran layers. Puffed rice, barley, ragi, oatmeal dry maize and whole wheat contain higher amount of fibre than other cereals.

6.1.1.5 Carbohydrate

The carbohydrates present in cereals are soluble carbohydrates and fibre. Cereals are rich in carbohydrates. Starch is the most important carbohydrates in all cereals. Carbohydrate content of cereal varies from 62.8% to 80.9%. Most of the cereals have more than 70% carbohydrates.

6.1.1.6 Energy value

Cereals are rich source of energy contributing 72–80% of the requirement. The energy value varies from 328 to 374 kcal. They are main source of energy.

6.1.2 Micro nutrients

Vitamins and mineral contents of varies cereals are given in Tables 6.2 and 6.3, respectively.

Table 6.2. Nutritive value of cereals - vitamin content/100 g.

Cereals	Carotene (μg)	Thiamine (mg)	Riboflavin (mg)	Niacin (mg)	Folic acid (μg)
Whole wheat/flour	64	0.49	0.17	5.0	12.1
Wheat flour refined	29	0.12	0.07	1.2	–
Wheat bread white	25	0.07	0.04	0.7	–
Wheat bread brown	60	0.21	0.07	1.4	–
Wheat semolina	31	0.13	0.08	1.3	2.2
Rice brown	4	0.21	0.16	2.4	36.0
Rice polished white	0	0.06	0.06	1.2	22.0
Hand pounded	2	0.21	0.16	3.9	60.0
Para boiled rice	–	0.21	0.05	3.8	30.0
Rice flakes	–	0.21	0.05	4.0	–
Rice puffed	–	0.21	0.04	4.1	–
Barley	10	0.47	0.20	4.7	–
Bajra	132	0.33	0.25	2.3	14.7
Jwar	47	0.37	0.13	3.1	14.0
Maize dry	90	0.42	0.10	1.8	14.0
Oatmeal	0	0.98	0.16	1.1	32.0
Ragi	42	0.42	0.19	1.1	5.2

Table 6.3. Nutritive value of cereals minerals content/100 g.

Cereals	Calcium (mg)	Phosphorus (mg)	Iron (mg)
Whole wheat/flour	48	355	4.9
Wheat flour refined	23	121	2.7
Wheat bread white	11	70.0	1.1
Wheat bread brown	20	200	3.0
Wheat semolina	20	90	1.1
Rice brown	40	280	2.0

Rice polished white	25	160	0.7
Hand pounded	65	190	3.2
Para boiled rice	95	143	1.3
Rice flakes	20	238	20
Rice puffed	23	150	6.6
Barley	26	230	3.7
Bajra	42	296	8.8
Jwar	37	222	6.6
Maize dry	10	348	2.3
Oatmeal	50	380	3.8
Ragi	344	283	3.9

6.1.2.1 Vitamins

Carotene: Cereals contain little amount of carotene except bajra and dry maize which have comparatively higher content. Cereals do not have ascorbic acid or vitamin C.

Thiamine: Cereals are important source of B vitamins. Thiamine content is higher in oatmeal, barley, whole wheat, dry maize and ragi than other cereals. Oatmeal has the highest content of thiamine followed by whole wheat flour.

Riboflavin: The riboflavin content of most of the cereals is less than 0.2% except bajra and barley, which have relatively higher content.

Niacin: Niacin content of cereals varies from 0.7 to 5 mg/100 g. Cereals containing 4–5% niacin are whole wheat, rice flakes, puffed rice and barley. Hand pounded and paraboiled rice retains better content of niacin than polished white or brown rice.

Folic acid: Folic acid content of hand pounded rice is higher than paraboiled, polished and brown rice. Other cereals which are fair source of folic acid are oatmeal, bajra, jwar and dry maize.

Cereal grain oils are rich in vitamin E. Most of the B vitamins are occurring in outer bran. Polishing or refining the grains reduced the content of B vitamins.

6.1.2.2 Minerals

Calcium: Millets such as ragi, bajra, jwar and oatmeals are rich in minerals. Calcium content of cereals is very poor except ragi which is very rich in calcium.

Phosphorus: Cereals are rich in phosphorus content. Oatmeal, whole wheat flour and dry maize have higher content of phosphorus. Some parts of phosphorus and calcium in cereals present in the form of phytin which are not available for absorptions.

Iron: The iron content of bajra and jwar is higher among the various cereals. Whole wheat flour has higher content of iron than refined wheat flour and other forms of wheat. Rice is poor in iron content. Phylates present in cereals reduces absorption of iron.

Other minerals such as copper (polished rice, wheat flour, bajra), magnesium (maize, whole wheat, barley, bajra, polished rice) and zinc are also found in small amount in cereals.

6.2 Pulses

Pulses are seeds of pod-bearing plant belong to the family Leguminaceae. The common pulses or legumes may be classified into three heads - grams, peas and beans. Pulses/edible leguminous seed are rich in protein. They are also good source of B vitamins and minerals. Tender pulses such as green peas, green Bengal gram and green field beans are fair source of ascorbic acid. The nutritive values of pulses are as follows.

6.2.1 Macro nutrients

The moisture, protein, fat, fibre, carbohydrate and energy values are given in Table 6.4.

Table 6.4. Nutritive value of pulses: macro nutrients.

Pulses	Moisture (g)	Protein (g)	Fat (g)	Fibre (g)	Carbohydrate (g)	Energy (kcal)
Bengal gram whole	9.3	17.1	5.3	3.9	60.9	360
Bengal gram dal	–	20.8	5.6	1.2	59.8	372
Bengal gram roasted	–	22.5	5.2	0.9	58.1	369
Black gram dal	10.9	24.0	1.4	0.9	59.6	347
Green gram whole	10.4	24.0	1.3	4.1	56.7	334
Green gram dal	–	24.5	1.2	0.8	59.9	348
Horse gram whole	11.8	22.0	0.5	5.3	57.2	321
Red gram dal	13.4	22.3	1.7	3.5	57.6	335
Cowpeas	13.4	24.1	1.0	3.8	54.5	323
Dry field beans	9.6	24.9	0.8	1.4	60.1	347
Dry peas	16.0	19.7	1.1	4.5	56.5	315
Roasted peas	–	22.9	1.4	1.5	58.8	340
Kidney bean	11.0	22.9	1.3	4.2	60.6	346

Lentil	12.4	25.1	0.7	0.7	59.0	343
Lathyrus pea	10.0	28.2	0.6	2.3	56.6	345

6.2.1.1 *Moisture*

Moisture content of pulses generally varies from 9% to 13%. Peas, cowpeas, lentil contains little higher amount of moisture than other pulses.

6.2.1.2 *Protein*

Protein content of pulses varies from 19.7% to 28.2%. Lathyrus pea (khesari dal) has higher content of protein followed by lentil, dry field bean, green gram and cowpeas. Protein content of pulses is double the amount of cereals. Pulse protein is mainly globulins and to some extent albumins in some species. Pulses are also good source of essential amino acids such as leucine, isoleucine, phenylalanine, threonine and valine but they are deficient in sulphur-containing amino acids particularly methionine and tryptophan.

6.2.1.3 *Fat*

Pulses are low in fat content. It varies from 0.5% to 5.6%. Bengal gram in various forms such as whole, roasted and dal has higher value as compared to other pulses. Horse gram whole, lathyrus pea, lentil and dry field beans have less than 1% fat. Pulses contain higher amount of poly unsaturated fatty acid and meet the requirements of essential fatty acids in the diet.

6.2.1.4 *Fibre*

Fibre content of pulses varies from 0.7% to 5.3%. Bengal gram, horse gram, green gram, dry peas and kidney beans have comparatively higher content of fibre than other pulses. Pulses which are very low or have less than 1% fibre are lentil and black gram dal.

6.2.1.5 *Carbohydrate*

Pulses contain 54.5–60.9% carbohydrates. Starch accounts the major portion of carbohydrates. Other forms of carbohydrates such as soluble sugar, fibre and unavailable carbohydrate are also present. The unavailable sugar present in pulses is oligosaccharides which are reduced considerably during fermentation, germination and cooking.

6.2.1.6 *Energy*

The energy value of pulses varies from 315 to 372 kcal/100 g. Bengal gram dal has comparatively higher energy value than other pulses. The energy value of pulses is similar to that of cereals caloric value.

6.2.2 Micro nutrients

Vitamin and mineral contents of pulses are given in Tables 6.5 and 6.6, respectively.

Table 6.5. Nutritive value of pulses: vitamin content/100 g.

Pulses	Carotene (µg)	Thiamine (mg)	Riboflavin (mg)	Niacin (mg)	Folic acid (µg)
Bengal gram whole	189	0.30	0.15	2.9	34.0
Bengal gram dal	129	0.48	0.18	2.4	32.0
Bengal gram roasted	113	0.20	0.15	1.3	22.0
Black gram dal	38	0.42	0.20	2.0	24.0
Green gram whole	94	0.47	0.27	2.1	–
Green gram dal	49	0.47	0.21	2.4	24.5
Horse gram whole	71	0.42	0.20	1.5	–
Red gram dal	132	0.45	0.19	2.9	19.0
Cowpeas	12	0.51	0.20	1.3	69.0
Dry field beans	–	0.52	0.16	1.8	–
Dry peas	39	0.47	0.19	3.4	4.6
Roasted peas	18	0.47	0.21	3.5	–
Kidney bean	30	0.54	0.18	2.1	–
Lentil	270	4.5	0.20	2.5	14.5
Lathyrus pea	120	0.39	0.17	2.9	–

Table 6.6. Nutritive value of pulses: minerals content/100 g.

Pulses	Calcium (mg)	Phosphorus (mg)	Potassium (mg)	Iron (mg)	Magnesium (mg)
Bengal gram whole	202	240	322	4.6	168
Bengal gram dal	56	330	386	5.3	138
Bengal gram roasted	58	310	–	9.5	–
Black gram dal	154	370	643	3.8	185
Green gram whole	124	280	583	4.4	171
Green gram dal	75	410	643	3.9	139
Horse gram whole	287	390	322	6.8	172
Red gram dal	73	260	482	2.7	133
Cowpeas	77	490	323	8.6	230
Dry field beans	60	450	402	2.7	–
Dry peas	75	300	980	7.0	124
Roasted peas	81	360	–	6.4	–

Kidney bean	200	-	-	5.1	-
Lentil	130	250	402	3.0	94
Lathyrus pea	110	500	-	5.6	-

6.2.2.1 Vitamins

1. *Carotene*: Carotene content of pulses is very low. Most of the pulses have 72–70 µg (microgram) of carotene (provitamin A).
2. *B vitamins*: Pulses are rich in B vitamins particularly thiamine, niacin and folic acid.

Thiamine: Thiamine content varies from 0.2 to 0.5 mg/100 g. Kidney bean, dry peas and dry field beans have comparatively higher content than other pulses.

Niacin: Niacin content varies from 1.3 to 3.5 mg/100 g. Kidney bean, roasted peas, lathyrus pea, Bengal gram and cowpea have higher content of niacin.

Riboflavin: Pulses are low in riboflavin content and dry pulses have no ascorbic acid content.

6.2.2.2 Minerals

Pulses contain calcium, phosphorus, potassium, iron and magnesium. Pulses also contain zinc.

Calcium: Calcium content varies from 56 to 287 mg/100 g. Horse gram whole, Bengal gram whole and kidney beans have higher contents of calcium.

Phosphorus: Phosphorus content varies from 240 to 500 mg/100 g. Lathyrus pea, cowpea, dry field beans and green gram dal have higher content of phosphorus. Major portion of phosphorus is present as phytates. Potassium content of dry peas, black gram dal and green gram dal is higher than the other pulses.

Iron: Iron content varies from 2 to 9.5 mg/100 g. Bengal gram roasted, cowpea, dry peace and whole horse gram are rich source of iron.

Magnesium: Magnesium content of pulses varies from 124 to 230 mg/100 g. Cowpea has the highest content of magnesium followed by black gram dal.

6.3 Fruits

Fruit is the ripened ovary and any other structure that is closely associated with it. Fruits are indispensable part of our diet. It is the cheapest and rich source of essential nutrients such as vitamins, minerals, fibres, organic acid, etc., which are vital for our health, balanced growth and normal functioning of human system. Regular consumption of fruits is needed to reduce the malnutrition and to guard against diseases caused by the deficiency of various nutrients. Fruits are therefore, considered as protective food and assume great importance in nutritional security of the people. The nutritional values of fruits are as follows.

6.3.1 Macro nutrients

The moisture, protein, fat, fibre, carbohydrate and energy values of fruits are given in Table 6.7.

Table 6.7. Nutritive value of fruits: macro nutrients.

Fruits	Moisture (%)	Protein (%)	Fat (%)	Fibre (%)	Carbohydrate (%)	Energy (kcal)
Almond	5.2	20.8	58.9	1.7	10.5	655
Amra	90.3	0.7	3.0	1.0	4.5	48
Aonla	81.8	0.5	0.1	3.4	13.7	58
Apple	84.6	0.2	0.5	1.0	13.4	56
Apricot fresh	85.3	1.4	0.3	1.1	11.6	48
Avocado	73.6	1.7	22.8	–	0.8	190
Bael	61.5	1.8	0.3	7.0	31.8	137
Banana	701	1.2	0.3	0.4	27.2	116
Ber	81.6	0.8	0.3	–	17.0	74
Barbados cherry	85.9	1.8	0.2	1.2	10.5	60
Black berry	87.2	1.3	0.5	3.8	6.7	37
Cape gooseberry	82.9	1.8	0.2	3.2	11.1	58
Carambola	91.9	0.7	0.2	0.8	7.5	28
Cashew apple	86.3	0.2	0.1	0.9	12.3	51
Cashew nut	5.9	21.2	46.9	1.3	22.3	596
Cherry	83.4	1.1	0.5	0.4	13.8	17
Chironji	4.5	14	32.8	5.0	17.2	585
Coconut fresh	36.3	4.5	41.6	3.6	13	444
Currant	18.4	2.7	0.5	1.0	75.2	316
Custard apple	70.5	1.6	0.4	3.1	23.5	104
Date	59.2	1.2	0.4	3.7	33.8	144
Durian	58.0	2.8	3.9	-	34.1	183
Fig	88.1	1.3	0.2	2.2	7.6	37

Grape	79.2	0.5	0.3	2.9	16.5	71
Grapefruit	88.5	1.0	0.1	–	10	45
Guava	81.7	0.9	0.3	5.2	11.2	66
Jackfruit	76.2	1.9	0.1	1.1	19.8	88
Jamun	83.7	0.7	0.3	0.9	14	62
Karonda	80.5	1.1	2.9	1.5	3.5	42
Kiwi	84.0	1.2	0.9	3.3	17.5	57
Lasoda	83.4	1.8	0.5	4.2	12.5	50
Lemon	85.0	1.0	0.9	1.7	11.1	57
Lime	84.6	1.5	1.0	1.3	10.9	59
Litchi	84.4	0.7	0.3	2.2	9.4	61
Loquat	88.2	0.6	0.3	0.8	10.0	43
Mahua flower	40.7	2.8	0.9	2.6	30.5	235
Mandarin orange	87.6	0.2	0.1	–	9.8	53
Mango	81.0	0.6	0.4	1.1	16.9	74
Monkey jack	60.5	0.5	0.3	4.8	14	50
Mulberry	86.5	1.1	0.4	0.7	10.3	49
Papaya	90.8	0.6	0.1	0.8	7.2	32
Passion fruit	76.3	0.9	0.1	9.6	12.4	54
Peach	86.0	1.2	0.3	1.2	10.5	50
Pear	86.0	0.6	0.2	1.0	11.9	52
Persimmon	80	0.7	0.2	0.9	17.9	76
Phalsa	80.8	1.3	0.9	1.2	14.7	72
Pineapple	87.8	0.4	0.1	0.5	10.8	46
Pistachio nut	5.6	19.8	53.5	2.1	10.2	626
Plum	80.9	0.7	0.5	0.4	11.1	56
Pomegranate	78.0	1.6	0.1	5.1	14.5	77
Raspberry	84.8	1.0	0.6	1	11.7	56
Sapota	73.7	0.7	1.1	2.6	21.4	98
Sea buckthorn	74.5	2.6	1.5	3.5	20.5	106
Strawberry	87.8	0.7	0.2	1.1	9.8	77
Sweet orange	86.6	0.9	0.2	–	10.6	52
Tamarind	20.0	7.5	0.4	6.0	67.4	283
Walnut	4.5	15.6	64.5	2.6	11	687
Wood apple	64.2	8.0	3.7	5.0	18.1	134

6.3.1.1 *Water/moisture*

Fresh fruits contain 70–90% water. Soluble substances dissolved in water are sugar, salt, organic acids and soluble pigments found in vacuoles. Fruits are perishable because of high moisture content. Moisture content of dry fruits are low that varies from 4% to 5%.

6.3.1.2 *Protein and amino acids*

Generally fresh fruits are low in protein content. Dry fruits such as cashew nut, almond, walnut, chironji, pecan nut and dry coconut are rich source of protein.

Protein contains amino acids. Fruits contain fewer amounts of free amino acids but they are of fundamental importance. Essential amino acids found in fruits are histidine in banana, arginine in grape and glycine in muskmelon. Non-essential amino acids present in fruits are proline in orange, alanine in mango, goose berry and date, aspartic acid in apple, lemon and banana and glutamic acid in tomato fruits.

6.3.1.3 *Fat*

Fresh fruits contain little amount of lipids or fat with exception of avocado and olive which are rich in fat. Fatty acid is the part of lipids. The unsaturated fatty acids have beneficial effects on human health. The unsaturated fatty acid such as linoleic acid is rich in palm and mahua oils.

6.3.1.4 *Fibre*

Fibre is only found in foods of plant origin. Fruits are rich source of fibre. Fruits are very rich in fibre content. Sea buckthorn, passion fruit, bael, guava, tamarind, pomegranate, cape goose berry, wood apple and fig have comparatively higher content of fibre than other fruits.

6.3.1.5 *Carbohydrates*

Carbohydrate serves as the storage material in most of the fruits. Starch present in most of the fruits disappeared during ripening of fruits leading to the build-up of sugars. Sugars are responsible for quality of fruits. The most commonly occurring sugars are glucose (date, grape, fig, mulberry, strawberry, etc.), fructose (date, grape, apple, pomegranate, pear, etc.) and sucrose (mango, banana, pineapple, apricot, peach, melons, etc.). Sugars are easily digestible and yielding energy quickly to the body.

6.3.1.6 *Energy value*

Fruits are low in calories or energy value. Dry fruits have generally higher calorie value than fresh fruits. The fruits which have relatively higher caloric value are cashew nut, almond, walnut, coconut, dried karonda, tamarind pulp, dates, dried grapes, avocado, apricot, banana, durian, bael and custard apple.

6.3.2 Micro nutrients

Vitamin and mineral contents of fruits are given in Tables 6.8 and 6.9, respectively.

Table 6.8. Nutritive value of fruits: vitamins content/100 g.*

Fruits	Carotene (μg)	Thiamine (mg)	Riboflavin (mg)	Niacin (mg)	Vitamin C (mg)
Almond	0	0.44	0.57	0.7	0
Amra	450	0.02	0.02	0.3	21
Aonla	9	0.03	0.01	0.2	600
Apple	0	0.03	0.03	0.2	2
Apricot	2500	0.04	0.13	0.6	10
Avocado	62	0.06	0.13	1.7	13
Bael	206	0.15	3.0	1.1	17
Banana	78	0.05	0.08	0.5	7
Ber	21	0.02	0.05	0.7	76
Barbados cherry	1000	0.03	0.06	0.5	2000
Black berry	7	0.10	0.12	2.0	9
Cape gooseberry	5000	0.05	0.04	0.3	49
Carambola	336	0.05	0.07	0.5	50
Cashew apple	23	0.02	0.05	0.4	180
Cashew nut	60	0.63	0.19	1.2	2.1
Cherry	0	0.08	0.08	0.3	7
Chironji	-	0.70	0.50	3.6	0
Coconut fresh	0	0.05	0.10	0.8	7
Currant	21	0.03	0.14	0.4	1
Custard apple	0	0.07	0.20	1.3	37
Date	600	0.90	0.30	0.8	3
Durian	15	0.08	0.05	1.0	35
Fig	162	0.06	0.05	0.6	5
Grape	3	0.04	0.03	0.2	1
Grapefruit	130	0.12	0.02	0.3	67
Guava	0	0.03	0.03	0.4	300
Jackfruit	992	0.15	0.13	0.4	25

Jamun	80	0.03	0.01	0.2	45
Karonda	771	–	–	–	18
Kiwi	17.5	0.02	0.05	0.5	100
Lasoda	–	0.09	0.12	0.2	35
Lemon	10	0.02	0.01	0.1	40
Lime	26	0.04	0.04	0.2	45
Litchi	14	0.03	0.08	0.5	45
Loquat	559	0.10	0.13	0.07	0
Mahua flower	525	0.28	0.20	1.1	50
Mandarin	1104	0.08	0.10	0.5	55
Mango	4800	0.08	0.08	0.09	30
Monkey jack	2460	0.08	0.06	0.3	17
Mulberry	57	0.04	0.13	0.5	20
Papaya	2020	0.04	0.25	0.2	57
Passion fruit	430	0.07	0.15	1.6	30
Peach	0	0.02	0.03	0.5	6
Pear	28	0.06	0.03	0.2	0
Persimmon	2268	0.03	0.01	0.0	33
Phalsa	750	0.05	0.03	0.3	35
Pineapple	18	0.20	0.12	0.1	42
Pistachio nut	144	0.67	0.38	2.3	–
Plum	166	0.04	0.10	0.3	5
Pomegranate	0	0.06	1.0	0.3	16
Raspberry	1248	0.12	0.48	0.8	30
Sapota	97	0.02	0.03	0.2	6
Sea buckthorn	12849	2.8	6.6	2.5	424
Strawberry	18	0.03	0.02	0.2	52
Sweet orange	242	0.05	0.07	0.3	50
Tamarind	70	0.4	0.09	0.7	17
Walnut	6	0.45	0.45	1.0	5
Wood apple	61	0.04	0.17	0.8	3

*4 μg carotene = 1 μg vitamin A.

Table 6.9. Nutritive value of fruits: minerals content/100 g.

Fruits	Calcium (mg)	Phosphorus (mg)	Potassium (mg)	Sodium (mg)	Iron (mg)
Almond	230	490	856	6	5.1
Amra	40	11	201	–	3.9

Aonla	50	20	185	–	4.5
Apple	10	14	94	3	1.0
Apricot fresh	20	25	89	–	0.54
Apricot died	55	71	1162	10	2.6
Avocado	20	80	485	–	1.3
Bael	90	50	375	–	0.9
Banana	17	50	141	2	0.9
Ber	80	9	165	–	1.8
Barbados cherry	34	37	230	–	1.1
Black berry	30	20	360	–	4.3
Cape gooseberry	14	67	130	–	2.0
Carambola	4	16	170	–	0.26
Cashew apple	20	10	190	–	0.5
Cashew nut	50	450	129	41	5.8
Cherry	24	25	285	–	1.3
Chironji	300	580	478	12.5	3.6
Coconut fresh	10	240	336	15	1.7
Currant	130	110	–	–	8.5
Custard apple	17	47	140	2	4.3
Date	70	80	537	13	10.6
Durian	10	50	432	2	1.0
Fig	200	30	680	2	4.0
Grape	20	30	249	4	0.5
Grapefruit	30	30	200	1	0.2
Guava	10	28	106	15	1.4
Jackfruit	36	41	448	2	2.0
Jamun	15	15	55	26.2	3.9
Karonda	21	28	–	–	39.1
Kiwi	33	44.5	380	3.7	1.2
Lasoda	42	65	180	–	1.2
Lemon	70	10	148	1	2.3
Lime	90	20	102	2	0.3
Litchi	70	310	171	1	0.7
Loquat	35	20	266	1	1.3
Mahua flower	45	22	–	–	1.1

Mandarin	26	30	166	2	0.1
Mango	14	16	168	1	1.3
Monkey jack	56	20	–	–	0.5
Mulberry	70	30	194	10	2.5
Papaya	17	13	211	5	0.5
Passion fruit	10	60	348	28	2.5
Peach	15	41	212	1	2.4
Pear	8	15	161	2	0.5
Persimmon	15	28	–	–	0.3
Phalsa	130	39	–	–	5.0
Pineapple	20	9	86	1	2.4
Pistachio nut	140	430	–	–	7.7
Plum	10	12	–	–	0.6
Pomegranate	10	70	171	4	1.8
Raspberry	40	110	–	–	2.3
Sapota	28	27	–	–	2.0
Sea buckthorn	38.3		150	4.1	1.2
Strawberry	30	30	–	–	1.8
Sweet orange	50	30	–	–	0.8
Tamarind	170	110	628	–	18
Walnut	100	380	–	–	4.8
Wood apple	130	110	–	–	0.6

6.3.2.1 Vitamins

1. Pro-vitamin A/carotene

Fruits rich in carotene are Sea buckthorn, cape goose berry, mango, apricot, papaya, monkey jack, raspberry, barbados cherry, jackfruit, phalsa, carambola and persimmon. Sea buckthorn is the riches source of carotene followed by cape gooseberry, mango, apricot, monkey jack, persimmon and papaya.

2. Vitamin B complex

Thiamine: Fruits rich in thiamine are jackfruit, barbados cherry, banana, cashew nut, walnut, almond, pineapple, khirni, tamarind, sea buckthorn. Sea buckthorn has highest value followed by date and dry fruits such as chironji, pistachio nut and cashew nut.

Riboflavin: Fruits rich in riboflavin are bael, wood apple, sea buckthorn, litchi, pomegranate, almond, pineapple and khirni. Sea buckthorn has the highest value followed by bael, pomegranate and almond.

Niacin: Fruits rich in niacin are almond, apricot, cashew nut, walnut, bael, dates, custard apple, passion fruit, and cape gooseberry. Chironji fruit has highest content of niacin followed by sea buckthorn and pistachionut.

Fruits are also good source of other B vitamins such as pyridoxine (banana, lime and durian), folic acid (mango, kiwi and strawberry) and pantothenic acid (apricot and grapefruit).

3. Vitamin C

Vitamin C or ascorbic acid content of fruits varies greatly. Barbados cherry is the riches source of vitamin C followed by aonla the Indian goose berry, sea buckthorn and guava. Other fruits which are good source of vitamin C are kiwi, ber, cashew apple, strawberry, litchi, citrus fruits, papaya and carambola.

Fruits are also rich source of vitamins E (Cashew nut, almond, pecan and walnut) and K (almond, cashew nut and walnut).

6.3.2.2 Minerals

Fruits are good source of most of the minerals needed by human body. Some of the fruits rich in various mineral are as follows.

Calcium: Calcium is rich in chironji, almond, fig, pistachionut, tamarind, phalsa, walnut, lime, bael and wood apple. Dry fruits generally have higher content of calcium than fresh fruits.

Phosphorus: Dry fruits such as chironji, pistachionut and coconut are rich source of phosphorus. Fresh fruits which are good source of phosphorus are klitchi, raspberry, tamarind and wood apple.

Potassium: Potassium rich fruits are dried plum, dried apricot, almond, dry coconut, chironji, dried fig, tamarind, dates, fresh coconut, kiwi, grapes, durian, jackfruits and cape goose berry. Dry fruits have content of potassium than fresh fruits. Dried apricot is the riches source of potassium followed by almond and tamarind.

Sodium: Fruits rich in sodium content are cashew nut, jamun, fresh coconut and passion fruit.

Iron: Iron rich fruits are jackfruit, karonda, jamun, tamarind, dates, almond, cashew nut, walnut, phalsa, fig, chironji and dried grapes/raisins. Karonda is richest source of iron flowed by tamarind and date.

Fruits are also rich in magnesium (almond, custard apple, passion fruit, tamarind and banana) and sulphur (custard apple, strawberry, banana, passion fruit and lime).

6.3.2.3 Other constituents of fruits

1. *Organic acids*: Organic acids are an important source of respiratory energy in fruit tissues. Fruits exert its alkaline effects on lowering the

acidity because they contain salts of alkaline and alkaline earth metals such as calcium, sodium and potassium. Organic acids and their salts are oxidized in the body to carbon dioxide which is eliminated in the kidney and lungs. This leaves the alkaline metals available for neutralizing the acid produced during digestion of protein and fatty fruits.

Fruits contain several organic acids, some of them present in large amount, some of them in traces and usually one acid predominates. For example, citric acid predominates in oranges, lime, lemon, grapefruit, galgal, mango, guava, goose berry, pineapple, pomegranate, sea buckthorn, karonda, etc., tartaric acid in tamarind and grapes and malic acid in apple, pear, plum, apricot, peach, banana, sweet lime, cherry, etc. Organic acids are stored in vacuoles.

2. *Pectic substances*: Pectic substances are derivatives of polygalocturonic acids. Parts of the carbohydrates present as cellulose and pectic substances in the cell walls. Pectin together with cellulose serves as integral part of the cell wall. Structure of pectin related with fruit texture. Water insoluble protopectin substances occur in unripe fruits gives the firm texture to the fruits. During ripening of fruits, protopectin decreases and simultaneously increase soluble pectin, thus, leading to softening of the fruit tissues.

Protopectin $\xrightarrow{\text{Protopectinase}}$ **Pectinicacid** $\xrightarrow{\text{Pectinmethyl esterase}}$ **Pectin**

Pectin forms gel on heating with sugar and acid and play an important role in preparation of jelly. Fruits rich in pectin contents are guava, jamun, wood apple, citrus, loquat, strawberry, etc.

3. *Pigments*: Pigments are responsible for colour of the fruits. Most of the pigments occur in plastids - a specialized bodies lying in the protoplasm of the cells. The chief pigments of the fruits are divided into two groups - water insoluble pigments such as chlorophyll and carotenoids and water-soluble pigments such as anthocyanins and anthoxanthins.

Chlorophyll: Chlorophyll is a green pigments responsible for green colour. It is found in chloroplast. Chlorophylls are of two types, i.e., chlorophyll a (intense blue green) and chlorophyll b (dull yellow green). They occur in a ratio of 3a:1b in plants. Chlorophyll dominates in most of the unripe fruits with exception of pineapple fruits where eyes changed from light to dark green at ripening.

Carotenoids: These are fat-soluble pigments responsible for yellow, orange and red colour. They occur in chloroplast. Carotenoids are present as α-carotene, β-carotene, γ-carotene, xanthophylls, criptoxanthins and lycopene. β-Carotene is the most valuable among all carotenoids in synthesis of vitamin A. The carotenoids present in fruits are:

- β-Carotene: Fruits rich in β-carotene are mango, papaya, apricot, sea buckthorn, cape goose berry, persimmon
- Violaxanthin: Jackfruit, peach and pineapple fruits are rich in violaxanthin.
- Lycopene: Found in pink grapefruit, watermelon and tomato.
- Xanthophylls: Citrus fruits are rich in xanthophylls.

Anthocyanins and anthocyanidins: These have some effects on human health in preventing heart disease, cancer initiation, diabetes, cataracts, blood pressure and allergies.

Anthocyanins are cyanidin-based compounds attached with sugar. It is highly soluble in water responsible for red, blue and purple colour. Fruits developed their colour at ripening due to pre-dominance of anthocyanins are jamun, cherries, red delicious apple, phalsa, blue grapes, plum, pomegranate, fig, blueberries and currants.

Anthocyanidins are also anthocyanins in which sugar is not attached in their structure. These are cyanidin (reddish blue), pelargonidin (red), delphinidin (blue), petunidin (violet), malvidin (red) and peonidin (blue) found in apple, blackberry, blueberry, cranberry, grape, plum, nectarin and strawberry.

Anthoxanthins: These also play role in human health as protectants of heart disease, cancer initiation and capillary.

Anthoxanthins are also flavonoids and cyanidin-based waste compounds. It is soluble in water, occurs in vacuoles and responsible for white or colourless and pale yellow pigments. Anthoxanthins are found in fruits of guava, banana, pear, custard apple and gooseberry.

Anthoxanthins are classified into flavones (retinol luteolin in guava), flavonols (kaempherol, quercetin in strawberry), flavonones (naringin in grapefruit) and flavanols such as catechin in strawberry and leucoanthocyanins in white grapes.

4. *Phenolics*: Phenolics present in fruits and other plants, protect and prevent numerous diseases such as cancer and cardiovascular disease. Phenolics are mostly by-products of aromatic amino acids which are important for disease resistance and determining colour and flavours. Poly phenols present in fruits are cinnamic acid derivatives such as chlorogenic acid (apple, peach, plum, cherry), p-coumaric acid (grape, pineapple, etc.), cafeic acid (grape, blackberry, strawberry, etc.) and flavonoids. Various glycosides have been isolated from fruits are called flavonoids. The important flavonoids found in fruits

are catechin (apple, grape, etc.), epicatechin (apple, date and apricot), quercetin (mango, apple, strawberry), tangeritin (loose skin orange), hesperidin and linolin (sweet orange), naringin (grapefruit) and citrin (citrus juices, lemon peel). Flavonoids act as antioxidants.

Tannins (apple, grape, pomegranate), anthocyanidin such as cyanidin (fig, apple, grape, plum), pelargonidin (strawberry) delphinidin (pomegranate), peonidin (plum), petunidin (grape) and malvidin (grape) are also phenolics found in fruits.

5. *Antioxidants and oxygen radical absorbance capacity (ORAC) value*: Fruits containing antioxidants stop the formation of free radical. Antioxidants have definite role in preventing of certain cancer, age-related eye disease, and coronary artery disease. Antioxidants in fruits increase the amount of hormones like substances – prostacydin that dialates blood vessels and lowers blood pressure. The fruits which are rich in antioxidants (have β-carotene, ascorbic acid, vitamin E and P) are aonla, apricot, bael, mango, kiwi, jamun, cherries, berries, etc.

   The ORAC measures the level of antioxidant protection capacity of foods. If product has high ORAC value, it has ability to neutralize many free radicals. Diets which are plentiful in high ORAC foods are associated with decreased disease risk. The fruits which have high ORAC value/100 g are given in Table 6.10.

Table 6.10. ORAC value of fruits.

Fruits	ORAC units/100 g
Blueberries	2400
Blackberries	2036
Strawberries	1540
Plum	949
Oranges	750
Coloured grapes	739
Cherries	670
Kiwi	602
Grapefruit	483

6. *Volatile compounds*: Volatile compounds are flavouring constituents responsible for aroma of the fruits. Fruit volatiles include ester, aldehyde, ketones, hydrocarbon, acetate, alcohol, etc. These are characteristics of each fruit. They present in small amount and gives aroma of the fruits. The flavouring compounds present in some fruits are

Ethyl-2 methyl butyrate in apple, eugenol in banana, limonene in citrus fruits, geraniol and linalool in grapes, ethyl acetate in pineapple, methyl and ethyl esters in pear, linalool in papaya, cinnamyl acetate in guava and lactones in peach.

6.4 Vegetables

A plant parts or its product eaten raw or cooked as main parts of a meal, side dish or appetizer is called vegetables. Vegetables can be classified on the basis of their parts used for vegetables such as leaves, stem, flower, fruits and roots. Vegetables as protective or regulatory growth make important contribution of vitamins, minerals and fibre in our diet. A wide range of vegetable are produced in our country. The nutritive values of vegetables are as follows.

6.4.1 Macro nutrients

Macro nutrients such as moisture, protein, fat, fibre, carbohydrate and energy value are given in Table 6.11.

Table 6.11. Nutritive value of vegetables: macro nutrients.

Vegetables	Moisture (%)	Protein (%)	Fat (%)	Fibre (%)	Carbohydrate (%)	Energy (kcal)
Amaranth	87.5	4.0	0.5	1.0	6.1	45
Ash gourd	96.5	0.4	0.1	0.8	1.9	10
Beet root	86.4	3.4	0.8	0.7	6.5	46
Brussels sprouts	85.5	4.7	0.5	1.2	7.1	52
Bitter gourd	92.4	1.6	0.2	0.8	4.2	25
Bottle gourd	96.1	0.2	0.1	0.6	2.5	12
Brinjal	92.7	1.4	0.3	1.3	4.0	24
Cabbage	91.9	1.8	0.1	1.0	4.6	27
Capsicum	86.2	2.9	0.6	6.8	6.1	41
Carrot	86.0	0.9	0.2	1.2	10.6	48
Cauliflower	90.8	2.6	0.4	1.2	4.0	30
Chili green	85.7	2.9	0.6	6.8	3.0	29
Chenopods leaves	89.6	3.7	0.4	0.8	2.9	30
Colocasia	73.1	3.0	0.1	1.0	21.1	97
Cucumber	96.3	0.4	0.1	0.4	2.5	13
Cluster bean	81.0	3.2	0.4	3.2	10.8	16

Drumstick	86.9	2.5	0.1	4.8	3.7	26
Yam	78.7	1.2	0.1	0.8	18.4	79
Fenugreek leaves	86.1	4.4	0.9	1.1	6.0	49
Field bean	86.1	3.8	0.7	1.8	6.7	48
French bean	91.4	1.7	0.1	1.8	4.5	26
Garlic	62.8	6.3	0.1	1.3	29.0	142
Knol khol	92.7	1.1	0.2	1.5	3.8	21.0
Lettuce	93.4	2.1	0.3	0.5	2.5	21.0
Muskmelon	95.2	0.3	0.2	0.4	3.5	170
Mustard leaves	89.8	4.0	0.6	0.8	3.2	34
Okra	89.6	1.9	0.2	1.2	6.4	35
Onion	86.6	1.2	0.1	0.6	11.1	50
Pea green	72.1	7.2	0.1	4.0	15.9	93
Pointed gourd	92.0	2.0	0.3	3.0	2.2	20
Potato	74.7	1.6	0.1	0.4	22.6	97
Pumpkin	92.6	1.4	0.1	0.7	4.6	25
Radish	94.9	0.5	0.1	0.6	3.2	16
Ridge gourd	95.2	0.5	0.1	0.5	3.4	17
Round gourd	93.6	0.5	0.3	0.8	3.4	21
Snake gourd	94.6	0.5	0.3	1.0	3.3	18
Spinach	92.1	2.0	0.7	0.6	2.9	26
Sweet potato	68.5	1.2	0.3	0.8	28.2	120
Tapioca	59.4	0.7	0.2	0.6	38.1	157
Tomato	94.0	0.9	0.2	0.7	3.6	23
Turnip	91.6	0.5	0.2	0.9	6.2	29
Watermelon	95.8	0.2	0.2	0.2	3.3	26

6.4.1.1 Water content

Water content of vegetables varies from 59% to 96%. Water constitutes more than 90% of the edible portion of the vegetables. Vegetable which have more than 95% moisture are cucumber, bottle gourd, muskmelon, watermelon and ridge gourd. Vegetables which are low in water content are tapioca, garlic, colocasia, sweet potato and peas.

6.4.1.2 Protein

Vegetables are low in protein content. Some vegetables which are relatively fair source of protein are beans, peas, garlic and brussel sprout.

6.4.1.3 *Fat*

Fat content of vegetables are very low that is less than 1% in most of the vegetables.

6.4.1.4 *Fibre*

Fibre content of vegetables varies from 0.4% to 6.8%. Among the various vegetables capsicum, green chilies, green peas, beans, pointed gourd and drumstick contain fairly large amount of fibres. Since fibre is not digested in the body, it is considered as a roughage which promotes motility of food through intestine.

6.4.1.5 *Carbohydrates*

Vegetables are not rich in carbohydrates except few such as cassawa (tapioca), potato, sweet potato, elephant foot yam and colocasia.

6.4.1.6 *Energy value*

Vegetables are generally low in caloric value which varies from 10 to 170 kcal. The energy value of muskmelon, tapioca, sweet potato, potato, colocasia and garlic are relatively higher than other vegetables.

6.4.2 Micro nutrients

Micro nutrient contents of vegetables such as vitamins and minerals are given in Tables 6.12 and 6.13, respectively.

Table 6.12. Nutritive value of vegetables: vitamin content/100 g.

Vegetables	Carotene (μg)*	Thiamine (mg)	Riboflavin (mg)	Niacin (mg)	Folic acid (μg)	Vitamin C (mg)
Amaranth	20,160	0.83	0.3	1.2	149	99
Ash gourd	–	0.06	0.01	0.4	–	1
Beet root	–	0.04	0.09	0.4	–	10
Brussels sprouts	126	0.05	0.16	0.4	–	102
Bitter gourd	126	0.07	0.09	0.5	–	88
Bottle gourd	–	0.03	0.01	0.2	–	–
Brinjal	74	0.04	0.11	0.9	34	12
Cabbage	120	0.6	0.09	0.4	23	124
Capsicum	690	0.55	0.05	0.1	–	137
Carrot	1890	0.04	0.02	0.6	15	3
Cauliflower	30	0.04	0.1	1.0	–	69

Chili green	2430	0.19	0.39	0.9	–	111
Chenopods leaves	1740	0.01	0.14	0.6	–	60
Colocasia	24	0.09	0.03	0.4	54	–
Cucumber	–	0.03	0.02	0.2	14.7	7
Cluster bean	198	0.09	0.03	49	144	48
Drumstick	110	0.05	0.07	0.2	–	120
Yam	260	0.06	0.07	0.7	17.5	–
fenugreek leaves	2340	0.04	0.31	0.8	–	52
Field bean	187	0.10	0.06	0.7	15.5	9
French bean	132	0.08	0.06	0.3	45.5	24
Garlic	–	0.08	0.4	0.5	–	–
Knol khol	21	0.05	0.09	0.5	–	85
Lettuce	990	0.09	0.13	0.5	–	10
Muskmelon	169	0.11	0.08	0.3	–	26
Mustard leaves	2622	0.03	–	–	–	33
Okra	52	0.07	0.1	0.6	25.3	13
Onion	–	0.08	0.01	0.4	6	11
Pea green	83	0.25	0.01	0.8	–	9
Pointed gourd	153	0.05	0.06	0.5	–	29
Potato	24	0.1	0.01	1.2	7	17
Pumpkin	2100	0.06	0.04	0.5	13	2
Radish	4	0.02	0.03	1.4	–	21
Ridge gourd	33	–	0.01	0.2	–	5
Round gourd	13	0.04	0.08	0.3	–	18
Snake gourd	96	0.04	0.06	0.3	15.5	–
Spinach	9440	0.03	0.26	0.5	123	51
Sweet potato	2200	0.08	0.04	0.7	–	24
Tapioca	–	0.05	0.10	0.3	–	25
Tomato	3010	0.12	0.06	0.4	14	27
Turnip	–	0.04	0.04	0.5	–	43
Watermelon	–	0.02	0.04	0.1	–	1

*4 µg carotene = 1 µg vitamin A.

Table 6.13. Nutritive value of vegetables: minerals content/100 g.

Vegetables	Calcium (mg)	Phosphorus (mg)	Potassium (mg)	Sodium (mg)	Iron (mg)
Amaranth	397	83	–	–	25.5
Ash gourd	30	20	211	2	0.8
Beet root	18.3	56	300	60	1.0
Brussels sprouts	43	82	400	12	1.8
Bitter gourd	20	70	382	14	1.8
Bottle gourd	20	10	–	–	0.7
Brinjal	18	47	229	3	0.9
Cabbage	39	44	281	7	0.8
Capsicum					
Carrot	80	530	482	47	22.0
Cauliflower	33	57	355	12	1.5
Chili green	30	80	–	–	12.0
Chenopods leaves	150	80	–	–	4.2
Colocasia	40	140	464	25	17
Cucumber	10	25	149	7	1.5
Cluster bean	130	57			4.2
Drumstick	30	110	463	6	5.3
Yam	50	34	422	22	0.6
Fenugreek leaves	395	51	–	–	16.5
Field bean	210	68	402	89	1.7
French bean	50	28	282	2	1.7
Garlic	50	70	–	–	2.3
Knol khol	20	35	199	12	0.4
Lettuce	50	28	329	9	2.4
Muskmelon	32	14	–	–	1.4
Mustard leaves	155	26	–	–	16.3
Okra	66	56	332	54	1.5
Onion	47	50	385	5	0.7
Pea green	20	139	346	2	1.5
Pointed gourd	30	40	–	–	1.7
Potato	10	40	249	18	0.7
Pumpkin	10	30	259	2	0.7
Radish	20	20	325	41	18
Ridge gourd	18	26	–	–	0.5

Round gourd	25	24	–	–	0.9
Snake gourd	26	20	–	–	0.3
Spinach	73	21	570	89	10.9
Sweet potato	46	50	373	10	0.8
Tapioca	50	40	10	2	0.9
Tomato	48	20	360	3	0.4
Turnip	30	40	243	6	0.4
Watermelon	11	12	115	1	7.9

6.4.2.1 Vitamins

1. Carotene (pro-vitamin A)

Vegetables which are rich in carotene contents are amaranth, spinach, beet green, chili green, tomato, sweet potato, fenugreek leaves, pumpkin, carrot, capsicum, colocasia leaves, coriander leaves, drumstick leaves, chenopod leaves and mustard leaves. Amaranth has highest content of carotene followed by spinach.

2. Vitamin B complex

Thiamine: Thiamine content of vegetables varies from 0.01 to 0.83 mg/100 g. Vegetables rich in thiamine content are amaranth, cabbage, capsicum, lima bean and peas green.

Riboflavin: Riboflavin content of vegetables varies from 0.01 to 0.39 mg/100 g. Vegetables rich in riboflavin are amaranth, spinach, garlic and green chili.

Niacin:

Niacin content of vegetables varies from 0.2 to 1.4 mg/10 g. Vegetables rich in niacin are radish, amaranth, cauliflower, brinjal, chili green, potato, elephant foot yam and cluster bean.

Pantothenic acid: Vegetables which have fair source of pantothenic acid are cauliflower, sweet potato, peas green, spinach, mustard green and knol khol.

Pyridoxine: Sweet potato, spinach and knoll khol are rich source of pyridoxine.

Folic acid: Folic acid content of vegetables varies from 6 to 149 mg/100 g. Amaranth, cluster bean, cucumber, colocasia, French bean, cabbage, carrot, brussels sprout, knol khol, mustard leaves, broccoli green, peas, okra are good source of folic acid. Amaranth and cluster bean have higher content of folic acid than other vegetables.

3. Vitamin C

Capsicum has the highest vitamin C content followed by cabbage, drumstick and green chili. Other vegetables which are good source of vitamin C are cauliflower, bitter gourd, amaranth, tomato, coriander leaves, brussels sprout, fenugreek leaves, knol khol and cluster bean.

Vegetables are also rich source of vitamins E and K. Vitamin E rich vegetables are corn, dried beans and dark green leafy vegetables. Vegetables rich in vitamin K are leafy vegetables (spinach, cabbage and kale), broccoli, cauliflower, green onions and brussels sprout.

4. Minerals

Vegetables are rich source of most of the mineral needed by the human body. Minerals found in vegetables are as follows.

Calcium: Calcium content of vegetables varies from 10 to 397 mg/100 g. Calcium-rich vegetables are amaranth, fenugreek, field bean, mustard leaves, cluster bean and chenopods leaves. Amaranth and fenugreek green leaves have higher content of calcium than other vegetables.

Phosphorus: Vegetables rich in phosphorus are carrot, colocasia, drumstick and green peas. Carrot is the richest source of phosphorus among various vegetables.

Potassium:

Vegetables rich in potassium are spinach, carrot, colocasia, drumstick, coriander leaves, okra, yam, onion, sweet potato, lettuce, bitter gourd, tomato, peas green, field bean and brussels sprout. Spinach has the highest content of potassium followed by carrot, colocasia and drumstick.

Sodium: Spinach, field bean, beetroots, okra and carrot are rich source of sodium. Other vegetables have low content of sodium.

Iron: The iron content of vegetables varies from 0.3 to 25.5 mg/100g. Vegetables rich in iron content are amaranth, fenugreek leaves, mustard leaves, spinach and coriander leaves.

Vegetables rich in magnesium are cauliflower, onion, garlic amaranth, capsicum, spinach and tapioca and sulphur are onion, garlic, okra, cauliflower, beetroot, bean, drumstick.

6.4.2.2 Other constituents

1. *Organic acids*: Organic acids present in vegetables are formic, succinic, citric, acetic and malic. The concentration of these acids is lower in vegetables than fruits. The pH of most of the vegetables is 5.0 to 5.6. Peas and potato have pH 6.1 to 6.3.
2. *Pigments*: The chief pigment of vegetables are chlorophyll, carotenoids, anthocyanins and anthoxanthins
3. *Chlorophyll*: This is a water insoluble pigments. Chlorophyll 'a' and chlorophyll 'b' have been isolated. Chlorophyll a is found in florets of blue green broccoli and chlorophyll b is in stalk. The chlorophyll pigment is present in leafy vegetables, beans, green chili, peas and capsicum.

4. *Carotenoids*: This is also water insoluble pigments but soluble in fats. The beneficial effect of carotenoids is protection against cancer. The carotenoid pigments present in vegetables are β-carotene, α-carotene, xanthophylls, cryptoxanthin and lycopene
5. *β-Carotene*: β-Carotene is valuable in the synthesis of vitamin A. Vegetables which are rich in β-carotene are carrot, melons, broccoli, lettuce, red capsicum, spinach and sweet potato.
6. *Xanthophylls*: Lutein, zeaxanthin and β-cryptoxanthins are important source of xanthophylls. Vegetables rich in these are sweet corn, spinach, okra, cantaloups, summer squash, turnip green and green capsicum.
7. *Lycopene*: Lycopene is insoluble in water and gives red or pink colour to tomato and offers potential health benefits. The lycopene content of tomato (Pusa, Shyamla) is 4.5 mg/100 g and carrot (Pusa, Rudhira) 10.7 mg/100g. The consumption of tomato-based food may reduce the susceptibility of lymphocytes DNA to oxidative damage. Tomato is processed for high lycopene serum concentration and reduced the risk of prostate cancer.
8. *Anthocyanins*: Anthocyanins give purple and red colour to vegetable leaves and fruits such as purple broccoli, purple cabbage, brinjal, purple sweet potato, purple radish, onion and rhubarb. The anthocyanins contents of vegetables such as brinjal, varies from. 32-48 mg/100 g and black carrot (Pusa, Asita) 339 mg/100 g. Nasunin and anthocyanin from brinjal inhibit brain cells lipids. Peroxidation cause by hydroxyl free radicals.
9. *Anthoxanthins*: Like anthocyanins, these are water-soluble and occur in vacuoles of plant cells. Anthoxanthin pigments are either white or pale yellow. Anthoxanthins give colour to cauliflower, white onion, spinach and other leafy vegetables. The colour of green leafy vegetables is masked by chlorophyll.
10. *Betalains*: Anthocyanin pigments are absent in plants of some family and are replaced by two pigments betacyanins and betaxanthins. These two pigments together are called betalains. High ratio of betacyanins to betaxanthins gives violet yellow to orange and red tuber colours. Betalains is also found in beetroot.
11. *Phenolics*: Phenolics are diverse group of chemicals and largest group of phytochemicals found in vegetables which have positive effects on human health. Phenolics mostly flavonoids represent the most important class of polyphenolics in vegetables. The important phenolics particularly flavonoids found in vegetables are flavonols and flavones. Flavonols include quercetin, kaempherol, fisetin and myricetin. Quercetin is the most important flavonoids present in

vegetables such as onion (97-101 mg/100 g), tomato, kale, lettuce and beans. Kaempherol, myricetin and fisetin are found in onion, lettuce, broccoli, snapbeans and peppers.

Flavones include luteolin and apegenin found in celery, spinach, parsley, kale and peppers. Isoflavonoids include diadzein and genistein have also been found in small quantity in okra, broccoli, asparagus and mushrooms. The total phenolics of some leafy vegetables are given in Table 6.14.

Table 6.14. Phenolic contents of some leafy vegetables.

Vegetables	Phenolics, µg GAE/g
Amaranth	1124
Onion	850
Chenopod	750
Fenugreek	418
Mustard leaves	234
Spinach	226
Lettuce	202

12. *Antioxidants and ORAC/CUPRAC values*: Antioxidants or phytochemicals present in vegetables play definite role to reduce the risk of several serious or chronic diseases including cancer, coronary heart disease, diabetes, cataract and Parkinson's disease. Vegetables contain a wide variety of biologically active, non-nutritive compounds such as antioxidants and phytochemicals which provide health benefits beyond basic nutrition. The valuable antioxidants of vegetables are carotenoids, ascorbic acid, vitamin E and flavonoids.

The potential antioxidants supplying vegetables are onion, garlic, broccoli, cauliflower, kidney bean and other beans, kale, spinach, bell pepper, carrot, tomato, beetroot, amaranth and chenopods.

The Oxygen Radical Absorbance Capacity (ORAC) and cupric ion reducing antioxidant capacity (CUPRAC) testing is a way to measure the level of antioxidants protection capacity of a food. Vegetables of high ORAC or CUPRAC value have ability to neutralize many free radicals. Hence, diets that are plentiful in high ORAC or CUPRAC value have beneficial effect on human health. The ORAC and CUPRAC values of some vegetables are given in Table 6.15.

Table 6.15. ORAC and CUPRAC value of some vegetables.

Vegetables	ORAC units	Vegetables	CUPRAC µm trolax/g
Brussels sprout	980	Amaranth	32.7
Broccoli flower	890	Chenopod	18.8

Red bell pepper	710	Spinach	17.8
Onion	450	Fenugreek	10.3
Corn	400	Lettuce	5.9
Brinjal	390	Mustard leaves	5.0

13. *Volatile/flavour compounds*:

Flavour compound of vegetables is important to their acceptance in diet. The natural flavours of the vegetables are due to mixture of ketones, alcohol, aldehydes, organic acid and sulphur compounds. Some vegetables have an astringent taste due to phenolic compounds.

Vegetables resulting strong as well as mild flavour due to sulphur-containing compounds such as di-sulphide in garlic, thiopropanal-s-oxide in onion and dimethyl sulphides in cabbage, cauliflower, brussels sprout and knol khol.

6.5 Spices and herbs

Spices are generally dried roots, barks, seed, fruits and flower used whole or crushed and powdered for adding flavour and colour to the food. Herbs are normally the fresh leaves, stem, seeds and flowers of the herbaceous plants, have culinary and medicinal value.

Spices have strong flavour than herbs. Spices are source of some nutrients, fibre, antioxidants, flavouring agents, natural colouring agents, oil and oleo resins. Spices acts as preservative, have antibacterial and antifungal properties and used in prevention of many diseases. The spices are classified on the basis of their parts used such as leaves of (fenugreek), flower parts of (clove and saffron), fruits of (chili and black pepper), seed of (coriander, cumin, fennel, aniseed) rhizomes of (ginger and turmeric), bulbs of (onion and garlic), kernel/aril of (nutmeg) and barks of (cinnamon and cassia). Spices have tremendous importance in daily life.

Herbs are the soul of flavour. Most commonly herbs used in India are mint leaves, coriander leaves and curry leaves. The nutritional values of important spices and herbs in terms of vitamins and minerals are given in Tables 6.16 and 6.17, respectively.

Table 6.16. Vitamins content of spices and herbs/100 g edible material.

Spices and herbs	Thiamine (mg)	Riboflavin (mg)	Niacin (mg)	Vitamin A (mg)	Vitamin C (mg)
Spices					
Green chili	0.19	1.18	0.5	Trace	111
Red chili	0.93	0.43	9.5	0.18	50

Chili powder	0.59	1.66	14.2	1.85	63
Onion	0.42	0.06	0.6	0.06	15
Garlic	0.68	0.08	0.7	0.05	12
Ginger	0.05	0.13	1.9	0.05	12
Turmeric	0.09	0.19	4.8	0.05	50
Mustard seed	0.65	0.45	8.5	0.06	22
Coriander seed	0.26	0.23	3.2	0.05	12
Cumin seed	0.73	0.38	2.5	0.05	17
Tamarind	–	0.07	0.7	0.03	3
Herbs					
Mint	0.05	0.16	1.0	400	27
Coriander leaves	0.05	0.06	0.8	1725	135
Curry leaves	0.08	0.21	2.3	1890	4

Table 6.17. Minerals content of spices and herbs/100 g edible material.

Spices and herbs	Calcium (mg)	Phosphorus (mg)	Iron (mg)
Spices			
Green chili	30	80	1200
Red chili	160	370	2300
Chili powder	100	320	10
Onion	300	290	Trace
Garlic	100	1420	10
Ginger	100	150	10
Turmeric	200	110	50
Mustard seed	300	790	10
Coriander seed	800	440	10
Cumin seed	900	450	50
Tamarind	200	110	10
Herbs			
Mint	200	80	15.6
Coriander leaves	140	60	10
Curry leaves	810	600	3.1

6.5.1 Vitamins

6.5.1.1 Vitamin A

Herbs are richer in vitamin content than spices. Curry leaves and coriander leaves are fair source of vitamin A.

6.5.1.2 *B vitamins*

Thiamine: Spices have better content of thiamine than the content of herbs. Red chili, cumin seed and garlic are the good source of thiamine.

Riboflavin: The riboflavin content of spices is also richer than the content of herbs. Chili powder and green chili have relatively higher content of riboflavin than other spices and herbs.

Niacin: Chili powder, red chilies and mustard seed are rich in niacin content. Niacin content of curry leaves is higher than mint and coriander leaves.

6.5.1.3 *Vitamin C*

Coriander leaves in herbs and green chili in spices are rich source of vitamin C. Turmeric and red chili have also fair content of vitamin C.

6.5.2 Minerals

6.5.2.1 *Calcium*

Calcium is rich in coriander and cumin seed in spices and curry leaves in herbs. Mustard seed and onion are also fair source of calcium.

6.5.2.2 *Phosphorus*

Garlic is rich source of phosphorus. Mustard seed, coriander seed and curry leaves are also good source of phosphorus.

6.5.2.3 *Iron*

Red chilies and green chili are an excellent source of iron. Turmeric and cumin seed are also fair source of iron.

6.5.3 Other constituents

6.5.3.1 *Fibres*

Among various spices, fenugreek, onion, chilies and garlic contains fairly large amount of fibres. Fibres play an important role in constipation and protecting various diseases and disorders.

6.5.3.2 *Antioxidants*

Several spices have antioxidant properties which prevents oxidation. Antioxidant component of spices are curcumin, anti-obesity factors from garcinia, piperine from black pepper, gingiberin from ginger, anticholesterol and anti-diabetic properties of garlic, onion and fenugreek. Antioxidants have definite roles in prevention of certain diseases and retarding oxidation.

6.5.3.3 Flavour

Spices are used for flavouring fruits and food beverages. Ginger is used as flavourants in alcoholic and non-alcoholic beverages. Cardamom is useful in flavouring bakery, tea and confectionery. Cinnamon and all spices are used for flavouring meet, sauces and sausages. Similarly cumin and fennel are also used as flavouring agents in foods.

6.5.3.4 Natural colour

Natural colour from spices attains great importance with the ban on artificial colour in food industry and increasing health awareness. Turmeric is widely used as food colouring agent in confectionery, poultry, marine and other processed products. Curcumin is successfully used in covering of dairy and bakery products. Red chili colour finds application in the processed meat products. Saffron contains water-soluble pigment crocin which give yellow to orange colour to the various food products. Kokam rind gives natural colouring agent anthocyanins.

6.5.4 Excess use of spices

Excess use of some spices has harmful effects. The active principle of some spices such as chili, black pepper and asafoetida contain strong pungency. Hence, excessive amount of these causes irritation of the mucous membranes and also it may be one of the causes for peptic ulcer in human beings.

6.6 Nuts and oil seeds

Nuts are seed or fruit containing kernel. These are concentrated food with little water or roughage. Nuts are rich source of protein, energy, minerals and B vitamins. Some nuts such as almond and hazelnuts are excellent source of vitamin E, an antioxidant. Nuts have dissoluble fat content and fatty acids particularly polyunsaturated. The important nuts are almond, cashew nut, walnut, pistachio nut, coconut, oil palm including olive.

Oil seeds are the major source of edible oil. These are also good source of protein, minerals, B vitamins and dissoluble fatty acid. The major oil seeds are groundnut, mustard, rape seed, sesame, linseed, safflower, sunflower and soya bean. The most important of these are groundnut, soya bean, mustard, rape seed and sesame. The nutritive value of nuts and oil seeds are as follows.

6.6.1 Macro nutrients

Macro nutrients such as moisture, protein, fat, fibre, carbohydrate and energy are given in Table 6.18.

Table 6.18. Nutritive value of nuts and oil seeds: macro nutrients.

Nuts and oil seed	Moisture	Protein (g)	Fat (g)	Fibre (g)	Carbohydrate (g)	Energy (kcal)
Almond	5.2	20.8	58.9	1.7	10.5	655
Cashew nut	5.9	21.2	46.9	1.3	22.3	596
Coconut fresh	36.3	4.5	41.6	3.6	13.0	444
Coconut dry		6.6	62.3	3.9	18.4	662
Pistachio nut	5.6	19.8	53.5	2.1	16.2	626
Walnut	4.5	15.6	64.5	2.6	11.0	687
Groundnut	8.5	26.7	40.1	3.1	26.1	567
Mustard seed	7.5	22.0	39.7	1.8	23.8	541
Gingelly seed	6.0	18.3	43.3	2.9	25.0	563
Soya bean	8.0	43.2	19.5	3.5	20.9	432

6.6.1.1 Moisture

The moisture content of nuts and oil seed varies from 4.5% to 8.0% except fresh coconut which contains 36% moisture. Water content of walnut is lowest.

6.6.1.2 Protein

Nuts and oil seeds are rich source of protein except coconut which is low in protein content. Soya bean as oil seeds has highest content of protein followed by groundnut.

6.6.1.3 Fat

Nuts and oil seeds are very rich in fats; hence, they are concentrated source of energy. The fat content varies from 19.5% to 64.5%. Nuts are high in polyunsaturated fatty acid linoleic and linolenic and low in saturated fatty acids, hence, useful in cholesterol lowering diets.

6.6.1.4 Fibre

The fibre content of nuts and oil seeds varies from 1.3% to 3.9%. The dietary fibre content of coconut both dry and fresh and soya bean are higher than other nuts and oil seeds.

6.6.1.5 Carbohydrates

Oil seeds are rich in carbohydrates. Groundnut has higher value (26%) than other nuts and seed. Almond and walnut have lower content of carbohydrate.

6.6.1.6 *Energy value*

Nuts and seeds are high in energy value. The energy value varies from 432 to 687 kcal/100 g. Walnut have highest energy value followed by dry coconut and almond.

6.6.2 Micro nutrients

The vitamins and mineral contents of nuts and oil seeds are given in Tables 6.19 and 6.20, respectively.

Table 6.19. Nutritive value of nuts and oil seed: vitamins content/100 g.

Nuts and oil seed	Carotene (µg)	Thiamine (mg)	Riboflavin (mg)	Niacin (mg)
Almond	–	0.24	0.57	4.4
Cashew nut	60	0.63	0.19	1.2
Coconut fresh	–	0.05	0.10	0.8
Coconut dry	–	0.08	0.01	3.0
Pistachio nut	144	0.67	0.28	2.3
Walnut	6.0	0.45	0.40	1.0
Groundnut	37	0.90	0.13	19.9
Mustard seed	162	0.65	0.26	4.0
Gingelly seed	60	1.01	0.34	4.4
Soya bean	426	0.73	0.39	3.2

Table 6.20. Nutritive value of nuts and oil seed: minerals content/100 g.

Nuts and oil seed	Calcium (mg)	Potassium (mg)	Phosphorus (mg)	Magnesium (mg)	Iron (mg)
Almond	230	856	490	257	5.1
Cashew nut	50	129	450	–	5.8
Coconut fresh	10	336	240	52	1.7
Coconut dry	400	700	160	30	7.8
Pistachio nut	140	–	430	–	7.7
Walnut	100	–	380	–	2.6
Groundnut	90	700	390	181	2.5
Mustard seed	490	–	700	–	7.9
Gingelly seed	1450	725	570	–	2.5
Soya bean	277	–	690	–	10.4

6.6.2.1 Vitamins

Carotene: Nuts and oil seeds are poor source of carotene or pro vitamin A. Soya bean contains comparatively higher content of carotene than other nuts and oil seeds.

B vitamins: Nuts and oil seeds are good source of B vitamins.

Thiamine: Nuts and oil seeds are good source of thiamine except coconut fresh or dry. Gingelly or sesame seeds have higher content of thiamine. Other nuts and oil seeds rich in thiamine content are ground nut, soya bean, pistachio nut and mustard seed.

Riboflavin: Almond, walnut, soya bean and gingelly seeds have relatively higher content and are rich in riboflavin.

Niacin: Nuts and oil seeds are rich source of niacin. Ground nut has higher content of niacin. Almond, gingelly seed and mustard seed are almost similar in niacin content. Nuts and oil seeds are deficient in vitamin C but these are rich source of vitamin E an antioxidant.

6.6.2.2 Minerals

Nuts and oil seeds are good source of various minerals such as calcium, potassium, phosphorus and iron.

Calcium: Gingelly seed is an excellent source of calcium. Dry coconut and mustard seed is also rich in calcium.

Phosphorus: Phosphorus content of nuts and oil seeds varies from 160 to 700 mg/100 g. Phosphorus content is relatively higher in mustard seed, soya bean, gingelly seed and almond.

Potassium: The potassium content varies from 129 to 856 mg/100 g. Almond, ground nut, dry coconut and gingelly seed are good source of potassium.

Magnesium: Almond and ground nut are rich in magnesium content. Coconut is a poor source of magnesium.

Iron: Iron content of nuts and oil seeds varies from 1.7 to 10.4 mg/100 g. Soya bean is an excellent source of iron. Other nuts and oil seeds rich in iron are mustard seed, dry coconut, pistachio nut and cashew nut.

6.7 Fats and oil

Fats and oil serve as a source of energy. They serve as carrier for the fat-soluble vitamins (A, D, E, K) and is also essential for the absorbance of carotene (pro-vitamin A). Fats supply essential fatty acids which are needed by the body. Vegetable oils are rich in vitamin E. Fats and oil play an important role in food preparation and nutrition.

The oils and fat of plant origin are coconut, palm oil, olive, groundnut, mustard, sunflower, gingelly oil, soya bean, sunflower and rice bran oil. The fat sources of animal origin are butter, lard and tallow. The nutritive value of plant- and animal-based oil and fats are as follows.

6.7.1 Plant-based fats and oil

The nutritive values in terms energy and vitamins and oil and their fatty acid are given in Tables 6.21 and 6.22, respectively.

Table 6.21. Energy value and vitamin content of plant-based fat/100 g.

Plant-based sources	Energy (kcal)	Vitamin A (μg)	Vitamin E (mg)
Vegetable oil and fat	900	–	10–140
Red palm oil	900	400–10,000	10–15
Margarine	775	700	10–50
Vanaspati	900	700	10–30

Table 6.22. Oil/fat content and their fatty acids.

Oil/fat sources	Oil content (%)	Fatty acids		
		Saturated (%)	Monounsaturated (%)	Polyunsaturated (%)
Plant sources				
Olive oil	15	14.8	74.5	10.0
Palm oil	45	46.3	43.7	10.0
Coconut oil	65	89.5	7.8	2.0
Mahua oil	48	47.5	38.0	14.0
Groundnut oil	40	20.9	49.3	29.9
Mustard oil	40	10.7	56.0	32.6
Soya bean oil	20	13.1	28.9	57.2
Rice bran oil	–	22.1	41.0	35.7
Gingelly oil	45	13.7	41.3	44.5
Safflower oil	–	10.7	13.7	75.5
Sunflower oil	35	9.1	25.1	66.2
Rape seed oil	40	25.1	–	–
Margarine	86	–	–	–
Vanaspati	100	–	–	6

6.7.1.1 Energy

Vegetable oils or fat provide 900 kcal energy/100 g.

6.7.1.2 *Vitamins*

Vitamin A: In plant sources, red palm oil is rich in vitamin A content (400-10,000 μg/100 g) followed by vanaspati or margarine (700 μg/100 g).

Vitamin E: Plant-based fats and oil are good source of vitamin E an anti-oxidant. Vitamin E content varies from 8 to 140 mg/100 g.

6.7.1.3 *Oil content and their fatty acids*

Oil content varies from 15% to 65%. Coconut has highest content of oil followed by mahua, palm oil and gingelly or sesame. Ground nut, mustard and rape seed are also good source of oil.

Saturated fatty acid content of coconut oil is highest. Mahua and palm oil are also higher in saturated fatty acid. Saturated fatty acid content in other oils is low.

Monounsaturated fatty acid content is highest in olive oil followed by mustard, ground nut, palm oil, gingelly, rice bran and mahua oil.

Poly unsaturated fatty acid are very rich in safflower, sunflower, soya bean and gingelly oils.

6.7.2 Animal-based fats and oil

The fat sources of animal origin are butter, ghee, lard (pork) and tallow (beef). The nutritive values of these fats and oil are given in Table 6.23.

Table 6.23. Nutritive value of animal-based fats.

Fat and oil	Fatty acid			Energy (kcal)	Vitamin	
	Saturated	Mono saturated	Poly saturated		A (μg)	E (mg)
Butter	69.4	2.5	4.0	775	700	2.4
Ghee	60			900	600	2.0
Lard	46.2	11.0	11.0	900	0	1.0
Tallow	54.9	4.2	4.2	900	0	2.0

Animal-based fat also contains 900 kcal/100 g energy except butter which has 774 kcal/100 g due to higher moisture content. Animal-based fats are poor source of essential fatty. They are very high in saturated fatty acids and also have cholesterol. The fats of animal origin such as butter and ghee content 700 μg and 600 μg/100 g of vitamin A, respectively. Animal-based fats are very low or poor (1–2 mg/100 g) in vitamin E content.

6.7.2.1 *Essential fatty acid*

The essential fatty acid contents of some fat and oils are given in Table 6.24.

Table 6.24. Essential fatty acid of fats and oil.

Fats and oils	Linoleic	Linolenic
Coconut oil	2.0	–
Mahua	14.9	–
Palm oil	10.0	–
Olive oil	10.0	–
Cotton seed oil	60.0	–
Corn oil	57.0	–
Ground nut oil	29.9	–
Rape seed/mustard	18.1	14.5
Safflower seed oil	73.5	–
Gingelly oil	44.5	–
Sunflower seed oil	66.2	–
Soya bean oil	51.0	8.1
Butter fat	2.5.0	–
Egg fat	22.0	2.9
Vanaspati	4.9	–

The rich sources of essential fatty acids (linolic) are safflower, sunflower, cottonseed, corn, soya bean and gingelly oils. Groundnut, mustard, rapeseed, mahua and egg fat are also a good source of essential fatty acid. Rape seed or mustard oil is rich in both linolic and linolenic essential fatty acids. Butter fat, coconut oil and vanaspati are the poor source of essential fatty acids.

6.8 Sugar and related products

6.8.1 Sugarcane

Sugarcane is the cheap source of sugar and jaggery. Sugar and jaggery (solid, powdered and liquid) are used as sweeting agents in many food products to increase their palatability. The various forms of sugar used other than jaggery are cube sugar used in tea, powdered sugar used in doughnuts and puris, brown sugar used in baked products, rock sugar used on festive occasion, diamond sugar used in confectionery and betel nut, icing sugar in cake icing and caster sugar used in bakery.

- Jaggery sugar may be liquid, solid and powdered prepared from sugarcane.
- Jaggery can also be prepared from date palm, palm and coconut fruit.
- Honey sugar is manufactured by bees. It has mixture of sucrose, glucose, maltose and fructose.

The nutritive value of sugarcane juice is given in Table 6.25.

Table 6.25. Macro and micro nutrients of sugar cane juice.

Macro nutrients	Value (%)	Micro nutrients: Vitamins	Value (μg)
Water	73–76	Thiamine	53.0
Sucrose	75–90	Riboflavin	31.0
Glucose	70–80	Niacin	9.0
Fructose	2–4	Pantothenic acid	2.2
Amino acids	0.5–2.5	Biotin	22.0
Fibre	11–16	Vitamin D	176.0
		Mineral	0.5%

Sugarcane juice is rich in sugar mainly glucose and fibre content. It has also little content of amino acids. Juice is rich contains B and D vitamins and minerals.

6.8.2 Nutritive value of sugar and related products

6.8.2.1 Macro nutrients

The macro nutrient contents of sugar and related products are given in Table 6.26.

Table 6.26. Nutritive value of sugar and related products: macro nutrients.

Sugar and related products	Moisture (%)	Protein (g)	Carbohydrates (g)	Energy (kcal)
White sugar	0.2	0.3	99.5	398
Solid jaggery	3.9	0.4	95.0	383
Liquid jaggery	30.0	0.15	60.0	312
Honey	20.0	0.10	79.7	320

1. *Moisture*: Liquid jaggery contains higher amount of moisture than honey. Similarly solid jaggery is higher in moisture content than white sugar. The moisture content of white sugar is very low.
2. *Protein*: Sugar and its related product in honey are poor source of protein.
3. *Carbohydrates*: White table sugar has highest content of carbohydrates (99.5% pure sucrose). Solid jaggery has high content of carbohydrate than liquid jaggery. Honey has about 80% carbohydrates which is higher than liquid jaggery.
4. *Energy*: The main contribution of sugar to the diet is energy. White cane sugar contains relatively higher caloric value (398 kcal) than jaggery. Solid jaggery has higher energy value than liquid jaggery. The energy value of honey is nearly similar to content of liquid jaggery.

6.8.2.2 Micro nutrients

The micro nutrients such as vitamins and mineral contents of sugar and related products are given in Tables 6.27 and 6.28, respectively.

Table 6.27. Nutritive value of sugar and related products: vitamin contents.

Sugar and related compounds	Carotene (μg)	Vitamin E (mg)	Thiamine (mg)	Riboflavin (mg)	Niacin (mg)	Vitamin C mg
White sugar	–	–	0.01	–	–	0
Solid jaggery	168	111	0.02	0.06	0.5	5.0
Liquid jaggery	–	–	14.0	–	–	7
Honey	0	–	0.01	0.04	0.2	0

Table 6.28. Nutritive value of sugar and related products: minerals content.

Sugar and related products	Calcium (mg)	Phosphorus (mg)	Iron (mg)
White sugar	12	–	0.15
Solid jaggery	80.0	40.0	0.69
Liquid jaggery	0.3	–	8.5
Honey	10.0	20.0	0.9

1. *Vitamins*: Solid jaggery has little amount of carotene nut rich in vitamin E an antioxidant. Liquid jaggery is rich in thiamine content. Other sugar and related products are poor source of B vitamins and vitamin C.
2. *Minerals*: Solid jaggery is a fair source of calcium, phosphorus and iron. It is preferred than white sugar due to its iron content, colour and flavour. Liquid jaggery is rich in iron. White sugar and honey are poor in mineral contents.

6.9 Food beverages

Beverages supply fluid to the body for refreshing, nourishing, stimulating, soothing and appetizing. Beverages are classified into two main groups non-fermented and fermented. Non-fermented beverages are divided into various sections such as fruit- and vegetable-based beverages, sugarcane juice, tea, coffee and cocoa, beverages and carbonated or aerated soft drink. Fermented beverages are wine, bear, cider, whisky, brandy, gin and rum.

6.9.1 Non-fermented beverage

6.9.1.1 Fruit-based beverages

The nutritive value of fruit-based beverages in terms of water, carbohydrate, energy value and mineral content is given in Table 6.29 and vitamins in Table 6.30.

Table 6.29. Nutritive value of fruit-based beverages.

Non-fermented beverages	Water (g)	Carbohydrate (g)	Energy (kcal)	Calcium (mg)	Iron (mg)
Fruit juice					
Mango	84.2	14.6	58	12	0.5
Orange	87.5	11.0	44	20	0.2
Pineapple	86.2	13.0	52	15	0.5
Grape	85.3	13.7	55	8	0.3
Apple	85.6	13.8	54	6	0.5
Coconut water	94.0	5.0	24	10	0.1
Coconut milk	89.8	2.0	76	20	0.2
Neera	84.7	14.3	57	40	1.0
Fruits squashes (diluted)					
Mango	83.0	15.6	62	8	0.3
Orange	83.2	15.2	61	5	0.2
Lemon	83.4	15.0	60	7	0.4
Pineapple	83.0	15.2	60	8	0.2

Table 6.30. Vitamin content of fruit-based beverages.

Non-fermented beverages	Carotene (μg)	Thiamine (mg)	Riboflavin (mg)	Vitamin C (mg)
Fruit juice				
Mango	1500	0.03	0.05	49
Orange	190	0.03	0.02	49
Pineapple	80	0.03	0.03	20
Grape	29	0.02	0.03	3
Apple	4	0.02	0.02	1
Coconut water	–	0.01	0.01	2
Coconut milk	–	0.02	0.01	1
Neera				

Fruit squashes (diluted)				
Mango	500	0.01	0.02	6
Orange	20	0.01	0.01	6
Lemon	–	0.01	0.01	5
Pineapple	50	0.01	0.01	5

1. *Moisture*: Moisture content of fruit juice varies from 89% to 94%. There is a little variation in water content of orange, pineapple, grape and apple juice. Water content of coconut water is higher (94%) than coconut milk, neera and other fruit juice. There is no variation in water content of mango, orange, lemon and pineapple squashes.
2. *Carbohydrate and energy*: Carbohydrate mainly sugar content of fruit juice varies from 5% to 14%. Sugar provides energy which varies from 24 to 76 kcal in fruit juices. Mango juice and neera the sweet dried from fresh sap of palm contains relatively higher amount of sugar than other fruit juices. Coconut water is a very popular low caloric beverage with 5% sugar.

   Diluted squash contains about 15% sugar which provides 60 kcal energy.
3. *Minerals*:

   Calcium: Neera juice contains relatively higher content of calcium than other juices. Coconut milk obtained from grated mature coconut kernel has some amount of calcium as the content of orange juice. There is little variation in calcium content of diluted fruit squashes.

   Iron: Iron content of fruit juices varies from 0.2 to 1.0 mg/100 g. Mango, pineapple and apple juices contain 0.5 mg iron/100 g. Neera juice has higher content of iron among various fruit-based beverages. Iron content of diluted squashes of various fruits ranged from 0.2 to 0.4 mg/100 g. Lemon squash has relatively higher value.
4. *Vitamins*:

   Carotene: Mango juice and diluted mango squash are rich in carotene. Other fruit beverages contain little amount of carotene.

   B vitamins: Fruit-based beverages such as juices and squashes are not rich in B vitamins such as thiamine and riboflavin content.

   Vitamin C: Mango and orange juices are rich in vitamin C content. Pineapple juice is also fair source of vitamin C. Apple is very low in vitamin C. Vitamin C content of diluted squashes varies from 5 to 6 mg/100 g.

6.9.1.2 *Vegetable-based juice and soups*

Tomato juice contains 93.5% moisture, 4-5% sugar, 17 kcal energy, rich in calcium carotene and vitamins C. Carrot juices are rich in carotene and minerals. Vegetable-based soups such as tomato soup and mixed vegetable soups are appetizers and are rich in vitamins and minerals. Mushroom soup is rich in protein and various minerals.

6.9.1.3 *Sugarcane juice*

It is very nutritious. It contains good amount of sugar that provides energy and has some amount B vitamins and D vitamins. It is also rich in iron content. Thus its nutritive value is higher than carbonated or aerated soft drink that lack or deficient in vitamins and minerals.

6.9.1.4 *Milk-based beverages*

Milk-based beverages such as flavoured milk with different colour and essence as rose milk and milkshake with fruit pulp is rich in proteins, vitamins and minerals.

Tea, coffee and cocoa

Tea, coffee and cocoa are commercially used beverages. These are stimulating beverage due to their caffeine content.

Fresh leaves of tea contains 4.3% caffeine, 22.0% polyphenols about 17% protein, 27.0% crude fibre, 0.5% starch and 5.6% ash. It has also little amount of B vitamins, carotene and vitamin C. The flavour of the tea beverage is influence by caffeine, polyphenols and essential oils. Polyphenols present in tea has antioxidant activity which deactivates cancer promoters and enzymes responsible for tumour growth.

The important constituents of coffee are bitter substances, flavour substances and caffeine. Caffeine is responsible for stimulating effects of the beverage. Caffeine present in the coffee bean varies from 1.2% to 2.5% according to the species. *Coffee arabica* produces largest and best quality of coffee bean which contains 1.0% to 1.2% caffeine. The flavour is largely due to 2-thiofuran and its methyl and ethyl esters. The aroma of coffee is partly due to the mercaptans present in roasted beans.

Cocoa beans contain 5% moisture, 11.5% protein, 9.0% starch and 54% cocoa butter. It also contains theobromine, caffeine and aromatic oils. Theobromine has stimulating properties like caffeine and also provides pleasant flavour to the milk.

Nutritive value of tea, coffee and cocoa beverage

The nutritive value of a cup of tea, coffee and cocoa are given in Table 6.31.

Table 6.31. Nutritive value of tea, coffee and cocoa/cup.

Nutritive value/cup of beverage	Beverage		
	Tea	Coffee	Cocoa
Protein (g)	1.0	1.8	7.2
Carbohydrate (g)	16.4	17.8	26.2
Energy (kcal)	79	98	2.3
Vitamin A (IU)	51	102	408
Calcium (mg)	34	68	270
Phosphorus (mg)	25	50	200

A cup of cocoa beverage has higher nutritive value in terms of higher content of protein, carbohydrate, energy value, vitamin A and mineral such as calcium and phosphorus than a cup of tea and coffee. This is due to addition of more milk in cocoa than tea and coffee.

A cup of coffee beverage contains little more nutrients than a cup of tea beverage due to more milk content resulting more protein and minerals. Caffeine an alkaloid substance present in coffee increases the capacity for physical exertion and it is also cardiac stimulant and diuretic.

The caffeine content of a cup of coffee (150 mL) is about 100 mg. An adult of normal health can consume moderate amount that is 2–3 cups coffee a day and hence, 200–300 mg caffeine. Excessive intake can cause problem such as insomnia. Brewing coffee has more caffeine content. Coffee can be decaffeinated which contains most of the characteristic of aroma of coffee.

A cup of tea beverage has little nutritive value that comes from added milk and sugar. The antioxidant activity of a cup of tea is about 200 mg flavonoids is much higher than a cup of orange juice. It is also much higher than spinach and many other vegetables. Excessive consumption of tea has the similar effects as excessive consumption of coffee. Tea also contains oxalic acid and hence, excessive use may lead to the formation of renal calculi.

6.9.2 Fermented beverages

Fermented beverages are stimulating and appetizing. They contain varying amount of alcohol. Alcohol in moderate dose stimulates gastric secretions and serves as source of energy. Alcohol in excessive amounts causes depressions and loss of consciousness. Alcoholic beverages are wine, malted beverage, beer and distilled liquor. The alcohol content and energy value of these beverage are given in Table 6.32.

Table 6.32. Alcohol content and energy value of alcoholic beverage.

Alcoholic beverages	Alcohol (%)	Energy (kcal)
Wines		
White wine	10	70
Red wine	10	65
Fortified wine	20	135
Beer		
Bitter	5	30
Mild	4	25
Cider		
Dry	4	35
Sweet	4	40
Toddy	5	35
Distilled liquors/spirit		
Whisky, brandy, gin, rum, vodka	35–40	220

6.9.2.1 Wine

The term wine strictly signifies fermented alcoholic beverage produced from grape juice without distillation. Different fermented fruit juices are often included and called fruit wines. Wines are of different types. Sparkling wines which contain excess of carbon dioxide due to secondary fermentation that occurs after bottling example champagne. Natural and still wines without excess of carbon dioxide. White wines prepared from coloured grapes using only juice. Red wines prepared by coloured grape using both juices and skin. Dry wines in which fermentation is up to utilization of all sugars. Sweet wines in which fermentation is stopped while some sugar remains. These wines have 10-14% alcohol. Fortified wines are of two types: port and sherry and Vermouth. In port and sherry, some alcohol such as grape brandy is added before completion of fermentation. Vermouth is prepared by addition of some spices and mixture and extract at different stages of fermentation. The fortified wines contain 20% alcohol. Table wine contains less than 14% alcohol and dessert wine contains 15–21%.

Wines are also prepared from other fruit juices such as cider (fermented apple juice). Other fruit juices such as guava, bael, aonla, jamun, etc., are also used for making cider. Perry wine prepared from pear fruit and *Madhuka* wine prepared from mahua flower. Toddy fermented sap of palm tree obtained by tapping or cutting the stalk of flower branches. This contains 4% alcohol. Honey wine is prepared from diluted honey known as mead.

Wines, generally contains 10–16% alcohol with an energy value of 65–70 kcal. Fortified wines contain up to 20% alcohol with energy value of 135 kcal.

6.9.2.2 Beer (malted beverage)

The term beer generally applied to the fermentation of barley malt. The most commonly cereals other than barley used are maize grit and flakes, broken rice, wheat, tapioca and sorghum. Beers are of various types depending upon strength of alcohol, colour, malt quality, mashing methods, amount of hopes and condition of fermentation.

The term like porter, ale, stout and lager are also used for bears. Beer, porter, ale and stout beverages is produced by top fermentation while lager beer is the product of bottom fermentation.

The alcohol content of various types of beer varies from 3% to 7%. Beers produced in India contains 4–5% alcohol and have caloric value of 25–30 kcal.

Cider contains 4–8% alcohol and have 35–40 kcal energy value. Toddy contains 4–7% alcohol with energy value of 35 kcal.

6.9.2.3 Distilled liquors

Liquors are obtained by steeping herbs, fruit, flowers or plants in distilled spirit. The distilled liquors are of various types such as whisky (scotch, malt whisky and scotch grain whisky), brandy, rum, gin and vodka. Scotch malt whisky prepared from malted barley and scotch grain whisky from barley malt and other malted cereal grains. Brandy is prepared from wine particularly distillate from grape wine. This can also be prepared from many fruit. Rum is an alcoholic beverage distilled directly from sugarcane juice and syrup molasses. Gin is a distilled spirit flavoured with juniper berries or some other aromatics. Vodka is a distilled liquor made by diluting neutral spirits obtained from wheat or other cereal grains and potato.

Distilled liquors generally contain 35–40% alcohol and have calorific value of 220 kcal.

7
Nutritive value of animal-based foods

Animal-based foods are milk and milk products, eggs, meats and fish. The nutritive values of these foods are discussed in this chapter.

7.1 Milk and milk products

Milk is the most complete of all foods. It is regarded as ideal food for nourishing infants and young children. This is also good supplementary food in the diet of adult. Milk and milk products are excellent source of protein, fat, carbohydrate, vitamins and minerals. Man uses milk of many animal sources such as cow, buffalo, goat, etc. Cow is the most important among these. About 45% milk produced is consumed as liquid milk and remaining 55% is converted into wide range of dairy products such as curds, chenna, cheese, khoa, condensed milk, butter/ghee and milk powder.

The nutritional value of milk varies with the species, breed and diet. The nutritive value of milk and milk products are as follows.

7.1.1 Macro nutrients

The macro nutrient content of milk and milk products such as moisture, protein, fat, carbohydrate and energy are given in Table 7.1.

Table 7.1. Nutritive value of milk and milk products – macro nutrients.

Milk and milk products	Moisture (g)	Protein (g)	Fat (g)	Carbohydrate (g)	Energy (kcal)
Cow's milk	87.5	3.2	4.1	4.4	67
Buffalo milk	81.0	4.3	6.5	5.0	117
Goat milk	85.2	3.7	5.6	4.7	84
Human milk	88.0	1.1	3.4	7.4	65
Curd (cow's milk)	89.1	3.1	4.0	3.0	60
Chenna (cow's milk)	57.1	18.3	20.8	1.2	265
Cheese	40.3	24.1	25.1	6.3	348
Khoa (buffalo milk)	30.6	14.6	31.2	20.5	421
Khoa (cow's milk)	25.2	20.0	25.9	24.9	413
Condensed milk	27.1	8.1	8.7	54.3	321

Evaporated milk	73.8	7.0	7.9	9.7	137
Skimmed milk powder	4.1	38.0	0.1	51.0	357
Whole milk powder	3.5	25.8	26.7	38.0	496

7.1.2 Moisture

The moisture content of cow milk is higher than buffalo milk. The moisture content of curd is higher than other milk products. Milk powder contains about 4% moisture.

7.1.3 Protein

Milk has good quality protein. Cow's milk contains 3.2% and buffalo milk 4.3%. Milk protein is rich in all essential amino acids. Casein constitutes about 80% of the total nitrogen in milk. Casein is a good source of essential amino acids. Lysin and threonine which are abundant in milk protein, supplement effectively cereals protein. Milk products such as chenna, cheese, khoa and dehydrated milk powders are in concentrated forms, hence, have higher amount of protein.

7.1.4 Fat

Milk fat or butter fat is of a great nutritive and economical value. The fat content of cow's milk is 4.1% and buffalo milk 6.5%. Milk products have high fat content except skimmed milk powder which is deficient in fat. Buffalo milk and its products have higher fat content than cow's milk and its products. Fat provides flavour to the milk. Milk fat is mainly composed of several glycerides. They contain high amount of fatty acids. Saturated fatty acids account for butyric and caproic acid 62% and unsaturated 37%. Out of unsaturated fatty acid, polyunsaturated is 3.8%. Milk of both cow and buffalo is a poor source of essential fatty acids. It contains 2.1% linoleic, 0.5% linolenic and 0.14% arachidonic. Milk also contains small amount of phospholipids and cholesterol.

7.1.5 Carbohydrates

Lactose is the chief carbohydrate of milk. Lactose present in milk is 4-5%. Lactose the milk sugar is preferred as a source of carbohydrate due to its controlled glycaemic effect. Condensed milk has relatively higher content of carbohydrates than skimmed milk powder and whole milk powder. Chenna and curds are very low in carbohydrate content.

7.1.6 Energy

Buffalo milk provides higher energy value than cow's milk. The energy value of whole milk powder is highest followed by khoa, skimmed milk powder and cheese. Curd is low in caloric value.

7.1.7 Micro nutrients

The vitamin and mineral contents of milk and milk products are given in Tables 7.2 and 7.3, respectively.

Table 7.2. Nutritive value of milk and milk products: vitamin content/100 g

Milk and milk products	Vitamin A (IU)	Thiamine (mg)	Riboflavin (mg)	Niacin (mg)	Vit. B_{12} (μg)
Cow's milk	174	0.05	0.19	0.1	0.14
Buffalo milk	160	0.04	0.10	0.1	0.14
Goat milk	55	0.05	0.14	0.3	–
Human milk	137	0.02	0.02	0.1	0.02
Curd (cow's milk)	102	0.05	0.16	0.1	0.13
Chenna (cow's milk)	366	0.07	0.02	–	–
Cheese	273	0.03	0.46	0.4	–
Khoa (buffalo milk)	315	0.21	0.39	0.4	–
Khoa (cow's milk)	497	0.23	0.41	0.4	–
Condensed milk	108	0.08	0.38	0.2	–
Evaporated milk	96	0.04	0.34	0.2	–
Skimmed milk powder	0	0.45	1.64	1.0	0.83
Whole milk powder	1400	0.31	1.36	0.8	–

Table 7.3. Nutritive value of milk and milk products: mineral content/100 g.*

Milk and milk products	Calcium (mg)	Phosphorus (mg)	Iron (mg)
Cow's milk	120	90	0.2
Buffalo milk	210	130	0.2
Goat milk	170	120	0.3
Human milk	28	11	0.2
Curd (cow's milk)	149	93	0.2
Chenna (cow's milk)	208	138	–
Cheese	790	520	2.1
Khoa (buffalo milk)	650	420	5.8
Khoa (cow's milk)	960	610	6.1

Condensed milk	260	210	0.1
Evaporated milk	250	210	0.1
Skimmed milk powder	1370	1000	1.4
Whole milk powder	950	730	0.6

* Gopalan, C., Rama Sastri, B.V. and Bala Subramanian, 2004.

7.1.8 Vitamins

7.1.8.1 Vitamin A

Milk contains both fat and water soluble vitamins. The vitamin A content of cow milk is 176 IU and buffalo milk 160 IU/100 g whole milk powder contains higher amount of vitamin A among various milk products. Khoa of cow's milk contains relatively higher content of vitamin A than khoa of buffalo milk.

7.1.8.2 B vitamins

Milk powder is good source of B vitamins. Milk is rich in riboflavin. Cheese and khoa are also good source of riboflavin. Milk is fair source of folic acid and vitamin B_{12}. Thiamine occurs in fair amount in milk. Niacin content is low and ascorbic acid is deficient in milk.

7.1.9 Minerals

7.1.9.1 Calcium

Milk and milk products are excellent source of calcium. Buffalo milk has higher content of calcium than cow's milk. Among the various milk products, skimmed milk powder contains highest amount of calcium followed by Khoa of cow's milk and whole milk powder. Khoa of cow's milk contains more calcium than khoa of buffalo milk. Cheese also has more calcium than chenna.

7.1.9.2 Phosphorus

Buffalo milk contains higher amount of phosphorus than cow's milk. Phosphorus content of skimmed milk powder is higher as compared with whole milk powder. Khoa of cow's milk contains more phosphorus than khoa of buffalo milk. Phosphorus content of cheese is also higher than chenna.

7.1.9.3 Iron

Iron content of milk is very low. Among various milk products, khoa of both buffalo and cow's milk has higher amount of iron due to concentrated forms.

7.2 Eggs

Egg is an ideal protective food due to its mineral, vitamin and essential amino acids. Egg protein has the highest biological value among proteins of various food sources. Though eggs of most of the birds are edible but the eggs of hen and duck are mainly used in India for human consumption. The eggs are of two types: fertilized eggs of the hen formed with fusion of sperm and unfertilized egg without the fusion of sperm called vegetarian egg. Leg horns are improved birds suitable for egg production and produce unfertilized eggs without mating with cock.

Egg is composed of shell, egg white and egg yellow or yolk. The nutritive value of egg white is different from that of egg yolk. Egg white has large amount of water (about 80%) and absence of fat than egg yolk which has low content of water about 50% and large amount of fat (about 33%) with fat and water-soluble vitamins. Both hen and duck eggs are rich in nutritive value. The nutritive values of eggs are given as follows.

7.2.1 Macro nutrients

The macro nutrients content of eggs are given in Table 7.4.

Table 7.4. Nutritive value of eggs - macro nutrients.

Macro nutrients	**Value (g)**	
	Hen egg	**Duck eggs**
Moisture	73.7	71.0
Protein	18.3	18.5
Fat	13.3	13.7
Energy (kcal)	173	180
Essential amino acids	Value g/16 g N	
Lysine	6.4	7.9
Methionine	3.1	4.9
Leucine	8.8	9.6
Tryptophan	1.7	1.4
Threonine	5.0	7.0
Phenyl alanine	5.8	6.2
Iso-leucine	6.6	5.5
Valine	7.3	7.5
Histidine	2.4	2.9
Cystine	2.4	1.7

7.2.1.1 Moisture

The moisture contents of hen and duck eggs are 73.7% and 71.0%, respectively.

7.2.1.2 Protein

Hen egg (whole) contains 13% protein and duck egg (whole) has 18% protein. The egg white has about 11% protein and egg yolk about 17%. Different type of protein is found in egg white but albumin constitute in higher amount. Egg protein is of excellent quality and contains all essential amino acids needed by human body. Among various essential amino acids, leucine content is highest followed by valine, iso-leucine and lysine. The lysine content of egg protein is higher than cereals and cystine content is higher than pulses and oil seeds. Therefore, protein quality of food can be enhanced by combination of egg with any of the cereals or mixture of cereals and pulses.

7.2.1.3 Fat

Eggs of hen and duck contain about 13% fat. Fat is found in egg yolk. The main fatty acid present in egg yolk is oleic, palmitic, stearic and linoleic. Presence of high unsaturated fatty acids in egg yolk fat is liable to undergo oxidation and result off flavour. Egg is also a rich source of lecithin, a phospholipid which forms a part of structure of living cell wall in the body. The egg yolk contains high amount of cholesterol (1085mg/100g). Hence, egg yolk is restricted to patient of cardiac and liver diseases.

7.2.1.4 Energy

Energy value of eggs of hen and duck is 173 and 180 kcal, respectively.

7.2.2 Micro nutrients

The micro nutrients such as vitamins and mineral content of eggs are given in Table 7.5.

Table 7.5. Nutritive value of egg – vitamin and mineral content/100 g.

	Eggs	
	Hen	Duck
Vitamins		
Vitamin A (IU)	2200	2100
Thiamine (mg)	0.40	0.12
Riboflavin (mg)	0.30	0.30
Niacin (mg)	0.10	0.20

Folic acid (μg)	78.0	80.0
Vitamin B_{12} (μg)	11.0	9.0
Minerals		
Calcium (mg)	60	70
Phosphorus (mg)	220	260
Iron (mg)	2.1	3.0
Sodium (mg)	129	135

7.2.2.1 Vitamins

The fat-soluble vitamins A, D, E and water-soluble vitamins, B vitamins such as thiamine, riboflavin, niacin, folic acid and B_{12} are found in egg in appreciable amounts. Egg is particularly rich source of vitamin A, thiamine, riboflavin, folic acids and vitamin B_{12}. Egg is deficient in ascorbic acid or vitamin C.

7.2.2.2 Minerals

Egg contains important minerals such as calcium, phosphorus, iron, sodium and zinc. Eggs of duck have relatively higher value of minerals than eggs of hen. Egg is a good source of iron, phosphorus, sodium and zinc but poor in calcium content.

7.3 Flesh foods

7.3.1 Meat

Meat is a good source of protein. Meat includes poultry (chicken, duck and turkey), calf or beef, buffalo meat, sheep meat (mutton), swine meat (pork) and goat meat (chevon). The nutritive values of various types of meat are as follows.

7.3.1.1 Macro nutrients

Macro nutrients such as moisture, protein, fat and energy content of various types of meat is given in Table 7.6.

Table 7.6. Nutritive value of meats – macro nutrients.

Meat	Moisture (g)	Protein (g)	Fat (g)	Energy (kcal)
Poultry meat				
Chicken	72.2	26.0	0.6	109
Duck	72.3	21.6	4.8	130
Goat meat	74.2	21.4	3.6	118
Mutton (sheep)	71.5	18.5	13.3	194

Beef (cattle)	74.3	22.6	16.0	114
Buffalo meat	78.7	19.4	2.6	86
Pork meat	77.5	18.7	35.0	114
Organ meat				
Liver goat	76.3	20.0	3.0	107
Liver sheep	70.4	19.3	7.5	150

1. *Moisture*: The moisture content of various meats varies from 71% to 78%. There is no difference in moisture content of poultry meat that is chicken and duck. Buffalo meat contains relatively higher contents of moisture. Goat meat including organ meat contains higher amount of water than sheep meats. There is little difference in water content of buffalo and pork meat.
2. *Protein*: The protein content of meat varies from 18% to 26%. Chicken meat has relatively higher content of protein than duck- and animal-based meats. Beef or cattle meat has also little higher content of protein than goat, sheep, buffalo and pork meat. Organ meat such as liver of goat and sheep contains about 20% protein. Meat proteins are good source of essential amino acids particularly lysine (7.5–8.7 g/16 g N) and leucine (7.2–9.2 g/16 g N) which can supplement cereal protein.
3. *Fat*: Pork meat contains higher amount of fat followed by beef (cattle) and mutton (sheep). In organ meat, goat liver has lower content of fat than sheep or mutton liver. Chicken meat has lowest fat content.
4. *Energy*: Caloric value of meat varies from 86 to 194 kcal. Mutton contains higher energy value than other meats. Chicken meat has lower caloric value than duck meat. The energy value of pork and beef is similar. In organ meat, sheep liver has higher calorie than goat liver. Meats are deficient in carbohydrates.

7.3.1.2 Micro nutrients

The micro nutrients such as vitamins and minerals content of meats are given in Table 7.7.

Table 7.7. Nutritive value of meat – vitamins and minerals.

Meat	Vitamins				Minerals		
	Vit. A (µg)	**Vit. B_1 (mg)**	**Vit. B_2 (mg)**	**Niacin (mg)**	**Ca (mg)**	**P (mg)**	**Iron (mg)**
Poultry meat							
Chicken	-	0.10	0.14	6.8	25	251	1.6

Duck	-	0.10	0.12	7.7	10	240	1.5
Goat meat	31	0.18	0.27	6.8	150	150	2.3
Beef (cattle)	18	0.15	0.04	6.4	10	190	0.8
Buffalo meat	–	–	–	–	3.0	189	–
Mutton (sheep)	9	0.18	0.14	6.8	150	150	2.5
Pork	0	0.54	0.09	2.8	30	200	2.2
Organ meat							
Liver goat			3.20	17.6	17	279	6.3
Liver sheep			1.70	17.5	10	380	6.3

1. Vitamins

- Vitamin A

The organ meats are good source of vitamin A. Goat liver contains higher content of vitamin A than the content of sheep liver. Other meats are very poor source of vitamin A or deficient in vitamin A.

- B vitamins

Thiamine: Thiamine content varies from 0.10 to 0.54 mg/100 g. Pork meat has higher value in thiamine content among various meats. Organ meats are also good source of thiamine. Thiamine content is poor in poultry meat.

Riboflavin: Riboflavin content varies from 0.04 to 3.2 mg/100 g. Organ meat particularly goat liver has higher content of riboflavin than the content of other meats. Sheep liver is also rich in riboflavin. Beef and pork are poor source of riboflavin.

Niacin: Meats are very good source of niacin. Organ meats that is liver contains higher amount of niacin than other meats. Niacin content of poultry meats, goat and sheep is 6-7 mg/100 g.

The organ meat is also rich in biotin, pantothenic acid and pyridoxine. It is the riches natural source of vitamin B_{12}.

2. Minerals

Calcium: Goat and sheep meats are very rich source of calcium. Other meats are poor in calcium content.

Phosphorus: Phosphorus content of flesh meats varies from 150 to 380 mg/100 g. Organ meats contain relatively higher content of phosphorus than the contents of other types of meats.

Potassium and sodium: Potassium and sodium content of meat varies from 244 to 333 mg/100 g and 55 to 90 mg/100 g, respectively.

Iron: Iron content of meats varies from 0.8 to 6.3 mg/100 g. Organ meats, liver of both goat and sheep contain higher content of iron among various types of meat.

7.4 Fish foods

Fish is also a good source of protein and minerals. Fishes are of various types. Commonly consumed fishes are cat fish, katla, rohu, pomfret, mackerel, sardine, shark, prawn, shrimp and chela. The nutritive values of these fishes are as follows.

7.4.1 Macro nutrients

Macro nutrient contents of various types of fishes are given in Table 7.8.

Table 7.8. Nutritive value of fish – macro nutrients.

Fishes	Moisture (g)	Protein (g)	Fat (g)	Energy (kcal)
Cat fish	77.1	21.4	2.0	86
Katla	73.7	19.5	2.4	111
Rohu	76.7	16.6	1.4	97
Pomfret black	74.5	20.3	2.6	111
Pomfret white	78.4	17.0	1.3	87
Mackerel	77.3	19.1	1.7	93
Sardine	78.1	21.0	1.9	101
Shark	76.0	21.6	0.4	93
Prawn	77.4	21.0	1.0	89
Chela fresh	76.6	14.6	4.3	103
Shrimp (dried)	6.0	68.1	88.5	349
Chela dried	9.7	54.8	17.0	392

1. *Moisture*: Moisture content of fresh fishes varies from 73% to 78%. Dry fishes such as chela and shrimp contain 9% and 6% moisture, respectively.
2. *Protein*: Fresh fishes contain protein from 15% to 21%. Fish protein is rich in essential fatty amino acids particularly lysine, leucine, valine, isoleucine and threonine. Lysine content varies from 7% to 9% which can supplement cereals protein. Dried small fishes such as chela and shrimp have higher content of protein (55–68%) due to its concentrated form.

3. *Fat*: Fat content of fishes is very low about 1–2% (except chela fish); hence, fishes are not good source of energy. Fishes also contain omega-3 fatty acids. Shark fish has lowest content of fat. Dried fishes have higher content of fat due to its concentration.
4. *Energy*: Fishes are generally low in caloric value. Energy value varies from 87 to 111 kcal. Dried fishes have higher energy value which varies from 349 to 392 kcal.

7.4.2 Micro nutrients

The vitamins and minerals contents of fishes are given Table 7.9.

Table 7.9. Nutritive value of fishes per 100gms – micro nutrients.

Fishes	Vitamins			Minerals		
	B_1 (mg)	B_2 (mg)	Niacin (mg)	Calcium (mg)	Phosphorus (mg)	Iron (mg)
Cat fish (wild)	0.210	0.072	1.907	14	209	0.23
Katla	0.20	0.25	0.8	530	235	0.9
Rohu	0.05	0.07	0.7	650	175	1.0
Pomfret Black	0.10	0.16	3.0	286	306	2.3
Pomfret white	0.12	0.15	2.6	200	290	0.9
Mackerel	–	–	–	429	305	4.5
Sardine	–	–	2.6	90	360	2.5
Shark	0.08	0.15	2.5	357	262	1.4
Prawn	0.01	0.10	4.8	323	278	5.3
Chela fresh	0.14	0.18	–	590	340	2.0
Shrimp (dried)	–	–	–	4384	1160	8.8
Chela (dried)	–	–	–	2950	1700	10.0

1. Vitamins

- Vitamin A

Fishes are the poor source of vitamin A. Fish oil is rich source of vitamin A. Cod liver oil contains high amount of vitamin A, that is, 10,000 to 24,000 μg/100 g and shark liver oil 9000 μg.

- B vitamins

Thiamine and riboflavin: Fishes are not rich in thiamine and riboflavin content.

Niacin: Fishes are fair source of niacin. Niacin content varies from 0.7 to 4.8 mg/100 g. Prawn has higher content of niacin among various fishes.

Fishes are also good source of vitamin B_{12} and vitamin D.

2. Minerals

Calcium: Fishes are rich in calcium. Calcium content varies from 10 to 650 mg/100 g in fresh fishes. Rohu contains highest content of calcium followed by chela and katla. Cat fish is poor source of calcium. Dried fishes have higher concentration of calcium than fresh fishes due to its concentration forms.

Phosphorus: Phosphorus content is highest in sardine fish followed by chela pomfret and mackerel. Dried fishes have higher concentration of phosphorus than the content of fresh fishes.

Iron: Iron content of fresh fishes varies from 1 to 5 mg/100 g. Fishes are poor in iron content except prawn which have relatively higher value. Dried fishes contain higher value than fresh fishes.

Iodine: Marine or ocean fishes are good source of iodine.

7.5 Nutritive value of other foods

Foods of other sources include mushroom of fungi origin and spirulina of algae origin.

7.5.1 Mushroom

Mushroom is a food of fungi origin. The use of mushroom as a food has been a delicacy since ancient time. Mushroom is a rich source of protein, vitamins and minerals. Protein content is higher than cereals, pulses and various fresh fruits. This has attracted attention of mankind. Commonly cultivated types of mushrooms are button mushroom, oyster mushroom and paddy mushroom. Among these, button mushroom is very popular and widely cultivated. The nutritive values of mushroom are as follows.

7.5.1.1 Macro nutrients

The macro nutrient contents of mushroom are given in Table 7.10.

Table 7.10. Nutritive value of mushroom – macro nutrients.

Nutrients	Value in fresh mushroom (g/100 g)
Macro nutrients	
Moisture (g)	88.5
Protein (g)	3.1
Fat (g)	0.8
Carbohydrate (g)	4.3
Fibre (g)	0.4
Energy (kcal)	43

Essential amino acid	Value in dried mushroom (g/100g)
Lysine	1.62
Methionine	0.39
Leucine	2.16
Tryptophan	3.94
Threonine	1.48
Phenylalanine	1.55
Isoleucine	1.55
Valine	1.63
Histidine	0.64
Cystine	0.18

7.5.1.2 Micro nutrients

The micro nutrients such as vitamins and minerals are given in Table 7.11.

Table 7.11. Nutritive value of mushroom – vitamins and minerals.

Vitamins	**Value in fresh mushroom (mg)**
Thiamine	0.09
riboflavin	0.31
Niacin	5.85
Pantothenic acid	2.85
Minerals	
Calcium	6.0
Phosphorus	110.0
Potassium	320.0
Sodium	5.0
Magnesium	9.0
Iron	1.5

Fats, carbohydrate and energy: Mushroom has low content of fat, carbohydrate and energy value; hence, suitable for diabetes and form an article of slimming diet or low caloric diet.

Protein: Fresh mushroom contains about 3% protein. The quality of protein is better than the protein of cereals and soya bean. The mushroom protein is easily digestible and its quality is intermediate between vegetable and meat protein.

Essential amino acids: Mushroom protein contains most of the essential amino acid in adequate quantity particularly tryptophan, leucine, lysine and valine.

Vitamins: Mushrooms are poor in pro-vitamin-A but are good source of B vitamins particularly riboflavin, niacin and pantothenic acid. Folic acid a blood building vitamin is also found in mushroom.

Minerals: Mushroom contents various minerals and rich in potassium and phosphorus. Calcium and iron are in low concentration.

7.5.2 Spirulina

Spirulina the blue green algae are known as health food. It is an excellent source of protein, vitamins and phytochemicals. Freshly harvested spirulina can be sun dried or spray dried for use. The nutritive values of spirulina in terms of macro nutrients and micro nutrients are given in Tables 7.12 and 7.13, respectively.

Table 7.12. Nutritive value of dried spirulina - macro nutrients.

Macro nutrients	Value (g)	Essential amino acids	(%)
Protein	65–71	Theonine	3.04
Carbohydrates	16	Lysine	2.99
Fat	6.7	Phenyl alanine	2.87
Fibre	9.3	Methionine	1.38
Energy (kcal)	346	Cystine	0.47

Table 7.13. Nutritive value of dried spirulina - micro nutrients.

Vitamins	Value	Minerals	Value (mg)
β-Carotene	320,000 μg	Calcium	658
Tocophenol/Vit. E	0.73 IU	Iron	47.7
Biotin	0.22 mg	Phosphorus	977
Folic acid	176 μg	Potassium	1140
B_{12}	65.7 μg	Sodium	796

1. *Protein*: Spirulina (spray dried) is very rich in protein content. It has more than 60% protein. The quality of protein is better than the protein of cereals and soya bean. Essential amino acids content of protein such as lysine, theonine and phenyl alanine are higher that is about 3%. It has also fair source of methionine and cystine.
2. *Vitamins*: Spirulina has very high content of β-carotene (provitamin A). It is much higher than carrot. It is also rich in vitamin E an antioxidant, folic acid, biotin and vitamin B_{12} (cyanocobalamin) and other B vitamins. It is one of the vegetarian source provides vitamin B_{12}.

3. *Minerals*: Spirulina is an excellent source of minerals. It is very rich in calcium, iron, phosphorus, potassium and sodium.

Spirulina also contains polyunsaturated fatty acid such as omega-3 fatty acids and most important essential fatty acid gamma-linolenic acid which helps in heart disease, premenstrual stress, arthritis and obesity.

The pigments present in spirulina (chlorophylls, carotenoids, xanthophylls and phycocyanin) can raise the activity of lymphocytes and prevent certain types of cancer by increasing immunity.

8

Dietary allowances in normal life cycle

The significance of nutrition at specific times of growth, development and aging is becoming very important. Nutrient requirement is the minimum amount of the absorbed nutrient which is necessary for maintaining normal physiological function of the body. Recommended dietary allowances (RDA) is a nutrient present in the diet which satisfy the daily requirement of nearly all individuals in a population. These requirements depend on several factors such as age (adult requires more than child), sex (male requires more calories than female), physical work (hard working persons requires more calories than sedentary workers) and physiological stress (more nutrient required in pregnancy and lactation period). Dietary allowances for different age groups, work and stress period can be classified into various groups. The life cycle of each person consist of five basic stages that are adulthood, pregnancy, infancy, childhood and adolescence. The Indian Council of Medical Research (ICMR) has made recommendation for the dietary allowances of the Indian population by physical activity, sex and age which are discussed in this chapter.

8.1 Dietary allowances during adulthood

Adulthood is the period during which growth level is maximum or there is not much of apparent growth. An adult Indian man is between 20 and 39 years of age, weighing 60 kg, free from diseases and is physically fit for active work. He is employed for 8 h in occupation on each working day for moderate activity or if not at work spends 8 h in bed, 4–6 h in sitting and moving and 2 h in walking or house hold activities. ICMR has taken a height of 163 cm. An adult Indian woman is between 20 and 39 years of age, weighing 50 kg, free from diseases and engaged for 8 h is general house hold work or office work or in any other moderate activity. She spends 4–6 h in sitting and moving and 2 h in walking or house hold activity apart from 8 h in bed. ICMR has taken a height of 151 cm for such women. Adequate amount of the all essential requirements need to be provided to adults through their diet for maintaining both physical and mental health.

The ICMR RDAs for both Indian men and women based on different activity levels which are given in Table 8.1.

Table 8.1 Recommended dietary allowances for an adult men and women/day.

Nutrients	Adult men			Adult women		
	Sedent	Moderate	Hard	Sedent	Moderate	Hard
Energy (kcal)	2320	2730	3490	1900	2230	2850
Protein (g)	60	60	60	55	55	55
Fat	25	30	40	20	25	30
calcium (mg)	600	600	600	600	600	600
Iron (mg)	17	17	17	21	21	21
Zinc (mg)	12	12	12	10	10	10
Magnesium (mg)	340	340	340	310	310	310
Vitamin A						
Retinol (μg)	600	600	600	600	600	600
β-carotene (μg)	2400	2400	2400	2400	2400	2400
Thiamine (mg)	1.2	1.4	1.7	1.0	1.1	1.4
Riboflavin (mg)	1.4	1.6	2.1	1.1	1.3	1.7
Niacin (mg)	16	18	21	12	14	16
Pyridoxine (mg)	2.0	2.0	2.0	2.0	2.0	2.0
Folic acid (μg)	200	200	200	200	200	200
Vitamin B_{12} (μg)	1.0	1.0	1.0	1.0	1.0	1.0
Ascorbic acid (mg)	40	40	40	40	40	40

The food stuffs required to meet nutritional requirements of adults are milk, meat, pulse, cereals, leafy and other vegetables, fruit, vegetable fat and sugar.

8.2 Dietary allowances during pregnancy

In pregnancy, human life begins and developed to birth. Maternal health is complex and affected by several factors which can affect the foetal growth. The reserves of several nutrients in well-nourished women before conception, begins her pregnancy can meet the needs of growing foetus without affecting her health. Well-nourished infant in the womb has better chance of entering life with good physical and mental health. Therefore, adequate nutrition before and during pregnancy has great potential for long-term impact on health.

The ICMR RDAs during pregnancy for Indian women are given in Table 8.2.

Table 8.2 Dietary allowances during pregnancy.

Nutrients	Requirement/d
Energy (kcal)	+350
Protein (g)	78
Fat (g)	30
Calcium (mg)	1200
Iron (mg)	35
Zinc (mg)	15
Magnesium (mg)	310
Vitamin A	
Retinol (µg)	800
β-Carotene (µg)	6400
Thiamine (mg)	+0.2
Riboflavin (mg)	+0.3
Niacin (mg)	+2.0
Pyridoxine (mg)	2.5
Folic acid (µg)	500
Vitamin B_{12} (µg)	1.2
Ascorbic acid (mg)	60

8.3 Dietary allowances during lactation

Mother nurses her baby hence, requires greater demand for her body. The nutritional requirement should meet her own daily needs for growing of infants and energy for mechanics of milk production. The RDAs by ICMR for lactating mother is given in Table 8.3.

Table 8.3 Dietary allowances for lactating women.

Nutrients	Requirement/d	
	0–6 months	6–12 months
Energy (kcal)	600	520
Protein (g)	74	68
Fat	30	30
Calcium (mg)	1200	1200
Iron (mg)	21	21
Zinc (mg)	12	12
Magnesium(mg)	310	310

Vitamin A		
Retinol (μg)	950	950
β-carotene (μg)	3800	3800
Thiamine (mg)	+0.3	+0.2
Riboflavin (mg)	+0.4	+0.3
Niacin (mg)	+4	+3
Pyridoxine (mg)	2.5	2.5
Folic acid (μg)	300	300
Vitamin B_{12} (μg)	1.5	1.5
Ascorbic acid (mg)	80	80

Food stuffs required to meet nutritional requirements of lactating mother are cereals, milk, meat, split pulses, vegetables, fruits, vegetable fat or oil and sugar.

Foods generally should be avoided during lactation period are seedy vegetables, leafy vegetables, potato, curds, cold food and whole pulses.

8.4 Dietary allowances during infancy

Infancy is a period of rapid growth. The infants grow and develop very rapidly during the first year of life. The nutritional requirements during early infancy are met by breast feeding. Breast milk has all nutrients that the baby needs for the first 4–6 months of life. Breast milk is bacteriologically safe and is quickly digested due to the enzyme lipase. The breast fed babies have little incidents of diarrhoea and other infections than artificially fed infants. After 4–6 months, nutritional needs have to be met by other supplements. The RDAs for infants are given in Table 8.4.

Table 8.4 Dietary allowances during infancy.

Nutrients	**Requirement/d**	
	0–6 months	**6–12 months**
Energy (kcal)	92/kg	80/kg
Protein (g)	1.16/kg	1.69/kg
Fat (g)	–	19/kg
Calcium (mg)	500	500
Iron (mg)	46 μg	5
Zinc (mg)	–	–
Magnesium (mg)	30	45
Vitamin A		
Retinol (μg)	350	350

β-Carotene (μg)	–	2800
Thiamine (mg)	+0.2	+0.3
Riboflavin (mg)	+0.3	+0.4
Niacin (μg)	710/kg	650/kg
Pyridoxine (mg)	0.1	0.4
Folic acid (μg)	25	25
Vitamin B_{12} (μg)	0.2	0.2
Ascorbic acid (mg)	25	25

Some of the supplementary food stuffs used to meet the nutritional requirement of infants are fruit juices and soups during 4–5 months of age, cereals cooked in water or milk during 5–6 months of age, boiled egg yolk, boiled and mashed potato and mashed banana with milk during 6–7 months of age, well-cooked vegetables and thin khichri during 7–8 months of age and soft boiled or scrambled egg custard with well cooked vegetables during 10–12 months of age.

8.5 Dietary allowances during childhood

Childhood is the period in which a lot of dietary changes occur from the age of two onwards. Nutritional needs and children appetites vary considerably according to the age, size, rate of growth and activity level. The physiological changes that occur in childhood are increase in body size such as height and weight and body composition such as water, muscle tissue, fat deposits and skeletal structure. Psychosocial changes also occur such as development of sense of individuality, increase in physical mobility, sense of independence imagination and curiosity.

Food and feeding is very important during this phase of life cycle to support food related habits and attitudes for life long. ICMR has RDAs during childhood which have been given in Table 8.5.

Table 8.5 Dietary allowances during childhood.

Nutrients	Age (years)		
	1–3	4–6	7–9
Energy (kcal)	1060	1330	1690
Protein (g)	16.7	20.1	29.5
Fat (g)	27	25	30
Calcium (mg)	600	600	600
Iron (mg)	9	13	16
Zinc (mg)	5	7	8

Magnesium (mg)	50	70	100
Vitamin A			
Retinol (μg)	400	400	600
β-Carotene (μg)	3200	3200	4800
Thiamine (mg)	0.5	0.7	0.8
Riboflavin (mg)	0.6	0.8	1.0
Niacin (mg)	8	11	13
Pyridoxine (mg)	0.9	0.9	1.6
Folic acid (μg)	80	100	120
Vitamin B_{12} (μg)	–	0.2	1.0
Ascorbic acid (mg)	40	40	40

The food stuffs required to meet the nutritional requirements are milk, meat, cereals, pulses, leafy and other vegetables, fruits, vegetable fat and sugar.

8.6 Dietary allowances during adolescence

Adolescence is the teenage of rapid growth and sexual maturity. This is very challenging period in human development which is characterized by sudden change in increase growth. The sudden change in growth requires an increase in supply of all nutrients. The growth period reaching its peak at the age of 12 and 14 in female and male, respectively, and ending at the age of 15 and 19 in female and male, respectively. The adolescence as an adult should consume a healthy diet compatible with long-term good health. The RDAs for adolescence are given in Table 8.6.

Table 8.6 Dietary allowance for adolescence/d.

Nutrients	Age (years)					
	Boys			Girls		
	10–12	13–15	16–17	10–12	13–15	16–17
Energy (kcal)	2190	2750	3020	2010	2330	2440
Protein (g)	39.9	54.3	61.5	40.4	51.9	55.5
Fat (g)	35	45	50	35	40	35
Calcium (mg)	800	800	800	800	800	800
Iron (mg)	21	32	28	27	27	26
Zinc (mg)	9	11	12	9	11	12
Magnesium (mg)	120	165	195	160	210	235

Vitamin A						
Retinol (μg)	600	600	600	600	600	600
β-Carotene (μg)	2400	2400	2400	2400	2400	2400
Thiamine (mg)	1.1	1.4	1.5	1.0	1.2	1.0
Riboflavin (mg)	1.3	1.6	1.8	1.2	1.4	1.2
Niacin (mg)	15	16	17	13	14	14
Pyridoxine (mg)	1.6	2.0	2.0	1.6	2.0	2.0
Folic acid (μg)	140	150	200	140	150	200
Vitamin B_{12} (μg)	0.2	0.2	0.2	1.0	1.0	1.0
Ascorbic acid (mg)	40	40	40	40	40	40

The food stuffs required to meet the nutritional requirements are milk, meat, cereals, pulses, leafy and other vegetables, fruits, vegetable fat and sugar.

8.7 Dietary allowances in old age

Aging is characterized by progressive loss of lean body mass and changes in most body system. The degenerative changes such as loss of cells become greater, once the body reaches physiological maturity. The loss of cells, lead to decreased efficiency and impaired or reduced organ function. The factors affecting food intake ability in elderly patient are physiological or physical, psychosocial and environmental. The presence and absence of these factors vary widely with individual. The dietary allowances suggested are given as follows.

Energy requirement for a person 51 years or old is reduced. Average calorie intake for these groups of elderly person is 2300 kcal/d for man and 1900 kcal for women. If total intake is less than 1500 kcal/d, then health problem arises.

There is decrease in skeletal tissue mass in aged person; hence, the store of protein provided by skeletal muscle is inadequate to meet the needs for protein synthesis. To meet the essential needs of dietary protein 1 g/kg IBW for males and 0.9 g/kg IBW for females is suggested.

Saturated fats should be reduced in total daily caloric intake. The intake of monounsaturated or polyunsaturated fat sources should be encouraged.

Calcium needs increase particularly for women over 50 years of age because there is more loss resulting in demineralization of bone and osteoporosis. The intake of 1500 mg is recommended.

Zinc deficiency is associated with older people who avoid flesh foods or other foods sources. Deficiency of zinc causes anorexia, delayed wound healing, ulcer development and impaired immune function.

The sodium intake should be reduced during old age. The dietary sodium intake should be approximately 1-2 g/d.

Vitamins particularly the antioxidant vitamins such as vitamin E, vitamin C and carotenoids should be encouraged to enhance the health of the old people. An increase in serum level of pyridoxine, folic acid and vitamin B_{12} has been found useful in protection against elevated serum homocysteine, an independent risk factor for cardiovascular diseases, depression and certain neurological deficits.

Daily fluid replacement is essential particularly in those who exercise regularly, consume large amount of protein, use laxatives or live in areas with high temperature. The suggested dietary allowances for man of 70 years age are 1975 kcal energy, 60 g protein, 400 mg calcium and 1 mg vitamin B_1 with antioxidant vitamins.

9 Dietary allowances in disorders/diseases

Dietary allowances for the treatment of various diseases or disorders need modification in the diet. This is required as the metabolism of the individual changes in different disorders with respect to one or more nutrition. Modifications are change in the diet in disorders or diseases may involve changes in different constituents such as elimination of food in the diet that causes allergic reaction, omitting spices and including bland diets, high or low carbohydrate diets, high or low fat diets, high or low calorie diets, high or low protein diets, high or low fibre diets and low purine and low sodium diets.

9.1 Modifications in diet

The type of modifications required in the diet in various diseases or disorders are briefly mentioned in the following sections.

9.1.1 Change in protein content

High protein diets such as double or twice the actual requirement is recommended in protein calorie malnutrition, peptic ulcer, cirrhosis of liver, celiac disease and nephrosis. Low protein or withdrawal of protein is necessary in hepatic coma and acute uraemia.

9.1.2 Change in vitamin content

Increase in vitamin content is essential in most of the therapeutic diets which partially lack in one or more vitamins. This can be achieved by the additions of synthetic vitamins.

9.1.3 Change in minerals content

High calcium diet is essential in treatment of osteomalacia and rickets. Restricted diet in calcium and phosphorus is required in renal calculi.

Low or restricted sodium diet is essential in the treatment of hyper tension and cardiac failure. Restriction in sodium chloride intake is essential in kidney diseases. Low purine diet is prescribed in the treatment of gout.

9.1.4 Change in fibre content

High fibre or rich fibre diet is prescribed for the treatment of constipation. Low fibre diets are essential in the treatment of gastrointestinal disorders like peptic ulcers, celiac disease, ulcerative, colitis, dysentery and diarrhoeas.

9.1.5 Change in carbohydrate content

High carbohydrate diet is desirable in Addison's disease such as hypoglycaemia. Adequate storage of glycogen is of considerable value in liver diseases. Low or restricted carbohydrate diet is essential in treatment of diabetes mellitus.

9.1.6 Change in fat content

High fat diet is generally used in the treatment of severe under nutrition. Low or restricted fat diet is necessary in the treatment of malabsorption syndrome, liver disease and steatorrhoea.

9.1.7 Change in calorie content

Diet in high calorie value is used for treating patients who are markedly underweight and suffering with fever, malabsorption, infections and hyperthyroidism. Low calorie diet is used for treating obesity hepatic coma, acute uraemia and cardiovascular disease.

The changes in diet pattern which are required in some specific disorders or diseases are given below:

9.1.8 Dietary allowances in protein calorie malnutrition

Diet rich in protein, adequate in calories and containing essential vitamins and minerals are prescribed for the treatment of this disorder. The high protein diet for an adult contains 120–150 g protein, 60–70 g fat, 250–300 g carbohydrate and 3000–3500 kcal. The food stuff required to meet the nutritional requirement is given in Table 9.1.

Table 9.1 High protein diet for an adult suffering from protein calorie malnutrition.

Food stuff	Requirement g/caput/d	
	Vegetarian	Non-vegetarian
Cereals	200–250	200–250
Pulses	100	100

Cow's milk	1000–1500	800–1000
Cheese	80–100	–
Meat fish		100–150
Egg		40–60
Nut	80–120	80–120
Fruits	100–200	100–200
Green leafy and other vegetables	120–200	120–200
Sugar/jaggery	30–50	30–50
Fats and oils	30–50	30–50

9.2 Dietary allowances in malnourished and underweight

High calorie diets are required for patient suffering from underweight or malnourished. The diet should contain 500 calories in excess of the daily needs. Protein intake should be 50% more than daily needs and it should be derived from milk and other animal foods. The high calorie diet contains 80–100 g protein, 60–80 g fats, 400–500 g carbohydrates and calories 3000–4000 kcal. The food stuffs required to meet the nutritional requirement are given in Table 9.2.

Table 9.2 High calorie diet for an adult suffering from malnourished and underweight.

Food stuffs	Requirement g/caput/d	
	Vegetarian	**Non-vegetarian**
Cereals	300–400	300–400
Pulses	80–100	80–100
Cow's milk	1000–1500	800–1000
Meat fish		50
Egg		30
Nuts	100–150	100–150
Fruits	200–300	200–300
Green leafy and other vegetables	200	200
Sugar/jaggery	100	100
Fats and oils	100	100

9.3 Dietary allowances in obese

Low calorie diets are required for persons suffering from obesity. Calories deficit diet such as 1100 kcal reduces body weight 1.0–1.5 kg/week. Food stuffs required to meet nutritional requirement for low calorie diet (1100–1300 kcal) are given in Table 9.3.

Table 9.3 Low calorie diet for an adult suffering from obesity

Food stuffs	Requirement g/caput/d			
	1100 kcal		1300 kcal	
	Veg.	Non-veg.	Veg.	Non-veg.
Cereals	80	80	100	100
Pulses	60	40	70	50
Skim milk	1000	500	1000	0
Cheese	50	–	50	–
Meat fish	–	50	–	60
Egg	–	60	–	80
Fruits	50	50	50	50
vegetables	450	450	450	450
Sugar/jaggery	50	15	20	20
Fats and oils	450	15	20	20

9.4 Dietary allowances in diabetes mellitus

This is chronic disorder in which blood glucose level is raised above 180 mg/100 mL of blood and glucose is excreted in urine. This is caused by a deficiency in production or secretion of hormone insulin. The factors responsible are heredity, age (more in person over 45 years), sex (both sexes but more in men the women), obesity (greater in obese person) and stress due to worry, infection and irregular meals. Diabetes is not a disease which can be cured but it can be kept under control by the patient with the help of proper nutrition. Diabetes if not kept under control a number of complications occur such as eye disorders leading to blindness, kidney dysfunction, thickening of arteries and loss of sensation in peripheral nerves. A fasting blood sugar level of 120 mg/dL or higher on two different days indicates that person suffers from diabetes. A proper nutrition plan is the foundation of successful diabetes management. Control of diabetes rests on three factors such as diet, exercise and insulin.

Dietary allowances for diabetic adults having normal body weight and moderate work contains 2500 kcal,100 g protein and 115 g fat for male adult and 2100 kcal, 90 g protein and 90 g fat for female adult. The food stuffs required to meet the nutritional requirement of diabetic male and female adults are given in Table 9.4.

Table 9.4 Diet for diabetic male and female adults.

Food stuff	Requirement g/caput/d			
	Male		Female	
	Veg.	Non-veg.	Veg.	Non-veg.
Cereals	150	150	150	150
Pulses	100	100	80	80
milk	1000	1000	700	700
Cheese	70	–	60	–
nuts	80	80	70	70
Meat/ fish	–	50	–	40
Eggs	–	40	–	40
Fruits	50	50	30	30
Green leafy and other vegetables	250	250	250	250
Vegetables oils	30	30	20	20

9.5 Dietary allowances in fever

Fever is caused by infection through microorganism. Increase in body temperature is due to heat production. Fever of short duration is colds, influenza, pneumonia, typhoid, chickenpox, etc.

Nutritional requirements will depend on the nature, severity and duration of the fever. Diet calorie and protein requirement are 50% more or excess of daily requirement. In carbohydrates, glucose is preferred over sucrose due to less sweet and rapidly adsorbed. Starch is present in cereals and cereal flours can be cooked into pudding along with milk, egg and sugar. Avoid fats such as butter, ghee and vegetable oils during the peak period of fever. These should be included when fever is controlled. The vitamins requirement can be met with intake of multivitamins. Mineral tablet such as calcium and phosphorus required will be met by taking 1 L of milk daily. The water intake should be in the form of fluids such as milk, fruit juice, glucose water, etc. About 3–5 L/d fluid diets should be given during the peak of the fever.

Diet for an adult suffering from acute fever contains calories 2700 kcal protein 35 g and carbohydrates 600 g. The food stuff required to meet nutritional requirement in acute fever are given in Table 9.5.

Table 9.5 Diet for an adult in acute fever.

Food stuffs	Requirement/caput/d
Barley water	1000 mL
Milk	1000 mL

Orange juice	500 mL
Glucose	200 g
Sugar	100 g
Dextri maltose	200 g
Multivitamin tablet	One

Dietary allowances for an adult after controlled fever contain calories 3000 kcal and protein 50 g. The food stuff required to meet the nutritional requirement of a patient during controlled fever are given Table 9.6.

Table 9.6 Diet for an adult during controlled fever.

Food stuffs	Requirement g/caput/d
Milled cereals products	200
Milk	1500
Fruit	100
Fruit juice	500
Glucose	100
Sugar	100
Dextri maltose	100
Butter	10
Multivitamin- mineral tablet	One

9.6 Dietary allowances in tuberculosis

This is an inflammatory disease of lungs associated with cough and mild fever lasting for a long time. Disease is of long duration hence, it is essential to provide high calorie-high protein diet in addition to treatment with drugs.

Diet contains calories 2900–3000 kcal and protein 100–115 g. The food stuffs required to meet the nutritional requirement for an adult suffering from to tuberculosis is given in Table 9.7.

Table 9.7 Diet for an adult suffering from tuberculosis.

Food stuffs	Requirement g/caput/d	
	Veg.	Non-veg.
Cereals and their products	300	300
Pulse	100	100
Nuts	50	50

Milk	1200	800
Egg	–	one
Meat	–	50
Fruits	200	200
Vegetables	250	250
Sugar	60	60
Butter/vegetable oils	40	40
Multivitamin tablet	One	One

9.7 Dietary allowances in gastrointestinal disorders

The gastrointestinal tract is involved with the digestion, absorption and utilization of food in our body. The function of the gastrointestinal tract is influenced by diseases or organs closely related to the digestive process. The gastrointestinal disorders include constipation, diarrhoea, peptic ulcer, ulcerative colitis, etc.

9.7.1 Constipation

Constipation is the retention of the faeces in the colon beyond the normal length of emptying time. It is infrequent, irregular and difficult passage of faeces. In other words, constipation is characterized by frequent and incomplete evacuation of the stools. Constipation is of two types, that is, atonic and spastic. Atonic constipation results due to loss of muscle tone in the colon which causes difficulty in evacuation of the stools. This is most common type occurs in the people leading a sedentary life, elder people, pregnant women and those person consuming mainly refined foods. Spastic constipation results due to an increase in the muscle tone which narrows the cavity and forward movement of faeces is retarded.

9.7.1.1 Dietary allowances in constipation

Diet rich in fibre is prescribed for patient suffering from constipation. Diet rich in fibre content helps to relieve constipation and retard the absorption of cholesterol and reduce its level in blood. Patients are also advised to take plenty of fluids as it helps to soften the stools. The diet for patient suffering from constipation contains calories 2400 kcal and protein 60 g. Food stuffs required to meet the nutritional requirement for a person suffering from constipation is given in Table 9.8.

Table 9.8 Diet for an adult suffering from constipation.

Food stuffs	Requirement g/caput/d	
	Veg.	**Non-veg.**
Whole cereals	350	350
Whole legumes	80	80
Pulse	50	50
Milk	600	400
Egg	–	30
Meat	–	40
Fruits	100	100
Vegetables	250	250
Leafy and other vegetables	400	400
Oils and fat	50	50
Sugar/jaggery	50	50

9.7.2 Diarrhoea

Diarrhoea is a condition in which loose, watery and unformed stools are passed frequently. Diarrhoea follows irritation and inflammation of the mucous membrane of the bowel. Diarrhoea may be acute or chronic.

9.7.2.1 Acute diarrhoea

Acute diarrhoea is characterized by sudden onset and frequent passage of watery and unformed stools. It lost from 1 to 3 days. The causes for acute diarrhoea are infection in the gastrointestinal tract by bacterial and parasitic through contamination of food and water, dietary factors such as food sensitivity and allergy, malnutrition such as protein energy malnutrition and deficiency of vitamins A and B and infection of cholera, typhoid, etc.

Dietary allowances in acute diarrhoea

In first 2 days, orally water containing 0.5% sodium chloride, 5% glucose and orange juice or oral rehydration solution (ORS) containing 3.5 g sodium chloride, 2.5 g sodium hydrogen carbonate/sodium bicarbonate, 1.5 g potassium chloride and 20 g glucose to be dissolved in 1 L of clean drinking water. About 150–200 mL fluid should be given to patient in every hour from 6 a.m. to 10 p.m. ORS is available in a dry pre-packaged form in the market.

From third day and onwards, diet should contain barley water mixed with equal amount of butter milk. About 200–250 mL should be given after every 2 h. Orange juice with glucose about 200 mL should be given once in 4 h. Other fluids which can be given are coconut water, carbonated beverages, and pulse water. Bread and pudding along with fruit juice should be given when the condition of the patient is improved. After this, the patient can consume bland diet.

The patient needs to progress from liquid diet or soft diet to normal diet gradually. Contamination of food must be prevented to avoid recurrence of diarrhoea.

9.7.2.2 Chronic diarrhoea

Chronic diarrhoea persists for a long time that is several weeks and patient may pass four to five unformed stools in a day. The causes for chronic diarrhoea are metabolic diseases such as diabetes, chronic alcoholism, colon cancer, liver cirrhosis, celiac disease, etc. The rapid passage of food through the intestinal does not allow enough time for absorption of nutrients and hence, nutritional deficiency symptoms may occur. Therefore, dietary allowance to compensate for the nutrient losses is very important.

Dietary allowance in chronic diarrhoea

A high protein intake that is increase in 50% is essential to build-up body tissue. Energy requirement should be increased 10-12% to overcome weakness and weight loss. Carbohydrate intake should be increased to meet energy requirement and fibre intake should be restricted to 1-2 g/d. Foods rich in calcium and iron and vitamins A and B complex should be provided.

The diet should be easily digestible. A soft, bland diet, low in fibre and fat should be given. Well-cooked, soft and semi-solid foods can be included. Foods permitted are washed pulses, refined cereals, well-cooked vegetables, fruits of low fibre such as papaya and banana, milk products such as curd and paneer, egg, chicken and fish.

Foods restricted or avoided are whole cereals, pulses, raw vegetables, fried foods, nuts, milk and milk-based beverages.

The patient suffering from chronic diarrhoea should drink plenty of fluids and eat food at frequent intervals. Patient should be given six to eight small meals in a day because patient may not be able to eat large meals at one time due to loss of appetite.

9.7.2.3 Peptic ulcers

Formation of chronic ulcer in the reason of gastrointestinal tract where the gastric juice comes in direct contact with the mucous membrane is called peptic ulcer. Mostly ulcers are found in the stomach, jejunum (gastric ulcers) and duodenum. Hypersecretion of acid is the primary cause of duodenal ulcers. In gastric ulcers, it is the weakened mucosal resistance to acid which causes ulcers. The factors which increase acid secretion are chemical stimulation, such as spices, seasonings, alcohol, acidic foods, etc. The other important causes are heredity, irritants such as strong tea, coffee and drugs, smoking and eating habits such as eating hurriedly. Peptic ulcer can occur at any age but the highest incidents are in middle adulthood that is between the age of 45 and 55 years.

Foods permitted in peptic ulcer are milled cereals such as rice, refined wheat flour and semolina, split legumes or pulses, milk, egg, tender vegetables, meat and fish in restricted amount, fruits, fats and oils and sugar. Foods which are not permitted are whole cereal and millets, legumes with husk such as Bengal gram, field beans, cow gram, dried peas, vegetables containing fibre, raw garlic and onion, spices, condiments, pickles, meat soup, fried foods, areca nut and tobacco.

Dietary allowances in peptic ulcer

Generally patients suffering from active peptic ulcers are undernourished and need an increased energy intake. A high protein intake is recommended to provide essential amino acids for tissue protein synthesis. The fat content should be moderate. Carbohydrates are required to meet the energy needs. The vitamin requirements are normal vitamin C content should be adequate for heeling of ulcers and better iron absorption. Foods rich in iron and calcium should be given. Dietary allowances for an adult suffering from peptic ulcer are given in Table 9.9.

Table 9.9 Diet for an adult suffering from peptic ulcer.

Food stuff	Requirement g/caput/d	
	Vegetarian	Non-vegetarian
Milled rice, bread, Refined wheat flour	200	200
Split legumes/pulses	50	50
Milk	1800	1500
Cheese	50	–
Egg	–	30
Meat/lean fish	–	60
Tender vegetables and potato	100	100
Fleshy fruits	100	100
Sugar/jaggery	60	60
Fats and oils	60	60

9.8 Dietary allowances in cardiovascular diseases

The cardiovascular diseases include coronary heart disease and atherosclerosis. Generally coronary heart diseases are due to coronary antheroma and atherosclerosis. This is a condition in which lipid is deposited in the intima of the blood vessel. Thus, high level of blood lipids is an important risk factor in the development of coronary heart disease. In atherosclerosis, there is narrowing of arterial walls due to deposit of fatty materials causes resistance to blood flow making the heart to pump harder thus increasing the blood pressure. The causes for development of atherosclerosis are high intake of saturated fat and cholesterol, high calorie intake, sedentary life, high level of cholesterol in blood and stress and strain.

The diet contains for an adult suffering from atherosclerosis and coronary heart disease is 1800–2000 kcal, fat rich in essential fatty acid 60 g and protein 50–60 g. The food stuffs required to meet the nutritional requirement are given in Table 9.10.

Table 9.10 Diet for an adult suffering from atherosclerosis and coronary heart disease.

Food stuffs	Requirement g/caput/d	
	Veg.	Non-veg.
Milled cereals	200	200
Skim milk fluid	1000	1000
Pulses	60	40
Cheese	60	20
Meat	–	50
Fruits	300	300
Leafy and other Vegetables	200	200
Vegetable oils	60	60
Sugar/jaggery	40	40

Foods avoided in atherosclerosis and coronary heart diseases are fatty fried foods, fatty sweets, nuts, salty sauces, sodium rich foods, soft and alcoholic drinks.

9.9 Dietary allowances in hypertension/high blood pressure

Normal blood pressure is less than 140 mmHg in systolic and less than 85 mmHg in diastolic. Systolic pressure of over 150 mmHg and diastolic pressure of over 95 mmHg is considered high blood pressure. This condition is known as essential hypertension. This is a common disorder in middle and old age groups of person. The cause may be heredity, stress and strain or obesity.

The diets should contain low sodium, low fat and low calorie. The diet prescribed for an adult suffering from hypertension is 2000 kcal, protein 20 g, fat 5 g, sodium 150 mg and chloride 200 mg. All fruits and fruit juices are permitted. The food stuffs required for an adult suffering from high blood pressure having 300 mg sodium content are given in Table 9.11.

Table 9.11 Low sodium diet for an adult in high blood pressure.

Food stuffs	Requirement g/caput/d	
	Vegetarian	Non-vegetarian
Milled cereals	300	300
Pulses	50	30
Skim milk fluid	400	200
Meat/fish	–	40
Fruits	300	300
Leafy and other Vegetables	200	200
Fruit juices - orange	400	400
Butter unsalted	10	10
Vegetable fat safflower/sesame	30	30
Sugar/jam	40	40

9.10 Dietary allowances in liver diseases

Liver is a multifunctional organ, which plays an important role in protein, carbohydrate and fat metabolism. Most of the end-products of the digestion of food are transported directly to the liver. The toxic substances such as drugs, dyes, mineral poison and decomposed bacterial products which are produced or enter via food in the body are detoxified in the liver. Therefore, the health of liver is a major factor in the quality of life. The diseases of liver include jaundice, hepatitis, cirrhosis and hepatic failure.

9.10.1 Jaundice

Jaundice is characterized by increased bilirubin levels in the blood. Bilirubin is a break down product of red blood cells. Bilirubin accumulates in the blood and imparts yellow colouration to the skin and sclera of the eyes. The urine also characterized with dark yellow due to the presence of bilirubin. Normal plasma bilirubin levels are 2–8 mg/L. A patient is said to have jaundice when plasma bilirubin rise above 20 mg/L. The cause of jaundice may be due to excessive break down of red blood cells, infra-hepatic obstruction, primary damage of parenchymal cells by viral infection and toxic drugs. The most common cause of jaundice is viral infection of liver. The primary aim is to protect the liver from further stress. Therefore, a nutritionally adequate diet is basic to avoid permanent damage.

Dietary allowances in jaundice

The diet for an adult suffering from jaundice should contain good quality protein (45 g), high carbohydrates (300–340 g), restricted moderate fat (20 g), calories 1600–1800 kcal and restricted sodium with vitamin supplement. The food stuffs required to meet the nutritional requirement of jaundice patient are given in Table 9.12.

Table 9.12 Diet for an adult suffering from severe jaundice.

Food stuffs	Requirement g/caput/d
Cereals	200
Skimmed milk	500
Potato	100
Leafy vegetables	50
Fruits (banana, papaya, mango)	200
Sugar/jam	60
Fats and oil	15
Multivitamin tablet	One

9.10.2 Hepatitis

Hepatitis is an infectious disease which is characterized by inflammation and degeneration of liver cells. Generally it is of two types, viral and drug induced; viral hepatitis is more common may be infective type called type A or serum hepatitis called type B. Infective type is mild and is due to a virus generally transmitted through faecel contamination of food and water. Serum hepatitis lead to serious hepatic damage and transmitted only the parenteral route through contaminated blood and through poorly sterilized needles. Both type A and B hepatitis are very similar except the mode of transmission of virus. Drug-induced hepatitis is due to a reaction of certain drugs such as penicillin, sulfa and toxic chemicals.

The symptoms of hepatitis are nausea, abdominal pain, vomiting, diarrhoea, loss of appetite, loss of weight, fever followed by enlargement and tenderness of the liver.

Dietary allowances in hepatitis

The main therapy in hepatitis consists of bed rest and nutritionally adequate diet. The points which should be considered for a patient suffering from hepatitis are as follows:

1. *Liquid diet*: Give full liquid diet in six small feed during early stages. The full liquid diets contain 75 g protein and calories 1875 kcal. The food stuffs required for full liquid diets are given in Table 9.13.

Table 9.13 Liquid diet for an adult suffering from hepatitis.

Food stuffs	Requirement g/caput/d
Strained cereals	25
Milk	200
Skim milk powder	25
Eggs	100
Spinach	150
Strained beans	50
Carrot	75
Tomato	75
Sweet orange	250
Papaya	100
Watermelon	100
Sugar	50
Butter/ghee	30

2. *Followed by soft fibre-restricted diet*: The soft fibre-restricted diet consist of well-cooked soft rice, kheer, dal, milk, eggs (scrambled), minced or ground meat/ fish, tender green cooked or blended vegetables, raw fruits/juices without skin, sugar syrup or honey and butter.
3. Give high calorie (2000–3000 kcal) and high protein (75–110 g) diet if there is heavy weight loss. High carbohydrate diets ensure adequate calories.
4. Low fat diet is given in beginning and gradually moves to make it normal.
5. Avoid spicy foods, rich deserts and vegetables with strong flavours.

9.10.3 Cirrhosis

Cirrhosis is a chronic disease of liver in which fibrous connecting tissue replaces the hepatic cells. It is the most serious and final stage of liver injury and degeneration. The disease is characterized by destruction of liver cells and distortion of normal lobules with fibrous tissue due to necrosis, fatty, filtration and fibrosis. Liver cirrhosis occurs due to various factors such as excessive alcoholic intake, attack of common viral, attack of common viral hepatitis, obstruction of bile ducts and exposure to certain drugs or toxic substances.

Chronic alcoholism is considered to be the most common cause since alcohol and its metabolic products, disturb liver metabolism and damage liver cells directly. There is an association between liver disease, chronic alcoholism and malnutrition.

The onset of disease is characterized with initial symptoms of gastrointestinal disturbance such as loss of hepatitis, nausea, vomiting, anorexia and epigastric pain. Appearance of jaundice is with increasing weakness, weight loss, oedema, gastrointestinal bleeding and anaemia due to iron deficiency. Macrocytic anaemia also occurs due to folic acid deficiency. Steatorrhea is a common symptom.

Dietary allowances in cirrhosis

The dietary allowances for patient suffering from cirrhosis consist of high calorie (2000–3000 kcal), 60% calorie should met with carbohydrates, high protein, restricted fat, restricted sodium intake (500–700 mg) and multivitamins tablet. Choline and methionine is useful if fatty infiltration of liver is present.

The food stuffs required to meet the nutritional requirement of cirrhosis patient are given in Table 9.14.

Table 9.14 Diet for an adult suffering from liver cirrhosis.

Food stuffs	Requirement g/caput/d	
	Veg.	**Non-veg.**
Cereals	250	250
Pulses	50	30
Milk low fat	800	500
Cheese	50	–
Meat and liver	–	100
Egg	–	60
Calcium caseinate	50	20
Fruits	200	200
Fruit juice	500	500
Vegetable	100	100
Fats and oils rich in essential fatty acid	20	20
Sugar	60	60
Glucose	60	60

9.10.4 Enlarged liver

This is known as hepatic failure. The function of the liver is severely reduced due to reduction in functional liver cells. The abnormalities of neurological and neuro muscular may result in coma. If it is not treated, it may lead to death. Diet should contain low amount of protein intake to reduce ammonia production. About 25 g protein should be given for few days and if improvement occurs, protein intake is increased 5–10 g every day until intake reaches 40–50 g/d. Ensuring intake of branched chain amino acid may improve protein profile. Calories 1500–2000 kcal should be provided through carbohydrates and fat. Tube feeling or parenteral nutrition is given if a patient is unable to take orally.

9.11 Dietary allowances in kidney diseases

Kidney plays a vital role in maintaining the bodies in normal state (homeostasis). The functions of kidney are filtration, maintenance of fluid electrolyte and acid-base balance, excretion, blood pressure regulation, production of a hormone (erythropoietin) and conversion of vitamin D to active form calciferol. Kidney diseases are glomerulonephritis, chronic glomerulonephritis, chronic renal failure, etc.

9.11.1 Glomerulonephritis

The term nephritis is used to indicate inflammation of the kidney. Inflamed capillaries in glomerulo called glomerulonephritis.

Dietary allowances for patient suffering from glomerulonephritis should be low in protein, restricted sodium and rich in carbohydrates. The diet should consist of calories 1800 kcal, protein 30 g, fat 60 g, carbohydrates 25 g, multivitamins 1 tablet. The food stuffs required to meet the nutritional requirement of nephritis patient are given in Table 9.15.

Table 9.15 Diet for an adult suffering from glomerulonephritis.

Food stuffs	Requirement g/caput/d
Cereals	250
Milk	400
Fleshy food	200
Fruit juices	150
Leafy and other vegetables	100
Fats and oils	60
Sugar/jam	80

9.11.2 Chronic glomerulonephritis

This is characterized by tiredness, oedema, increased blood pressure, severe albuminuria and frequent urination. The dietary allowances for the patient suffering from chronic glomerulonephritis should have high protein, high carbohydrates, salt free and moderate fat with restricted fluid intake. The diet consists of calories 2000 kcal, protein 100 g, fat 60 g, carbohydrates 230 g and salt free. The food stuffs required to meet the nutritional requirement of chronic glomerulonephritis patient are given in Table 9.16.

Table 9.16 Diet for an adult suffering from chronic glomerulonephritis.

Food stuffs	Requirement g/caput/d	
	Veg.	**Non-veg.**
Cereals	200	200
Pulses	70	50
Cow's milk	800	400
Meat and fish	–	100
Egg	–	50
Cheese	50	–
Nuts	100	100
Fruits	200	200
Green leafy and other vegetables	150	150
Fats and oils	40	40
Sugar/jaggery	40	40

9.11.3 Chronic renal failure

Kidney losses its function gradually and continue, the glomerular filtration rate begins to reduce resulting to chronic renal failure. In this condition, both glomerulo and tubules are heavily damaged. The dietary modification should be initiated when glomerular filtration rate drops from normal 125 mL/min to less than 30 mL/min. When glomerular filtration rate reduces to 3 mL/min, the diet control is not enough and dialysis or kidney transplant is essential to save the life of the patient.

The dietary allowances for the patient suffering from chronic renal failure should be low in protein content 20 g, calories 2000 kcal, fat 40 g, carbohydrate 400 g and restricted salt. The food stuffs required to meet the nutritional requirement of patient is given in Table 9.17.

Table 9.17 Diet for an adult suffering from chronic renal failure.

Food stuffs	Requirement g/caput/d
Cereals	200
Milk	200
Egg	30
Fruit juice	1000

Vegetables	100
Butter/vegetable fat	40
Glucose	200
Sugar	50

9.12 References

1. Anita, F.P. 1986. *Clinical Dietetics and Nutrition*, 3rd edn. Export University Press, Bombay.
2. Anthikad, J. 2014. *Nutrition and Biochemistry for Nurses*, 2nd edn. Jaypee Brothers Medical Publishers (P) Ltd, New Delhi.
3. Brain, F.A. and Cameron, A.G. 1989. *Food Science, Nutrition and Health*. Edward Amold, London.
4. Cataldo, C.B., Whitnery, E.N. and Linds, K.D. 2003. *Nutrition and Diet Therapy Principles and Practices*. West Publishing Co., St. Paul, MN.
5. Chadha, K.L. 2002. Diversification to horticulture for food, nutrition and economic security. *Indian J Hort* 59: 209-229.
6. Davidson, S.R., Passmore and Brock, J.F. 1986. *Human Nutrition and Dietetics*, 8th edn. Churchill Livingstone, London.
7. Garrow, J.S.S., James, W.P.T. and Ralph, A. 1999. *Human Nutrition and Dietetics*, 10th edn. W.B. Sounders, Philadelphia, PA.
8. Goodhart, R.S. and Shills, M.E. 1994. *Modern Nutrition in Health and Disease Dietotherapy*. Lea and Febiger, Philadelphia, PA.
9. Gopalan, C. 2000. *Nutritive Value of Indian Foods*. National Institute of Nutrition, Indian Council of Medical Research, Hyderabad, India, pp. 47-77.
10. Gopalan, C., Ramashastri, B.V. and Balasubramaniam, S.C. 2000. *Nutritive value of Indian Foods* (Revised). National Institute of Nutrition, Hyderabad, India.
11. Gopalan, C., Ramashastri, B.V. and Balasubramaniam, S.C. 2004. Nutritive value of Indian Foods. National Institute of Nutrition ICMR, Hyderabad.
12. Kaur, C., Bijoj, G., Deepa, N., Singh, B. and Kapoor, H.C. 2004. Antioxidant status of fresh and processed tomato. *J Food Sci Technol* 41(5), 479-486.
13. Kumar, S. and Singh, I.S. 2013. Physico-chemical studies of various cultivars of aonla fruit. *Prog Hort* 45, 80-82.
14. Khanna, K., Gupta, S., Passi, S.J., Seth, R., Mohna, R. and Puri, S. 2005. *Text Book of Nutrition and Dietetics*. Elite Pub. House Pvt. Ltd., New Delhi.
15. Lakshmi, B. and Vimla, B. 2000. Nutritive value of dehydrated green leafy vegetable powder. *J Food Sci Technol* 37, 465-471.
16. Lutz, C.A. and Karen, R.P. 1995. *Nutrition and Diet Therapy*, 4th edn. Davis, F.A., Philadelphia, PA.
17. Linda, F. 2001. *Classic Vegetarian Cooking*. Barnes and Noble, New York.
18. Meena, S.S., Lal, G., Mehta, R.S., Kant, K. and Anwar, M.M., 2010. Seed spices for home remedies. *Indian Hort* 55, 6-8.
19. Mohan, L.A. and Arlin, M.T. 1992. *Krase's Food Nutrition and Diet Therapy*, 8th edn. W.B. Saunders, London.
20. Mudambi, S.R. and Rajagopal, M.V. 2009. *Fundamentals of Foods, Nutrition and Diet Therapy*. New Age International (P) Ltd. Publishers, New Delhi, India.

21. Patwardhan, V.N. 1960. *Dietary Allowances for Indians - Calories and Protein*. Indian Council of Medical Research, New Delhi.
22. Peter, P.I. and Peter, K.V. 2011.*Choosing the Right Fruit for Wellness*. World Wellness Open University, Chennai, India.
23. Rao, N. and Milk, R. 2001. Milk nutrition. *Indian J Dairy Sci* 35(2), 13-14.
24. Robinson, C.H., Marilyn, R.L., Wanda, L.C. and Anne, E.G. 1996. *Normal and Therapeutic Nutrition*, 17th edn. Macmillan Publishing Co., New York.
25. Shils, M.S., Benjamin, C.A., Catherine, R. and Robert, J.C. 2005. *Modern Nutrition in Health and Disease*, 10th edn. Lippincott, Williams and Wilkins, Baltimore, MD.
26. Shrilakshmi, B. 2013. *Food Science*. New Age International Publishers, New Delhi.
27. Singh, B. and Pandey, A.K. 2011. Enhancing market access of fruits and vegetables through nutritive and neutraceutical value. *Indian Hort* 56, 20-23.
28. Singh, I.S. 2001. Minor fruits and their uses. *Indian J Hort* 58, 178-182.
29. Singh, I.S. 2011. *Food Processing*. Westville Publishing House, New Delhi.
30. Singh, I.S. and Kumar, S. 2015. *Vegetable Crops - Production, Handling and Processing*. Westville Publishing House, New Delhi.
31. Singh, I.S. and Singh, V. 2015a. *Production, Handling and Processing of Spices*. Westville Publishing House, New Delhi.
32. Singh, I.S. and Singh, V. 2015b. *Fruit Crops - Production, Handling and Processing*. Westville Publishing House, New Delhi.
33. Singh, I.S. and Wahid Ali. 1992. Bael: a panacea. *Indian Hort* 37, 35.
34. Swaminathan, M. 1985. Essentials of Food and Nutrition. Bangalore Printing and Publishing Co. Ltd., Bangalore.
35. Swaminathan, M. 2012. *Hand Book of Food and Nutrition*. The Bangalore Printing & Publishing Co. Ltd., Bangalore, India.
36. Townsend, C.E. and Roth, R.A. 2003. *Nutrition and Diet Therapy*, 8th edn. Delmar Publishers, Venice, FL.
37. Warries, P.D. 2000. *Meat Science. An Introductory Text*. CABI Publishing, Wallingford, U.K.
38. Williams, S.R. 1990. *Essentials of Nutrition and Diet Therapy*, 5th edn. Times Mirror/ Mosby College Publishing, St. Louis, MO.
39. William, S.E. 1999. *Basic Nutrition and Diet Therapy*, 1st edn. Elsevier Science, New York.

Part II
Food Science

10

Food sources

Food is the basic necessity of life. Food is a nutritious organic substance solid or liquid which is eaten to meet the requirements of the body for energy, growth, development, reproduction and maintenance of health. Plants and animals are the major sources of food. Most of the foods have plant origin such as cereals, pulses, nuts and oil seeds, fruits, vegetables, spices and herbs. Even animals which are food sources derive their food from plant origin. Foods of animal sources are milk and milk products, meat, poultry, eggs and fish. Some foods such as beverages are of both plant (tea, coffee, cocoa, fruit and vegetables) and animal (milk based beverages) origin. Both plants and animals are also the source of fat and oils. Some foods which are not of plant and animal origin are mushroom (fungi origin), spirulina (algae origin) and inorganic substances such as salts and baking soda. The important sources of foods are as follows:

1. Plant-based food sources
2. Animal-based food sources
3. Food of other sources

10.1 Plant-based food sources

10.1.1 Cereals

Cereals are the grasses which come under the monocot family Poaceae, and are harvested for their starch rich grains. Cereal grains are composed of endosperm, germ and brawn. When compared to other type of crops cereals are the largest energy providers and are grown in greater quantities worldwide. When considered the nutrient value of cereals as a whole grain, they are rich in vitamins, minerals, carbohydrates, fats, oils and proteins. However, after refined by removal of brawn and germ the remaining endosperm parts contains mainly starch. Cereals are classified into two groups:

- Fine cereals: wheat, barley, rice
- Coarse cereals/millets: jwar, bajra, maize, ragi

10.1.2 Pulses and legumes

Pulses are the seeds of certain plants of the legume family, which produce seeds or grains that grow within pods such as lentils, beans, peas and chick peas. Pulses are legume crops that are grown for their dry seeds to be used as food or grain. Pulses are an extremely healthy food due to their high protein content related to other vegetables. People eat the pulse seeds whole, dehulled or as flour. Some of these are red gram (pigeon pea), Bengal gram, black gram, green gram, cowpeas, dry peas, rajma, soya bean, etc.

10.1.3 Fruits

Fruits may be defined as mature ovary with or without accessory tissue usually containing seeds. At maturity, the ovary swells and become fleshy (juicy) or the ovary wall shrivels and becomes dry. Fruits are important source of vitamins, minerals, fibre and sugars. They are low in calories and naturally sweet. Fruits and their juices are good sources of water too. Fruits can be classified in various ways such as botanical classification, classification according to edible parts, respiratory patterns and perishability.

10.1.3.1 Botanical classification of fruits

All fruits may be classified into three major groups on the basis of the number of ovaries and the number of flower involved in their formation. These are simple fruits, aggregate fruits and multiple fruits which are given in Table 10.1.

Table 10.1 Botanical classification of fruits.

Name	Description	Examples
A. Simple fruits	Two types: fleshy and dry	
Fleshy fruits	Result from the ripening of a simple or compound ovary in flower with only one pistil. These fruits are berries, hesperidium, pepo, drupe and pome.	–
Berries	Berry is a fleshy fruit formed from one compound ovary containing few to many seeds.	Guava, grape, papaya, banana, date palm, bael, chiku, karonda, avocado, pomegranate, passion fruit, jamun, kiwi, currant, blueberries, raspberries, tomatoes, brinjal, etc.
Hesperidium	These are specialized berries with thick leathery covering or rind.	Citrus fruits such as lemon, lime, grapefruit, sweet orange and mandarin-orange.
Pepo	A fleshy fruit formed from a compound inferior ovary have hard/ tough outer wall or rind.	Watermelon, pumpkin, cucumber, squash.

Drupe	A fleshy indehiscent single-seeded fruit with stony endocarp. These are referred as stone fruits.	Mango, ber, phalsa, plum, apricot, cherry, almond, coconut, peaches, nectarines, olives, litchi.
Pome	A fleshy fruit formed from an inferior compound ovary have thick fleshy receptacle.	Apple, pears, quince, choke berry, juneberry, loquat.
Dry fruits	Dry fruits have dry pericarp at maturity. They may be dehiscent or indehiscent.	–
Dehiscent	A fruit that opens naturally to release the enclosed seed.	–
Indehiscent	A fruit that does not open to release the seeds. These are mostly one seeded fruit with hard coat.	Cashew nut, walnut, chest nut, pecan, chironji, almonds.
B. Aggregate fruits	An aggregate fruit is a fruit that develop from the merger of several ovaries that were separate in a single flower. Aggregate form a simple fleshy fruits.	Strawberry cluster of achiness blackberry, raspberry cluster of drupe, custard apple cluster of berry.
C. Multiple fruits	Fleshy fruit formed from several to many separate flowers. These flowers have superior ovary. These fruits are two types: sorosis and syconium.	–
Sorosis	Such fruits may resemble to aggregate fruit but is not formed from single flower.	Pineapple, papaya mulberries, pomegranate, jackfruit, rose apple, passion fruit.
Syconium	A fruit made up of a fleshy hollow receptacle bearing inside many small separate flowers which may produce seed like nutlets.	Fig.

10.1.3.2 Classification according to edible parts

Classification on the basis of edible parts or structures has been given in Table 10.2.

Table 10.2 Fruit classification on the basis of edible parts/structure.

Edible parts	Examples
Pericarp and thalamus	Date, custard apple, cape gooseberry
Pericarp and placenta	Guava
Mesocarp	Mango, papaya, chiku
Mesocarp and epicarp	Ber, phalsa, peach, plum

Mesocarp and endocarp	Banana, bael
Fleshy aril	Litchi
Juicy aril	Pomegranate
Fleshy thalamus	Apple, pear
Receptacle	Fig, strawberry
Bracts, perianth and seed	Jackfruit
Bracts and perianth	Pineapple
Peduncle and cotyledon	Cashew nut
Juicy placental hair	Oranges
Endosperm	Coconut

10.1.3.3 Classification on the basis of respiratory pattern

Fruits can be classified into climacteric and non-climacteric groups on the basis of respiratory pattern. These are given in Table 10.3.

Table 10.3 Classification of fruit on the basis of respiratory pattern.

Type	Description	Examples
Climacteric fruit	Climacteric fruits are defined as fruits that exhibit climacteric peak or rise at ripening. Fruits emit ethylene along with increased rate of respiration during ripening. Such fruits are harvested at hard green stage but fully mature and ripened after harvest.	Mango, banana, papaya, guava, avocado, date, chiku, bael, jackfruit, tomato, apple, pear, apricot, plum, muskmelon, chilies.
Non-climacteric fruits	Non-climacteric fruits are defined as fruits that do not exhibit climacteric peak or rise at ripening. Fruits produce very small amount of ethylene and no increased rate of respiration during ripening. Such fruits are harvested at ripe stage and do not ripe after harvest	Oranges, grape, pineapple, litchi, jamun, watermelon, strawberry, cherry, raspberry, lime, blackberry, lemon, pomegranate.

10.1.4 Vegetables

Vegetable is any part of a plant that is consumed by humans as food, as part of a meal. Vegetables are classified on the basis of their parts used for vegetables. Some vegetables fit into more than one category when several different parts of the plant are edible. Examples are beetroot and radish where both roots and leaves are eaten. Vegetables classified on the basis of their plant parts used are given in Table 10.4.

Table 10.4 Vegetables classified on the basis of edible parts.

Parts used	Description	Examples
Leaves	The edible leaves of plants	Cabbage, spinach, amaranth, lettuce, fenugreek leaves, coriander leaves, brussels sprout, watercress, radish leaves, chenopods, bok choy.
Stem	The edible stalks of plants when the stalk is the main part of the vegetables.	Amaranth, celery, lotus, asparagus.
Flower	The edible flowers of vegetables.	Cauliflower, broccoli, artichoke, choy sum, courgette, squash flowers, pumpkin flowers.
Fruits	Vegetables that are fleshy and contain seeds.	Tomato, brinjal, capsicum, okra, cucumber, drumstick, pumpkin, ash gourd, bottle gourd, ridge gourd, bitter gourd, plantain, squash.
Pods and seeds	Legumes apart from sweet corn, seeds grow in pods which are sometimes eaten along with seed.	Peas, snow pea, sweet corn, beans (green beans, French beans, broad beans), tender Bengal gram and red gram.
Bulb	Usually grow just below the surface of the ground and produce a fleshy, leafy shoot above ground. Bulbs normally consist of layers or clustered segments.	Onion, garlic, leaks.
Tuber	Vegetables which grow underground on the root of a plant.	Potato, sweet potato, tapioca, yam.
Roots	Usually a long or round shaped tap root.	Carrot, colocasia, beetroot, turnip, radish.

10.1.5 Spices and herbs

Spices are the barks, berries, fruits, roots and stems of all kinds of plants. Most often these are of tropical origin such as cloves, nutmeg, and pepper. Curry is a mixture of spices has strong fragrance when dried as powder.

Herbs are the fragrant leaves of plants that do not have woody stems such as thyme, oregano, pepper mint, etc. Herbs are more fragrant when fresh. Spices classified on the basis of plant parts used are given in Table 10.5.

Table 10.5 Classification of spices based on plant parts used.

Plant parts used	Examples
Spices	
Leaves	Coriander, fenugreek, cinnamon
Flower	Clove, saffron
Fruit	Chili, cardamom, black pepper, all spice
Seed	Ani seed, cumin, fennel, coriander, ajwain
Rhizome	Ginger, turmeric
Roots	Horse radish, angelica
Kernel	Nutmeg
Barks	Cinnamon, cassia
Herbs	Mint leaves, coriander leaves, curry leaves, soya leaves

10.1.6 Nuts and oil seeds

Nuts are a dried indehiscent one seeded fruit with hard seed coat. The important nuts are almond, walnut, cashew nut and pistachio nut.

Oil seeds are major source of oils. They are annual seed plant such as ground nut, soya bean, sunflower, gingelly seed (sesame), rape seed and mustard seed.

Some oil-bearing trees are also source of oil such as oil palm, olive, coconut and mahua.

10.1.7 Fats and oil

Plant-based fats and oils consumed by man are mustard and rape seed oil, ground nut oil, peanut butter, soya bean oil, sesame oil, sunflower oil, rice bran oil, olive oil, coconut oil, palm oil and mahua oil. Fats and oils are concentrated source of energy. They provide more energy than protein and carbohydrates. Fats and oil also an excellent source of fat soluble vitamins. Oils are also rich in protein and essential fatty acid (linoleic) necessary for human health.

10.1.8 Sugar and related products

Sugar cane (*Saccharum* species) and sugar beet (*Beta vulgaris*) are the important source of sugar. In sugar cane, sugar is stored in the stem of the plant and in sugar beet in roots of the plant. Other significant source of sugar is honey.

1. *Cane sugar*: Sugarcane is a chief source of sugar which gives energy. It contains 12-15% sugar (sucrose-glucose and fructose). Sugar from

sugarcane is obtained in three forms which are widely used as an article of food. They are as follows:

Gur: This is a raw sugar called jaggery. About 50-60% of sugarcane production is used for making gur. Gur contains 65-80% sucrose, 10--15% invert sugar and 2.5% ash.

Khandsari: This is an open pan sugar called refined sugar. About 5% sugarcane production is used for making khandsari. Only small quantity is produced.

White sugar: This is a sugar of vacuum pan. Most common sugar and widely used. About 25-30% sugarcane production is utilized for white sugar production.

2. *Beet sugar*: Sugar beet or beetroot is also a rich source of sugar. Beet sugar is produced in one stage process from beet to refined sugar. It is produced as raw sugar and then refined.

10.1.8.1 Forms of sugar

Various forms of sugar are available for use in food preparation.

1. *Cube sugar*: This is agranulated sugar moulded in cubes. Mostly used for sweetening tea and coffee.
2. *Powdered sugar*: This is an icing sugar prepared by pulverizing granulated sugar and used in bakery or confectionary.
3. *Brown sugar*: Brown sugar contains molasses and flavour substances used in baked products.
4. *Rock sugar*: This is a big slabs prepared by boiling sucrose solution to desired consistency. This is used on festive occasions.
5. *Diamond sugar*: Diamond sugar is a small rectangular crystal used with beetle nut and confectionary.

10.1.9 Beverages

A wide variety of plant-based beverages are consumed by human beings. Beverages have function of refreshing, nourishing stimulating, soothing and appetizing. Plant-based beverages are classified into two groups: non-fermented and fermented.

10.1.9.1 Non-fermented beverage

Non-fermented beverages are non-alcoholic. These are several types such as plantation crop based (tea, coffee, cocoa, coconut), fruit based (juices, RTS, nectar, crush, squash, syrup, cordial, barley water, juice concentrate, juice powder), vegetable based (tomato juice, carrot juice and soups), sugarcane-based juice, and carbonated beverage (synthetic drinks). The descriptions of these beverages are given in Table 10.6.

Table 10.6 Plant-based non-fermented beverages.

Non-fermented beverage	Description
Plantation crop-based beverages	Plantation crop-based beverages are tea, coffee, cocoa, coconut.
Tea	Most popular refreshing beverage. It is prepared by pouring boiling water over dry processed leaves.
Black tea	Manufactured by withering, rolling, fermentation and drying. The beverage prepared from black tea is less bitter and astringent than green tea and has rich aroma and flavour.
Green tea	Green tea is made by steaming the leaves to prevent colour followed by rolling and drying. The beverage prepared from green tea has greenish yellow colour and is bitter and astringent.
Coffee	Mainly used as beverage. It is aqueous extract prepared from roasted and powdered beans. The value of coffee as beverage is due to alkaloid substance caffeine, flavour substance such as sulphur compounds and bitter substance such as polyphenol/tannin.
Espresso coffee	It is prepared by a brewing finely ground coffee with a mixture of steam and hot water by a special machine a cup at a time.
Soluble coffee	It is spray dried strong coffee brew.
Decaffeinated coffee	Most of the caffeine is removed from the bean by chemical process to obtain decaffeinated coffee. It has good flavour.
Cocoa	Cocoa is used as beverage. Cocoa used for beverage. Contain 20% cocoa fat. Cocoa beverage is normally prepared with milk.
Coconut	
Coconut water	Tender coconut water is very popular which contains about 5% sugar and little amount of vitamins and minerals.
Coconut milk	Obtained from grated mature coconut kernel that contains small amount of protein, B vitamins and minerals.
Fruit-based beverages	
Juices	Juice may be pure with natural sugar or sweetened which has 10% total soluble solid and 85% juice. Wide variety of fruits are used for making juices such as pineapple, apple, guava, mango, mandarin orange, litchi, pomegranate, grape, etc.

RTS	Ready-to-serve beverage contains at least 10% fruit juice and 10% total soluble solids. Fruit used for making RTS beverage are mango, guava, bale, pineapple, litchi, papaya, plum, jamun, bael, etc.
Nectar	A type of fruit beverage which contains at least 20% fruit pulp/juice and 13–15% soluble solids. Nectar can be prepared from papaya, mango, guava, litchi, apricot, peach, etc.
Squash	A type of fruit beverage which contains at least 25% juice and 45% total soluble solid. It also contains about 1% acidity and 350 ppm sulphur dioxide. Fruit suitable for squash making are mango, mandarin orange, lime, lemon, guava, pineapple, bael, papaya, litchi, jack fruit. Phalsa, jamun, pomegranate, plum.
Crush	A type of fruit beverage contains at least 25% juice/pulp and 55% total soluble solid with 1% acidity. Crush can be prepared from lime, lemon, mandarin orange, mango, etc.
Syrup	A type of fruit beverage contains at least 25% fruit juice/pulp and 66% total soluble solids with 1.3% acidity. Suitable fruits for making syrup are pomegranate, phalsa, karonda, jamun, aonla, lime, lemon, etc.
Cordial	Cordial is a sparkling clear sweetened fruit juice from which pulp and other suspended materials are completely eliminated. Cordial contains at least 25% juice and 30% total soluble solids with about 1.5% acidity. Cordial can be prepared from lime, lemon, guava, grape, phalsa, etc.
Barley water	A type of fruit beverage contains at least 25% juice, 30% total soluble solid and 0.25% barley, starch with 1% acidity. Lime and lemon can be used for preparing barley water.
Juice concentrate	This is a fruit juice which are concentrated by removal of water either by heat or by freezing. Fruit juice contains at least 32% total soluble solid. Fruit juice concentrate is used for preparation of beverages including carbonated beverage. Juice concentrate can be prepared from orange, apple, pineapple, grape, etc.
Juice powder	This is a fruit juice which has been dried into powder. It is instantly soluble even in cold water. Banana, bael, mango, orange and guava can be used for making juice powder.
Vegetable based	
Juice	May be natural or sweetened. Juice contains 5% juice with 0.5% salt and 1% sugar and 0.4% acid. Tomato and carrot are used for making juice.
Soup	Vegetable soups are appetizers, rich in vitamins and minerals and provide nourishment. Tomato, mixed vegetable and mushroom are used for making soups.

Sugarcane-based juice	Sugarcane juice contains 9% sugar, small amount of B vitamins and iron
Carbonated beverage	Carbonated beverages based on synthetic colouring and flavouring agents. The popular carbonated drinks are Pepsi, Coco Cola, 7-up, Thumps up, Limca, Mountain dew and Spirit.

10.1.9.2 Fermented beverages

Fermented beverages are alcoholic beverages. These are several types such as wine, malted beverage and distilled liquors which are briefly mentioned in Table 10.7.

Table 10.7 Fermented beverages.

Fermented beverages	Description
Wine	Alcoholic beverage prepared by fermentation of grape juice. Wines are different types such as champagne, sparkling, still wines, fortified wines, white wines, red wines, dry wines, sweet wines, table wines and dessert wines.
Champagne	Produced in district champagne (France).
Sparkling	Contains excess of carbon dioxide due to secondary fermentation that occurs after bottling.
Still wine	Without excess of carbon dioxide. It contains 8-10% alcohol.
White wine	Prepared by coloured grape using only juice.
Red wines	Prepared by coloured grapes using both juice and skin.
Dry wines	Fermentation until all the sugar is used.
Sweet wines	Fermentation stopped while some sugar remains.
Table wines	Contain less than 14% alcohol.
Dessert wine	Contain more than 14% alcohol.
Fortified wines	Fortified wines contain 20% alcohol. They are two types.
Port and sherry	Fortified wine differs from natural wine in that some alcohol such as grape brandy is added to them before the completion of fermentation.
Vermouth	Fortified wine prepared by the addition of spices mixtures or their extracts at various stages during fermentation.
Other wines	Wines are also made from juice of other fruits.
Cider	Fermented apple juice contains 4-5% alcohol. Other fruits used for making cider are guava, bael, aonla, jamun, etc.
Perry wine	Made from pears
Madhuka wine	Alcoholic beverage prepared from mahua flower.

Toddy	Toddy is fermented sap of palm tree obtained by tapping/ cutting stalk of young flower branches. It contains 4% alcohol.
Mead	Honey wine made from diluted honey.
Malted beverages	
Beer	The term is normally applied to a beverage prepared by the fermentation of barley malt. The most commonly used cereals other than barley are maize grit and flask, broken rice, wheat, tapioca and sorghum. Beers produced in India contains 4–5% alcohol. Beers are of various types.
Porter beer	Porter is heavier and darker drink made with longer dried, roasted or caramelized malt with less hopes. It is produced by top fermentation.
Stout beer	It is like porter except it has heavier malt flavour and dark colour. It is produced by top fermentation.
Ale beer	Prepared like lager beer but stronger in hops character and contains higher alcoholic content. It is produced by top fermentation.
Lager beer	Lager beer is a product of bottom fermentation.
Saki beer	Japanese beer prepared from rice which contains 14–17% alcohol.
Sonti beer	Rice beer or wine of India. The mould *Rhizopus sonti* and yeast are involved in fermentation.
Plaque beer	Latin-American beer containing 6% alcohol result from natural fermentation of agave juice or century plant.
Ginger beer	Mildly alcoholic, acid beverage prepared from fermentation of sugar solution flavoured with ginger.
Pilsener beer	The beer containing little remaining fermented carbohydrate.
Bock beer	Dark beer with high alcohol content.
Distilled liquors	Liquors are product obtained by steeping herbs, flowers, fruits, plant or distilled spirits. Distilled liquors normally contain 40% alcohol. Distilled liquors are of various types
Whisky	Prepared by the fermentation and distillation of cereal grains.
Scotch malt whisky	Prepared from malted barley scotch grain.
Scotch grain	Prepared from barley malt and other unmalted cereal grains.
Rye and maize whisky	It is prepared in the United States
Brandy	Brandy is prepared from wine particularly distillate from grape wine. It can also be prepared from any fruit. Brandy is stored in oak casks and allowed to age as long as 20 years.

Rum	It is an alcoholic beverage distilled directly from. Fermented sugarcane products such as juice and syrup of molasses. Distilled rum is stored in barrels for aging or improving its flavour. The strength of alcohol is adjusted 40% before bottling.
Gin	Gin is a distilled spirit flavoured with juniper berry or some other aromatics. Alcohol content is 60%. No aging is required.
Vodka	Vodka is distilled liquors made by diluting neutral spirit obtained from wheat or other cereal grains or potato.
Traditional alcoholic beverages	Traditional alcoholic beverages are arrack, fenny, chang, koomak and Takju.
Arrack	Product obtained by distillation of fermented toddy and contains about 35% alcohol.
Fenny	Traditional distilled alcoholic beverage of India prepared from cashew apple in Goa.
Chang	Traditional alcoholic beverage of North-Western prepared from cooked rice and other cereals.
Koomak	Traditional alcoholic beverage of Thailand, prepared from boiled glutinous rice with spices
Takju	Traditional alcoholic beverage of Thailand prepared from barley, wheat and corn.

10.2 Animal-based food sources

Animal food plays an important role in the diet of man. Nutritionally, they are important source of protein of good quality and excellent source of vitamins and minerals. In addition, animal foods are in general more distinctive in flavour and texture and often more palatable than foods of plant origin. Foods of animal sources are as follows:

- Milk and milk products
- Egg
- Meat and poultry
- Fish

10.2.1 Milk and milk product

Milk is a complete mixture of lipids, proteins, carbohydrates, other organic compounds and inorganic salts dispersed in water. The valuable component of milk is fat and protein. It is universally regarded as an ideal food for nourishing infants and young children and supplementary food in the diet of adults. Man uses milk of many animals such as cow, buffalo and goat. The cow is the most important of all these animals. Milk products are divided into two groups: non-fermented and fermented. Non-fermented products are whole milk powder, skimmed milk powder, condensed milk, whey protein concentrate, khoya, rabri, channa and ice cream. Milk-based beverages such as flavoured milk, milkshake, milton and eggnog. Fermented milk products are butter, cheese, curd and shrikhand.

10.2.2 Eggs and eggs products

Highly nutritious food containing protein, fat, vitamin A, B complex and D. Egg white is rich in protein and B vitamins, while egg yolk is rich in fat, protein, vitamin A, B complex and D. Eggs of most of birds are edible, but in India, eggs of hen and duck are mainly used for human consumption. It is an ideal protein food due to the presence of essential amino acids. Egg products are egg powder and egg albumin flaks.

10.2.3 Flesh foods

Flesh foods are meat of various types, such as beef, mutton, lamb, pork, poultry meat and fish.

10.2.3.1 Meat and meat products

Meat refers to muscle of warm-blooded four-legged animals. Meat provides high quality protein of biological value. It is an excellent source of vitamin B complex and good source of iron and phosphorus. Liver is rich in vitamin B_{12}, vitamin A and iron. Animals mainly utilized for food are cattle (bovine), sheep (ovine), swine (porcine) and goat (chevon). Meat products are fat such as lard (pork fat) and tallow (beef fat) sausages, pickles canned meat, smoked meat, etc. The various types of meat are as follows.

1. *Beef*: Meat of cattle over 1 year old. Beef carcass is classified into various types according to the age and sex. These are: stear [A bovine (cattle) male animal castrated at very young age.], stag [A male bovine (cattle) animal castrated after maturity.], heifer [A female bovine (cattle) animal which has not born a calf.], cow [A female bovine (cattle) animal which has born calf.], calf [A male or female bovine (cattle) animal generally 3–8 months of age at the time of slaughter Flesh has pale pink colour].
2. *Mutton*: Flesh of ovine (sheep) animal sheep carcasses are classified into three groups according to the age. These are lamb, yearling mutton and mature mutton.

3. *Lamb*: Flesh of young ovine (sheep) animal of both sexes having age of 12 months or below. Flesh is pinkish colour.
4. *Yearling mutton*: Flesh of young ovine (sheep) animal having age of 12–20 months old. Carcasses have harder and whiter bones than lamb.
5. *Mature mutton*: Flesh of both male and female ovine (sheep) having age of 20 months at the time of slaughter. Colour is lighter to dark red.
6. *Pork*: Pork is the meat of swine. Swine animals having 3–12 months slaughtering age give good quality pork due to lesser fat. Pork generally have higher content of fat than other meat.
7. *Chevon*: Meat of goat, it has pink colour.
8. *Organ meat*: Organ meats are liver, kidney, brain and head and products. Value-added products are sausages, canned meat, smoked meat, cured meat, pickled meat and dehydrated meat.
9. *Poultry*: The word poultry is applied to all domesticated birds as food. These include chicken, turkey, ducks and geese. Among these, chicken and turkey are most commonly used for their meat. Poultry is one of the sources of animal protein having good quality.

Chicken: Chicken is classified as broiler (chicken of 8–12 weeks age of either sex), rooster (chicken of 3–6 months of age), stag (male chicken under 10 months of age), hen (chicken of 5–7 weeks), stewing chicken (mature female chicken more than 10 months of age) and cock (mature male chicken over 10 months of age).

Turkey: Turkey is classified into various age groups such as rooster (less than 16 weeks), young hen (female of 5–7 month age), young tom (male 5–7 months of age) and old turkey (15 months of age).

Duck: Small ducklings are used.

Geese: Young birds are used.

10.2.4 Fish and fish products

Fish is rich in protein of high nutritive value. It is fair source of B vitamins. Large fish are rich in phosphorus but are deficient in calcium. Small fish eaten with bones are rich source of calcium the beneficial effect of dietary is attributed to the fatty acid composition of the fish. Major production of fish in India is from marine sources, marine fishes are from tuna, cuttle, sardines, mackerel, cat fish, etc. The main catch fish Iceland sources are rohu, mirgal, catla, murrel, hilsa, ribbon brown duct, etc. Fish products are canned fish, pickle, fish protein concentrate, fish liver oils, sausages and dried salted fish.

Edible fish is classified into two groups: fin fish and shell fish.

10.2.4.1 Fin fish

Fin fish are those which have bony skeleton. Such fish mostly come from salt water and to some extent from lake and Iceland water. They may be white and oily. White fishes may be round (cod, whiting, haddoch) or flat (plaice, sole). Oily fishes are mackerel and herring.

10.2.4.2 Shell fish

This is mainly salt water fish which include both mollusks and crustaceans. Mollusks have no legs and outer shells are harder. Such fishes are oysters, clamps, mussels and scallops. Some have shells in one piece such as snails, winkles and cockles. Crustaceans have legs with outer shells partly jointed. Such fishes are prawns, shrimps, lobster and crabs.

10.3 Food of other sources

10.3.1 Fungi-based food

10.3.1.1 Mushroom

Mushroom is an umbrella-shaped edible fungi belonging to Basidiomycotina. Mushrooms are not like a green plant and lack chlorophyll; hence, they depend on the preformed food for their nutrition. The use of mushroom as a food has attracted attention of mankind due to richness of protein, vitamins and minerals in addition to preventing chronic diseases with the presence of antioxidants and fibre. Most popular forms of edible mushrooms cultivated artificially are as follows.

1. White button mushroom (*Agaricus bisporus*): Button mushroom derives its name from the shape of button. The fruiting body consists of stem (stipe) and umbrella-shaped cap (pileus) grows in cool climate or in low temperature.
2. Paddy straw mushroom (*Volvariella volvacea*): Straw mushroom is a fast growing fungus with slander fleshy stipe and grey cap. It is grown in summer.
3. Oyster mushroom (*Pleurotus sajor-caju*): This is a soft mushroom that has white colour in hot weather and grey in cold weather with short stipe, fan like when young and gradually becomes deeply lobed to form branches. It is grown at moderate temperature (22-28°C).

The white button mushroom is more acceptable to the consumer which has higher price and extensively cultivated throughout the world.

10.3.2 Algae-based food

10.3.2.1 Blue-green algae (spirulina)

Blue green algae is the most nutrient dense food currently known as health food. It has also some medicinal uses. The algae are cultivated in open outdoor tents with well-defined medium. Freshly harvested spirulina can be sundried or spray dried for use or can be incorporated in any recipe. It is an excellent source of proteins and vitamins such as β-carotene, thiamine, riboflavin, pyridoxine, vitamin B_{12}, ascorbic acid, biotin and vitamin E. It is only vegetarian source providing vitamin B_{12}. Pigments present include phycocyanin, chlorophyll, carotenoids and xanthophylls. The quality of protein of spirulina is better than cereals and soya protein. One gram spirulina contains carotenoids equivalent to 1 kg of vegetables or fruits. One serving of spirulina (10 g) is considered better than one serving of one egg or 200 mL of milk in nutritive value. The β-carotene content of spirulina is 18 times more than carrot which is known for its higher value. Spirulina, apart from being rich in nutrients, contains phytonutrients such as gamma linolenic acid (polyunsaturated fatty acid) sulpholipids, phycocyanins and antioxidant vitamins.

10.4 Food accessories

Food accessories are edible materials used to improve flavour, taste and appearance of the food. These are also known as food adjuncts. The materials include in this class of food items are spices and herbs, salts and vinegar, tamarind, kewra and vanilla essence, orange and strawberry essence and natural colouring agents.

11

Nutritional benefits maximization

Food preparation is an important step in meeting nutritional needs of the people. With limited food resources, it is important to get maximum food value out of every bit of food. This can be achieved by enhancing the nutritive value of foods, preventing the loss of nutrients in food preparation and avoiding food losses/wastage.

11.1 Enhancing nutritive value of food

Nutritive value of foods can be enhanced by various means such as fermentation, sprouting, combination and fortification.

11.1.1 Fermentation

Fermented foods are generally, more nutritious than their unfermented counter parts. The foods of some natural fermentation are fermented cereal products (nan or bhatura, dosa, idli, appam, ambali, rabdi, kulcha, jalebi, dhokla, etc.), fermented vegetable products (sauerkraut and other pickles), fermented milk products (yoghurt, butter milk, cultured cream, butter, ghee, etc.) and fermented meat and fish products (sausages, fish paste, fish sauce). The other fermented products such as coffee beans made by lactic acid bacteria, cocoa made by yeast with acetic acid bacteria, wines and vinegar made by bacteria producing acetic acid and beer, wine whisky, brandy made with yeast fermentation. The important point is that the several end-products of such food fermentation particularly acids and alcohol do not allow the growth of disease-producing or pathogenic microorganism which are present in to foods.

The reasons for fermented foods which are more nutritious are as follows:

- Microorganism,
- Liberation of nutrients
- Splitting of cellulose

Microorganisms break down more complex compounds and synthesize several complex vitamins (B_2, B_{12} and vitamin C); hence, the content of these vitamins are higher in fermented foods.

Liberation of nutrients particularly in grains and seed locked inside the plant structures and cells by indigestible material. Coarse milling is not enough to release the full nutritional value even cooking. Fermentation breaks down the indigestible protective coating and cell wall. Therefore, physically and chemically making the structure more permeable to cooking water and human's digestive juices.

Splitting cellulose and hemicellulose in plant material that can be utilized in the human digestive tract otherwise human cannot digest into simple sugars.

11.1.2 Fortification

Fortification is a technique to add nutrients to particular food for enhancing nutritive value. Nutrients selected for fortification in food either should have deficiency or absent which are supposed to contain them. Moreover food selected for fortification should have acceptability and consumed by large section of people. Iodine in salt, vitamins A and D in hydrogenated fats, mixing of gram or soya or coarse grain flour in wheat flour (fortified flour) and fortified fruit-based beverages are examples of food fortification.

11.1.3 Combination

Combination of two or more food items can enhance the quality or nutritional value of foods. Similarly the excess of one food item can compensate the deficiency of another food items. Cereals or pulses cannot provide adequate proteins to our body due to lack of one or the other essential amino acids. Therefore, judicious combination of pulse, cereals and other plant-based food has quality proteins of desirable pattern of essential amino acids.

Nutritionally beneficial combination of foods is our traditional dishes such dal–roti, khichri, rice–dal, chola bhatura, idli–sambar, etc. The other nutritionally beneficial combination have been worked out by various origination or agencies for various group of person such as infants, growing children's, pregnant women's, lactating mother, and disordered person to improve their nutritional status.

11.1.4 Sprouting

Sprouting increases the vitamin content particularly B and C vitamins. Dry grain and pulses generally do not contain vitamin C but vitamin C is formed in grain and growing sprout when they are allowed to germinate or sprout. Sprouting also increases the B vitamins content. The technique of sprouting involves soaking of pulses or grain in water for 24 hour and then wrapping them in a damp cloth. Grains germinate within 2–3 days and sprouts grow to the size of about 1 cm. The germinated grain can be used raw or with very short cooking.

The grains commonly used to sprout are Bengal gram and whole green gram. Sprouted green gram contains higher content of vitamins C (three times more) than sprouted Bengal gram.

11.2 Preventing the loss of nutrients in food preparation

Foods are source of various nutrients such as vitamins, minerals, protein, carbohydrates and fibres in our diet. The food should be nutritive and palatable that we prepare. Therefore, perfect balance of nutritional quality and palatability is very important in prepared foods. Loss of nutrients, occur during preparation or processing of foods. These losses may be quantitative and qualitative due to removal of edible parts, cuttings, washing, cooking, heating, etc.

Quantitative losses occur in form of discarding edible parts such as stems in leafy vegetables (amranth, colocasia, fenugreek and chenopods) due to lack of knowledge for their use. In processing industry, sometimes raw material is rejected that may be of 50%. Nutrients are also lost in the form of processing waste such as peels, pomace, seeds, core, cuttings, etc. This varies from 20–40%.

Qualitative losses occur in nutrients particularly vitamins and minerals due to leaching and heating or cooking. Vitamins C is the most heat labile and its loss is 25–30%. Thiamine is water-soluble vitamins and lost 20% in cooking. Washing cereals like rice causes loss of thiamine. Loss of water-soluble vitamins may go up to 60% due to leaching and heating. There is destruction of vitamin A and carotene in water due to oxidation by air. Frying or roasting of vegetables causes considerable loses of vitamin A/carotene.

Minerals are also lost by leaching up to 35%. Maximum quantity of calcium and phosphorus is lost during cooking when excess cooking water is discarded. Losses of iron, sodium, potassium and magnesium occur by leaching when excess of water used in cooking is discarded. Availability of lysine and other amino acids become less in heat processed proteins than that of from the unprocessed proteins due to Maillard reaction.

Some simple practices which can be followed for retaining the nutritive value or minimizing the loss of nutrients in food are as follows:

- Wash fruits/vegetables before cutting.
- Salad vegetables should be prepared just before serving.
- Use acid foods such as lime juice, tomatoes, vinegar and curds as salads dressing which helps to retain the vitamin C content of salad.
- Cook vegetables on low flames as much as possible and keep them covered while cooking to reduce the loss of nutrients.
- Do not overcook and avoid the use of soda as it increases the loss of vitamin C, thiamine and riboflavin.

- Cut vegetables, just before cooking and put into heated oil used for seasoning.
- Cut vegetables just before cooking and put into boiling water if it is to be cooked in water.
- Use minimum amount of water for cooking, if the vegetables are to serve as such.
- Cook tubers and root vegetables such as beetroot, colocasia, potato and sweet potato whole with skin to retain nutrients and flavour.
- While preparing soups, cook slowest cooking ingredient first and then other ingredients which take less time.
- Cut fruits just before eating.
- Rice is cooked in just as much water as it needs to cook. Do not use extra water which needs to be thrown away.
- Do not discard water used in cooking to avoid the loss of calcium, phosphorus, iron, sodium and potassium when excess of water used in cooking.
- Avoid the exposure of cut surface in some fruits and vegetables such as potato, brinjal and apple otherwise it may become brown.
- Flavouring ingredients such as spices, etc., put to the oil used for seasoning as they are soluble in fat.

11.3 Avoiding food losses/wastage

Foods are perishable commodities. Some foods such as fruits, vegetables, milk, eggs, meat and fish are highly perishable. They begin to deteriorate shortly after harvest, gathered and slaughtered. Food losses can occur at any stage of operation from harvesting to consumption. The food losses are excessive. About 28–48% of the fruits and vegetables, 10–12% food grains and 10–12% of milk, meat, poultry and fish are lost every year. The need of the hour is to avoid or minimize these losses in various foods because the cost involved in preventing the losses is always cheaper than the cost of production. Therefore, measures should be adopted to avoid the losses in various foods.

11.3.1 Fruits and vegetables

The nature of losses observed in fruit and vegetables are loss in weight (leafy vegetables, potato, onion and most of the fleshy fruits), shrinking and wilting (most of the fruits and leafy vegetables), change in colour (browning of litchi, yellowing of cauliflower heads, spinach and lettuce), change in texture (over ripe fruits and brittleness in leafy vegetables), change in taste (unpleasant odour of the fruits and sweetness in potato), physical injury such as bruising, abrasion, compression, impact, punctures and tears in various fruits and vegetables, sprouting (onion, potato, garlic, ginger), toughening (green beans, okra, sweet corn), greening (potato and sweet potato) and rotting (various fruits and vegetables due to pathogenic disorders).

The losses occur at various stages such as pre-harvest (3–5%), at harvest (3–6%), sorting/grading (1–2%), packaging (4–6%), transport (5–7%), storage (4–8%), handling (3–6%) and distribution (5–8%). Thus total losses occur 28–48% and consumer availability is 52–72%.

The points of losses at the level of producer and consumers can be avoided or reduced by adopting following measures:

- Careful harvesting which includes stage of harvesting, timely harvest, use of clean and smooth containers and use of right kind of harvesting tools/equipment.
- Pre-cooling or rapid cooling after harvest in rapidly respiring commodities such as mango, grape, litchi, tomato, etc.
- Curing is most effective way of reducing weight loss and decay before storage in vegetables such as potato, sweet potato, yams, onion and garlic. Dates also require curing.
- Sorting helps to remove diseased fruits and vegetables and prevent decay losses.
- Cleaning or sanitation is essential to control spread of diseases. Washing particularly leafy and root vegetables helps to reduce dirt and spray residue.
- Appropriate bulk and consumer packaging help to reduce transpiration and respiration rate and extend storage life.
- Active packaging such as oxygen scavenging, antimicrobial packaging, ethylene control packaging, moisture control packaging and gas permeability control packaging avoid the losses and extend storage life of fruits and vegetables.
- Safe storage such as evaporative cool storage at farm level, modified atmospheric storage and cold storage are effective methods for retention of freshness, extending, shelf life and reducing losses in various fruits and vegetables.
- Use of cool chain to maintain low temperature at different stages of handling helps to avoid losses and retain quality in various fruits and vegetables.

11.3.2 Milk

About 10–12% milk is lost every year. The nature of losses in milk is scum formation, over boiling, scorching, curdling, formation of gaseous product, proteolysis of casein and microbial spoilage or contamination. Measures to minimize the losses are as follows:

- Use clean containers to collect and store the milk.
- Freshly drawn milk is cooled immediately to 4°C.
- Process the milk consisting three units of operation that is clarification, homogenization and pasteurization by holding or HTST method or UHT method.
- Store HTST milk for 2–3 weeks at 1.6–4.4°C and UHT milk for 1 month at 1.6–4.4°C.

11.3.3 Eggs

The nature of losses in eggs occurs in three forms that is physical damage, chemical changes and bacterial decomposition. The nature of physical damage are shell damage or broken eggs, egg which becomes less viscous and spread rapidly, size of air cell increased due to loss of moisture, egg yolk flattened when broken on plate and water passes from egg white to egg yolk due to breakage of vitelline membrane.

The nature of losses occur in the form of chemical changes are loss of water, loss of carbon dioxide, change in egg pH from 7.6 to 9.7, change in pH of egg yolk (slightly acidic pH of 6–6.2 becomes alkaline in deteriorated egg), break down of protein, increase in amount of free ammonia, increase in water-soluble inorganic phosphorus, increase in free fatty acid in yolk fat and off flavour of egg due to invasion of microorganisms and change in fat and protein. Bacterial decomposition spoils the eggs during storage or as the eggs ages. Measures to avoid the losses are as follows:

- Discard the broken eggs.
- Refrigerate the eggs immediately at 4–7°C and can be stored in home refrigerator for 1 or 2 weeks.
- Purchase the eggs for 1–2 weeks consumption.
- Eggs can be stored in cool storage for 6 months at −1.5°C to 0°C and 85–90% humidity.
- It is best to cook and serve immediately.
- Do not leave egg dishes at room temperature for more than 1 h.

11.3.4 Meat

The nature of losses in terms of changes are stiffness of carcasses after 24 h in beef, accumulation of waste products particularly lactic acid in muscle due to anaerobic glycolysis, quality attributes such as texture becomes hard, water holding capacity reduced, colour changes from pink to dark red and flavour reduced. Spoilage occurs due to microorganisms such as live trichinas. Measures to reduce losses are as follows:

- Ageing or holding meat at 0.5°C to –20°C in cold room for 2 weeks for softening, palatability and improving flavour.
- Tenderization by using cold storage, enzymes such as papain, bromelain, ficin and salt such as sodium chloride and sodium bicarbonate.
- Curing for preservation, flavour, colour and tenderness by using curing agents such as common salt, sugar, spices and sodium nitrate.

11.3.5 Fish

Spoilage occurs after 3–6 h of catching. About 10–15% of fish is spoiled during catching and further handling. Shrimps and chela are highly perishable. The nature of losses observed is physical, microbiological and biochemical.

The physical losses are tearing of fish in belly regions and bursting of belly walls leads to look unsightly. Microbiological nature of losses is due to large number of bacteria on the surface of slime and digestive tract. When fish is skilled these bacteria multiply rapidly and affect the quality of fish. Biochemical nature of losses is due to loss of glycogen in killed fish and development of odour and rancidity. Measures to minimize the losses are as follows:

- Fish can be stored only for 2 days in coldest part of the refrigerator.
- The losses in terms of colour, texture, flavour and nutritive value can be prevented by maintaining freezer temperature –18°C or lower.
- Fish can be stored for a week in cold or refrigerated room at 0°C with wrapping of ice crystals.

11.3.6 Hints to avoid food losses at home

Some useful suggestions to avoid the food losses at home are as follows:

- Plan meals in advance at least for a week.
- Use food items which are likely to spoil first or highly perishables.
- Use excess or left over food as early as possible.
- Check store first before purchase.
- Purchase the correct amount needed for consumption.

12

Food selection

Food beyond nutrients, contribution provide health benefits when they are eaten on a regular basis in adequate amount. Food selection is an important aspect for deciding the kinds or variety, amount, cost, suitability, quality, nutritive value and ease of preparation. This is a first stage in ensuring better nutrition for the family. The criteria used for selection of various foods prior to purchase are discussed in this chapter.

12.1 Selection of plant-based foods

12.1.1 Selection of cereals

Cereals largely used in our country are wheat, rice, bajra, barley, maize and ragi. Cereals are the best and cheapest source of energy; hence, they form major portion of most dietaries around the world. The choice of cereals largely depends upon availability, cost and dietary habits. The criteria used for selection are as follows:

- Grain should be clean and free from dirt, gravels, etc.
- Cereals should not be infected with moulds, fungus and insects.
- Wheat varieties suitable for making good quality chapaties are C306, UP-262, Sujata, Raj 4038, PBW 533, etc.
- Plump looking kernels which are not shrivelled and broken should be selected for purchase.
- Wheat should be free from insects and chaff.
- Cereals flour should be free from moulds, insects and lumps.
- Select rice for purchase at least 1 year old for better cooking.
- Select fragrant and long grained variety of rice such as basmati for making *pulao* and fried rice and short variety of rice or broken rice for *khichri*, *idli* and *pongal.*
- Parboiled rice is considered cheaper and has better or more nutrients than milled rice.
- In coarse grains, *Jowar* flour is used for making *roti* called *Bhakri* and excellent *dosa*, and maize flour is used for making delicious chapaties.
- Ragi is an excellent source of calcium and used as breakfast cereals or porridge.

12.1.2 Selection of pulses

Pulses used in our country are red gram *dal*, black gram *dal*, green gram *dal*, Bengal gram dal, lentil Bengal gram whole, green gram whole, beans (field and French), cowpeas, peas and soya beans. They are the main and cheap source of protein and rich in essential amino acid lysine. They also provide B-complex, vitamins, iron and calcium. The choice of these pulses depends more upon the cost of various varieties, availability and preference of a family. The tips used for selection of pulses are as follows:

- Select grains of uniform size and soundness without any broken pieces.
- Pulses should not contain any foreign seed or mixture.
- Pulses should be clean and free form trash, gravels, dirt, sand and stones while purchasing.
- Pulses should not be infected with insects. Pulses should be dry while purchasing otherwise mould/fungus may grow on it.
- Lentil and red gram dal are suitable for sambars and rasams. Lentil is at lower cost.

12.1.3 Selection of fruit

Fruits are good source of vitamins, minerals and dietary fibre. Fruits are perishable and retain their freshness for a short time. Fruits are easily spoiled if stored at room temperature due to action of microorganisms. The criteria for selection in general is based on freshness, uniform size, variety, bright colour, degree of ripeness and freedom form defects such as bruises, scratches, shrivel, decays etc. Standards for selection of fruits vary with the specific commodity are as follows.

12.1.3.1 Apple

Bright colours according to the variety, uniformity, firm fruit and crisp. Small sour fruits can be selected for jelly, sauce, etc.

12.1.3.2 Banana

Fullness of finger, slightly hard finger, free from bruises and crown rot. Do not refrigerate banana.

12.1.3.3 Sweet orange

This is tight skin orange. Mosambi is a popular variety. Select mature, firm fruits of 35% colour break, heavy in relation to fruit size and free from blemishes and soft or moulded spot. Thin skin oranges contain more juice.

12.1.3.4 *Mandarin orange*

This is loose skin orange. Nagpur orange and kinnow are the popular varieties. Select firm mature fruits of 40–50% colour break with thin skin, heavy in relation to fruit size and free from any blemishes or spot.

12.1.3.5 *Lime*

Kagzi lime is a popular variety. Select yellow limes with at least 50% colour break and thin and shiny skin. Avoid large size fruit which have thick skin.

12.1.3.6 *Grape*

Should be shining, plumpy, uniform colour, firmly attached to the stem and free from discolouration and bruises.

12.1.3.7 *Guava*

Common fruit rich in vitamin C. Select light yellow fruits having good flavour. Fruit should be medium sized, firm and free from bruises, spot and fruit flies.

12.1.3.8 *Litchi*

Select bright, uniform pink colour of right variety such as Shahi, Bedana, etc. Fruit should be in bunches, free from browning and cracking.

12.1.3.9 *Mango*

A common fruit in our country is a rich source of β-carotene. Select the fruit of right varieties at hard green stage or firm ripe, free form blemishes and spots. Varieties having thin stone are more pulpi or juicy should be selected.

12.1.3.10 *Papaya*

Fruit is rich source of carotene. Papaya for table purpose should be firm and turning yellow colour, no milk on tapering and free from blemishes. Carbide ripen fruits should not be purchased and papaya should not be refrigerated.

12.1.3.11 *Pineapple*

Fruit should be heavy in relation to their size, fragrant with orange yellow colour. Fruit should be plumpy with square base and free from any injury. Giant kew and queen are the suitable varieties.

12.1.4 Selection of vegetables

Vegetable makes the food attractive due to their texture, flavour and colour. Vegetables are called protective food like fruits as they are also rich in minerals and vitamins. Vegetable are highly perishable and retain their freshness for short time even under ideal conditions. Most of the vegetables are seasonal. Vegetables used in family depend on habit and taste. The desirable characters for selection of various vegetables are as follows.

12.1.4.1 Leafy vegetables

Leafy vegetables include amaranth, spinach, bathua, fenugreek, colocasia leaves, mustard leaves, coriander and mint leaves. Leafy vegetables are good source of minerals such as iron and calcium and vitamins particularly A and C. Select leafy vegetables which are tender, dark green, crisp, clean and free from holes in the leaves, spot, dirt, insects and free from flowers. Do not buy wilted or shrivelled and insects eaten vegetables.

12.1.4.2 Cabbage

Should be fresh, green, compact or tightly packed. Leaves should not be yellow, withered and have insect holes.

12.1.4.3 Cauliflower

Compact curd with snow white colour and surrounded by turgid green leaves. Avoid to purchase spread out curd have yellow colour.

12.1.4.4 Carrot

Select firm, fresh, crisp smooth, sweet carrot with deep yellow to orange colour. Avoid to buy flabby or soft and wilted carrot.

12.1.4.5 Radish

Top should be turgid and green, roots tender, smooth, crisp and free from pithy tissues.

12.1.4.6 Tomato

Should be smooth, firm with good shape and size. The colour should be pink or red according to the variety. It should not be soft and free from holes, white spots and cracks. Select large, round and fleshy tomatoes for salad or slicing and sauce.

12.1.4.7 Brinjal

Brinjal should be firm, glistering and smooth with black or purple or white colour according to the variety. Select deep purple colour with small to medium size. Calyx and stem should be fresh green.

12.1.4.8 Capsicum

Should be tender and firm with fleshy walls. Capsicum should have clear glossy dark green colour and free from blemish or decay.

12.1.4.9 Beans

Beans have different colours and shapes according to the variety. Beans should be tender, good even colour, pods should be straight, string less and free from wilting.

12.1.4.10 Peas

Pods should be fresh tender, well filled or plumpy, smooth and turgid with deep green colour. Seeds should be grass green and well rounded.

12.1.4.11 Okra

Okra should be bright green, fresh, firm and tender. It should not be badly misshapen and free from blemishes.

12.1.4.12 Pointed gourd

Should be green and hard with whitish green colour. Do not buy yellow and soft pointed gourd.

12.1.4.13 Bitter gourd

Select green or white variety with no yellow skin, should be very firm, and should not be fibrous.

12.1.4.14 Bottle gourd

These should be fresh, tender firm with green colour. Do not buy thick and rough skinned gourd which is over mature.

12.1.4.15 Potato

Select potato of smooth surface and elongated to round shape. Potato should be free from external defects such as greening, sprouting, growth cracks, scab, physical and sun burn.

12.1.4.16 Onion

Bulb should be firm and well covered with dry scales and neck should be dry and thin. Flesh edible scales should not be exposed. Colour may be brown, reddish purple yellow or white depending upon the variety. White onion is good for making pickle.

12.1.5 Selection of spices and herbs

Spices add flavour to everyday meals. Spices impart distinctive flavours to the food as they contain essential oils. Essential oils give their characteristic flavour which appeal to the sense of smell and taste and making the food more palatable. Herbs are the soul of flavour. Mint, coriander, curry and soya leaves are herbs most commonly used in Indian cooking. Mint and coriander are rich in carotene and calcium and are also used in the form of chutney. The points used in selection of spices and herbs are as follows:

- Spices should be free from dirt, grit and gravels.
- Spices should be free from moisture, fungus and artificial colour.
- Buy whole spices and get them ground yourself to avoid adulteration.
- Store them in tightly closed container to a dry place.
- Do not store powder spices longer as they loose aroma.
- Herbs are easily grown from seeds and can be grown in your garden or pots or window boxes to get fresh leaves.
- Do not buy shrivelled or wilted leaves of coriander and mint.

12.1.6 Selection of sugar and related products

Sugar, jaggery and honey are used as sweetening agents in beverage and other food products. The different forms of sugar and other sweetening agents used in India are white crystalline sugar, cube sugar, icing sugar, brown sugar, liquid sugar, glucose, jaggery and honey. Honey is manufactured by bees. The points used in the selection of these are as follows:

- Select crystal sugar or sugar cube for tea, coffee, etc.
- Select icing sugar for cakes, biscuits and other baked products.
- Select liquid sugar for soft drinks.
- Select honey for beverage and medicinal products.
- Buy large crystal sugars which are purer than small crystal sugar.
- Sugar should be free from lumps, dirt and adulterants.
- Honey manufactured by bees should have natural colour, texture and flavour and free from adulteration.

12.2 Selection of fats and oils

The fats used in our foods are ghee, butter, vegetable oils and vanaspati or hydrogenated vegetable oils. Out of these which are liquid at room temperature called oils and which are solid at room temperature called fats. Hydrogenated oil means a process by which oils are rendered solid at room temperature.

Hydrogenated oils are cheaper than ghee. The choice of fats and oils depends on the type of food preparation, the family needs, regional preference and food budget. The criteria for selection of these are as follows:

- Ghee is preferred for delicate flavour in preparation of puree, sweet, etc.
- Butter is selected for use as spread, frying dal and baked products.
- Oil is selected as frying medium and used for seasoning vegetables.
- The essential fatty acids and derived essential fatty acids together called polyunsaturated fatty acid which helps in healthy functioning of the heart. Safflower oil, soya bean oil, maize oil and sesame oil are very rich in polyunsaturated essential fatty acid than saturated fats like ghee and vanaspati.
- The selected criteria for fat and oils should be based on characteristic aroma, natural colour, clarity and freedom from dirt, dust and mixture with other oils and rancid odour.

12.3 Selection of animal-based foods

12.3.1 Selection of milk and milk products

Cows and buffalos are the two main sources of milk in our country. Buffalo milk is richer in fat (7–9%) than cow's milk (4.5%). The milk may be standardized or pasteurized. The various products of milk are cream, butter, ghee, curds, paneer, khoa, milk powders, etc. The selection criteria for milk and their products are as follows.

- Select pasteurized milk as it is safe and does not spoil fast.
- Cream should be fresh and free from sour taste and smell.
- Butter should be firm, have fresh flavour and packed in a hygienic package when buying from market.
- Ghee should have its natural delicate flavour.
- Do not depend totally on ghee as a medium of cooking as it deprives the body from essential fatty acid which required in the diet and present in vegetable oils.
- Select curd which is fresh with a delicate sour flavour and it should not be very sour and pungent.
- Setting curds at home is hygienic is much cheaper than the curd purchased from the market.
- Paneer should be moist and free from fungus or any unnatural smell.
- Paneer should be almost white in colour and have no discolouration.
- Select or purchase khoa which is firm and free from any unpleasant odour or smell.

12.3.2 Selection of eggs

Eggs are much more eaten in India than flesh foods. The reason may be due to improved production and reorganization of nutritional value. Irrespective of size and colour, all eggs are similar from nutritional point of view. The selection criteria for eggs are as follows:

- Buy egg fresh, clean and unbroken shell.
- One of the ways to judge good and spoiled egg or stale egg is to place the egg in water. Good egg or fresh egg will sink in water and spoiled egg will float.
- Large eggs are preferred for table use.
- If there is no refrigeration facilities buy egg at a time only for 2–3 days in winter and a day during summer or monsoon.
- Egg should be fresh before use and storage.

12.3.3 Selection of fish

Fish is an excellent source of protein and provide calcium, phosphorus, iron, vitamin A and niacin. Nutritionally they are rich and easily digestible. The criteria for selection of fishes are as follows:

- Select fresh fish which is bright in colour with clear un-sunken eyes, red gills, stiff body or firm flesh and tight scales.
- Press the skin of the fish with the finger. If the impression remains, it is of poor quality and do not purchase.
- Spoiled fish has dull skin, slimy, pale colour, loose scales, dull and grey eyes and dark grills. Do not buy such fishes.
- Be sure to purchase fish which has been refrigerated and stored on ice and is not slippery to touch.
- Select fish according to the use. Whole fish or fillet for baking and steak for frying or boiling.
- The cleaning waste index in fish is high (25–30%) and in some fishes like prawn, lobsters, crab, etc., are very high (60%), hence, needs or requirements to be taken according to the edible portion.
- Consuming fish if not properly stored or processed can cause stomach upset resulting in severe stomach pain and diarrhoea, hence, can be taken.

12.3.4 Selection of meat or flesh foods

There is large variety to choose non-vegetarian food. The choice of flesh food is governed by cost and conviction. People have different preference for different flesh foods. Some eat fish but no meats or poultry and some eat beef but no pork. Some of the flesh foods are very expensive in our country. The kinds and form of meats available in our country are poultry meat, mutton, beef and pork. Some of the selection criteria for flesh foods or meats are as follows.

12.3.4.1 Poultry

Poultry includes chicken, ducks, geese and turkeys. In India, chicken meat is very popular. The birds raised under special condition which keeps meat tender are called broiler. They are slaughtered and soled as dressed chicken. Buy large broiler which is economical due to the wastage in terms of bones on weight basis is less. The skin of the chicken should be soft and tear easily. The breast bone should bend easily. Country chicken is more tasty but avoid to buy old or large country chicken which has tougher meat. Chicken meat prices vary according to the cut and quality. Selection should be made on the basis of intended use in preparation.

12.3.4.2 Mutton

Mutton is a goat meat which is very common but in west, it is called sheep meat. Select meat of young goat which has pinkish colour and has almost no fat. Avoid dark red coloured meat which has deposits of fat. This is an indication of older goat meat.

12.3.4.3 Beef

Meat from a mature cow and buffalo is called beef and from young animal called veal. Select the meat of veal which is pinkish and cooks easily as compared to beef which has darker colour.

12.3.4.4 Pork

Pork is a meat from pigs and is popular in some of the northern parts of the country and more in colder parts. Select the meat of young pig which has greyish white to pink muscle as compared to deep rose in old pigs. The flesh should be firm and fine grained and bones are soft. Always buy pork from government licensed shop. Pork be always well cooked before eating otherwise it is risky since pork contain a parasitic round worm produces a disease called trichinosis. High temperature in cooking destroy the organism.

12.4 Selection of beverages

Beverages are liquid for drinking which refresh the person and supplement their fluid requirement. Beverages, commonly used in India are tea, coffee, fruit-based soft drink (juices, RTS, squash, cordial, etc.), milk-based beverage (milkshakes) and aerated or carbonated soft drink (thumps, coca cola, sprite, dew, etc.). The selection criteria for some the beverages are as follows:

- Select whole leaf for light cup of tea with full of flavour and select granular tea for a strong cup of tea.
- Buy tea or coffee which is sealed in air tight package or container.
- Avoid buying loose tea/coffee from market.
- Select or buy unroasted coffee bean and roast it yourself before grinding for use.
- In cold drinks, select fruit-based beverages which have some nutritional value particularly vitamins and minerals.
- Milk-based cold drinks called milkshakes are very refreshing have nutritional value and are very good for children.
- Many varieties of aerated or carbonated synthetic drinks are available in the market. From nutrition point of view, these soft drinks have no nutritional value. Moreover, colour and sweetness such as saccharin used in carbonated or aerated drink is harmful to health. Hence, preference should not be given to such aerated soft drinks.

13 Food storage

Unless food is properly stored or preserved, much of it would be unfit for human consumption. Therefore, it is not important only to raise production but also to avoid wastage by proper storage so that every bit of food produced is utilized for human consumption. If the goal of nutrition, high eating quality, wholesomeness and economy are to be achieved, storage of food requires as much care as its purchase in the market. The main objectives of the storage are to increase the period of consumption, check losses, reduce glut, regulate supply and to obtain better price. Foods when properly stored, retain their freshness longer, have better nutritive quality and acceptability. Some practical hints for storage of commonly used foods are as follows.

13.1 Fruits

Fruits continue to respire even after harvest and have life. It is difficult to stop the process but it can be minimized. Therefore, principle of storage is to control the rate of respiration, the rate of transpiration, the rate of ripening, undesirable biochemical changes and microbial infections. Fruits are classified on the basis of their perishability. Dry fruits have very low perishability called low perishable and can be stored longer. Citrus fruits and apple have moderate perishability called semi-perishable fruits and have moderate storage life. Mango, banana, guava, grape, papaya, litchi, peach, plum and strawberry have high perishability and have less or short storage life.

There are various methods of storage of fruits such as evaporative cool storage, zero energy cool chambers, modified atmospheric storage, cold storage, controlled atmosphere (CA) storage and hypobaric storage.

13.1.1 Evaporative cool storage

This is one of the simple and effective methods for short-term storage of fruits and vegetables. This reduces shrivelling, extend storage life and prevent losses during marketing and storage. Such type of storage maintains high relative humidity with temperature nearer to wet bulb and thus reduces the weight loss considerably in stored fruits. It is one of the low-cost technologies for storage of fruits.

13.1.2 Zero energy cool storage

Based on principle of evaporative, zero energy cool chambers have been developed. This is low cost, simple and short-term storage of fruits.

13.1.3 Modified atmospheric storage

Modified atmospheric storage is the development of modified atmosphere around the product through permeable film. Fruits or vegetables are enclosed in a sealed plastic film which is permeable gases producing higher concentration of CO_2 and lower concentration of O_2. MAS technology retard maturation, ripening and senescence during storage by resting respiration. It reduces incidence of diseases and level of ethylene. The technique does not require high investment and can be adopted without refrigeration facilities. The recommended percentage of O_2 and CO_2 in MA storage for important fruits is given in Table 13.1.

Table 13.1 Optimum level of O_2 and CO_2 in MA storage for important fruits.

Fruits	O_2 (%)	CO_2 (%)
Banana	2–5	2–5
Mango	2–5	5–10
Orange and lemon	5–10	0–10
Grape fruit	3–10	5–10
Papaya	2–5	5–8
Pineapple	2–5	5–10

13.1.4 Cold storage

Most reliable and widely adopted for bulk storage of fruits and vegetables for a long period. This is a low temperature storage involves the principles of maintaining low temperature which reduces the rate of respiration, thermal composition, delays ripening and extending storage life for long period. Temperature and relative humidity is controlled in such type of storage. However, it is energy intensive and expensive. The temperature, relative humidity and storage life of some important fruits are given in Table 13.2.

Table 13.2 Storage life of various fruits in cold storage.

Commodity	Temperature (°C)	Relative humidity (%)	Storage life
Apple	1–4	90–95	3–10 months
Apricot	–0.5 to 0	90–95	2–3 weeks
Avocado	4–13	85–90	2–4 weeks

Banana green	13–14	90–95	1–4 weeks
Cherries Sour	0	90–95	1 week
Cherries Sweet	–1 to 0.5	90–95	2–3 weeks
Coconut	0–1.6	80–85	1–2 months
Custard apple	5–7	85–90	4–6 weeks
Dates	0	75	6–12 months
Fig fresh	–0.5 to 0	85–90	1 week
Grapes	–1.1 to 0.5	90–95	3–6 months
Guava	7–10	90	3–6 months
Jackfruit	13	85–90	3–6 weeks
Kiwi fruit	0	90–95	3–5 months
Lime	9–10	85–90	6–8 weeks
Lemons	10–13	85–90	2–3 weeks
Loquats	0	90	3 weeks
Litchi	1.6	90–95	3–5 weeks
Mangoes	13	85–90	2–3 weeks
Olive fresh	5–10	85–90	4–6 weeks
Orange	3.3–8.8	85–90	4–8 weeks
Papaya	7–13	85–90	1–3 weeks
Peaches	–0.5	90–95	2–4 weeks
Pears	–0.5	90–95	2–7months
Plums	–0.5 to 0	90–95	2–5 weeks
Pomegranate	5	90–95	2–3 months
Pineapples	7–13	85–90	2–4 weeks

All fruits are washed thoroughly before been placed in cold storage or refrigeration. Soft fruits keep better if spread out on a flat surface. Citrus fruits can be kept fresh longer by covering them with a wax paper so that a more moist atmosphere is provided. Ripen, bananas are not stored at low temperature because of a colour change in the skin.

Products such as fresh, canned or fruit juice keep the vitamin content better if poured into container covered and refrigerated canned foods retain higher level of vitamin C and B_1 if they are stored at low temperature.

13.1.5 CA (controlled atmosphere) storage

The CA storage works on principle of maintaining an artificial atmosphere in storage room which have a higher concentration of CO_2 and lower concentration of O_2 than normal atmosphere. This reduces the rate of respiration and extends storage life or delays aging. However, it is important to control Co_2 level sense at very high level of CO_2 anaerobic reaction leads to fermentation and development of alcohol. This method of fruit or vegetables storage is very effective when combined with low temperature storage. The recommended conditions for storage of some fruits and vegetables under CA storage are given in Table 13.3.

Table 13.3 Storage conditions of some fruits and vegetables under CA.

Commodity	Temperature range (°C)	CO_2 range (%)	O_2 range (%)
Apple	0–5	1–2	2–3
Banana	12–15	2–5	2–5
Kiwi fruit	0–5	5	2
Strawberry	0–5	15–20	10
Nuts and dry fruits	0–25	0–100	0–1
Tomato mature green	12–20	0	3–5
Tomato partially ripe	8–12	0	3–5
Lettuce	0–5	0	2–5

13.1.6 Hypobaric storage

This is also known as reduced atmospheric pressure/subatmospheric storage/low pressure storage and vacuum storage. The principle of such storage is to remove ethylene gas from the storage atmosphere and lowering the partial pressure O_2 which leads to slow ripening, hence, fruits can be kept longer. It is a type of CA storage with emphasis on reducing the pressure of O_2 and ethylene gas. Low oxygen reduces the respiration rate and low ethylene delays the ripening, as a result fruits are store for long time. In such storage, fruits like apple, pear, mango, banana, pineapple, guava, avocado and lemon fruits have better storage life. This system is used in transportation of fruits also. Low pressure of O_2 (102 mmHg) reduces the growth of pathogenic disorders such as *Rhizopus nigricans*, *Aspergillus niger*, *Botrytis species* and *Alternaria* species.

13.2 Vegetables

Most of the fresh vegetables retain their top quality for only a few days even under ideal condition of temperature and humidity. Vegetables also respire continuously after harvest. Some vegetables have higher storage life such as dry vegetables, potato, dry onion, garlic, pumpkin, yam, ash gourd, etc. Vegetables such as cauliflower, peas, spinach, tomato, cabbage, green beans, brinjal, gourd, etc., are highly perishable and have less storage life. Green leafy vegetables are washed and drained thoroughly because too much moisture can increase the possibility of spoilage/decay. They are packed in ventilated plastic bags or waxed paper and stored under refrigeration. Vegetable such as peas should be stored with pods only. Waxing of vegetables particularly tomato, brinjal and chilies can increase the storage life. In home, vegetables such as root vegetables, tubers and bulbs including potato, sweet potato, onions and carrots can be stored in a cool dark and dry place where there is air circulation.

Vegetables can be stored better in evaporative cool storage or zero energy cool chambers, modified atmospheric packaging (MAP) and cold storage.

13.2.1 Modified atmospheric packaging

Storage life of vegetables is extended under MAP in which respiration of the commodities is made use of to modify the atmosphere composition inside the package. The storage life of some vegetables by using MAP at ambient condition and at optimum low temperature is given in Table 13.4.

Table 13.4 Storage life of vegetables under MAP conditions.

Vegetables	At ambient conditions	At optimum low temperature
Carrot	14	42
Capsicum	18	21
Green chillies	8	28
Tomato	15	30

13.2.2 Cold storage

Vegetables can be stored longer in cold storage or low temperature storage. The recommended temperature, humidity and storage life of various vegetables in cold storage are given in Table 13.5.

Table 13.5 Storage life of various vegetables in cold storage.

Vegetables	Temperature (°C)	Humidity (%)	Storage life
Amaranth	0–2	95–100	1–2 weeks
Asparagus	0–2	95–100	2–3 weeks
Brinjal	12	90–95	1 week
Beans green	4–7	95	1 week
Cabbage	0	98–100	3–4 months
Cauliflower	0	95–98	2–4 weeks

Carrots	0	98–100	4–6 weeks
Cucumbers	10–13	95	1–2 weeks
Garlic	0	65–70	6–7 months
Ginger	13	65	6 months
Melons	7	90–95	2 weeks
Mushroom	0	95	2–4 weeks
Okra	7–10	90–95	1 week
Onion greens	0	95–100	3–4 weeks
Onion dry	0	65–70	6–8 weeks
Peas green	0	95–98	1–2 weeks
Peppers sweet	7–13	90–95	2–3 weeks
Potato (seed)	2–4	90–95	9–10 months
Potato (Table CIPC treated)	8–12	90–95	9–10 months
Potato (Processing CIPC treated)	8–12	95–98	9–10 months
Pumpkins	10–13	50–70	2–3 months
Radishes	0	95–100	2–4 weeks
Spinach	0	95–100	1–2 weeks
Sweet potato	13–15	85–90	4–7 months
Tomato mature green	18–22	90–95	1–3 weeks
Tomato firm ripe	13–15	90–95	1 week
Water melons	10–15	90	2–3 weeks

Vegetable products particularly pickles and packed canned products can be stored about a year.

13.3 Cereals and pulses

Cereals are the most important food stuffs consumed throughout the world. About 10% production of food grain lost due to improper storage and unscientific storage practices. Cereals have not been given much importance for proper storage facilities as given to produce like potato. If proper storage facilities are popularized through education and incentives, considerable amount of losses can be avoided in food grain.

Cereals are dried completely, packed in air tight containers such as bins, jute bag and gunny bag and stored in a cool and dry place. Wheat in bulk is stored in metal bin closed tightly. Rice is stored in a metal bin in a cool and airy place. Polished rice has better keeping quality than hand pounded rice. Dry maize grain is stored in gunny bag.

About 60–70% food grains remain in rural area and rest 30–40% come in urban area. Thus construction of rural godown or ware house for storing farmers produce on rental bases is very vital to reduce losses, maintain quality and achieve better price of the produce.

Cereal product such as wheat flour is best stored in metal bins. Freshly ground flour and maidas can be stored for 1–2 months. Semolina can be roasted lightly and stored in airtight containers. Bread and other baked products should be cooled completely before storing. Bread box should be well ventilated. It is better to kept in refrigerator to prevent mould. Cakes can be wrapped in cellophane cover and keep in refrigerator to maintain the freshness. Biscuits, macrons and other baked product are best stored at room temperature in airtight tin containers.

Pulses, such as red gram, Bengal gram, green gram, black gram, dry peas, etc., are stored in gunny bags or beans in a room or ware house.

13.4 Milk

Milk should be refrigerated as soon as possible after delivery or purchase. Fresh milk must be boiled thoroughly, cooled and stored under refrigeration with a covered container. Milk must be kept covered to protect it from dust, bacteria and undesirable flavour. Pasteurized, cooled and packed milk has better storage life. In home storage, where there is no refrigeration, milk may be boiled thrice a day in summer and twice a day in winter. The milk should be kept in cool and dark place or away from sunlight. Milk exposed to sunlight losses vitamin B_2 (riboflavin) and flavour within a short time.

Pasteurized, cooled and packed milk has better storage life. Pasteurized milk with high temperature short time technique can be stored 1–2 weeks at 1.4–7.2°C and 2–3 weeks at 1.6–4.4°C. Pasteurized milk with ultra-high temperature technique can be stored for a month at 1.6–4.4°C.

Dried milk should be stored at ordinary room temperature in airtight container. Once the container is opened and exposed to room temperature, it may be spoiled unless it is stored at low temperature. To increase the storage life of dry milk, containers should be tightly closed and stored at low temperature. Sweetened and evaporated milk in sealed cans can be stored at room temperature. Once the can is opened is should be at once transferred to a glass bottle or stainless steel container to prevent spoilage. Further this can be stored in a dry and ventilated place or under refrigeration at a temperature of 4°C.

13.5 Eggs

Bacteria and moulds spoil the eggs during storage; hence, eggs should be kept refrigerated (4–7°C) until used. To retain its best quality, eggs should be stored or placed in such a way that the broad end of the eggs are up which prevents movement of the yolk. Eggs pickup odours and flavours from other foods; hence, this should be kept covered to prevent absorption of undesirable flavour. Avoid washing eggs whenever possible because it removes protective film and cause them to become more porous.

Eggs are stored for future use in cold storage. It can be stored for 6 months in cold storage at −1.5°C to 0°C and 85–90% relative humidity. Frozen eggs are substituted for fresh egg in commercial food preparation.

13.6 Fish

Large number of bacteria on the surface slime and digestive tract is found on living fish. When fish is killed, these bacteria multiply rapidly and affect the quality of fish. Fish can be stored in refrigerator in coldest part for 2 days. Freezer temperature of −18°C or lower is necessary to prevent loss of colour, texture, flavour and nutritive value. Fish can be stored at 0°C in cold or refrigerated room for a week with wrapping of ice or ice crystals.

13.7 Meat

Meat should be stored under refrigeration slightly above freezing temperature, that is, 0.5–2°C to inhibit the growth of microorganism. Fresh meat should be wrapped loosely in wax paper or cellophane and placed in the coldest part of refrigerator (defreezer). Ground meat/minced meat are highly perishable and this should be also stored in defreezer. Freezing is one of the best methods of preserving freshness, flavour, colour, texture and eating quality; hence, goat, sheep, poultry and fish meat can be stored or preserved by freezing technique.

Foods when properly stored retain their freshness longer have better nutritive quality and acceptability. Therefore, for better storage and longer shelf life, foods should be stored in a proper place according to their requirements.

14
Food spoilage

Spoilage of food is a major problem and it occurs at any stage of food production, transport, storage, marketing and processing or preparation. Food spoilage refers to decay and decomposition of undesirable nature. Foods undergo chemical and physical changes when spoiled and become hazardous and unfit for human consumption. Most of the foods deteriorate, some are faster than others. On the basis of ease of spoilage, foods are classified into three categories that are highly perishable, semi-perishable and low perishable.

Highly perishable foods can be kept at room temperature for only few hours or 1–2 days before spoiling. These foods require refrigeration. Such foods are plant based such as fleshy fruits, leafy vegetables, including mushroom, milk, flesh foods and eggs.

Semi-perishable foods can be stored for a couple of weeks or even a month or two without any detectable signs of spoilage. Temperature and humidity of the environment again affects the shelf stability of such foods. Proper handling and storage can result in fairly long storage without spoilage. The examples of such foods are cereals, pulses, oil seed, wheat flour, Bengal gram, semolina, vermicelli, fruits such as apple, pomegranate, citrus and dry fruits and vegetables such as potatoes, sweet potato, yam, colocasia, onion, garlic and ash gourd.

Lowperishable foods can be kept for months or years without spoiling unless handled and stored carelessly. Such foods are rice, dry beans, sugar, spices and oils.

The major causes of food spoilage are microbial spoilage (bacteria, moulds and yeast), enzymatic spoilage, chemical spoilage, physical/mechanical spoilage and spoilage causing insects, parasite and rodents.

14.1 Microbial spoilage

Microorganisms are considered to be the primary cause of food spoilage. These are found everywhere in soil, air, water and fresh and processed foods. Microbial growth is referred as the increase in quantity of cellular constituents and structures and is followed by an increase in size or number of cells or both. The common forms of microorganisms are bacteria, moulds and yeast.

The primary sources of microorganisms in the food are given in Table 14.1.

Table 14.1. Source of microorganisms.

Sources	Microorganisms
Soil	
Plant surfaces, soil dust, soil particles carried by running water	*Bacillus*, *Clostridium*, *Escherichia coli*, *Enterobacter*, *Pseudomonas*, *Proteus*, *Acetobacter*, etc.
Water	
Surface water: stream, pools, stored water such as lake, pond, tanks and ground water wells.	*Pseudomonas*, *Chromobacterium*, *Proteus*, *Micrococcus*, *Bacillus*, *Streptococcus*, *Es. coli*, coliform or water-borne bacteria
Air borne	
Air containing dust, droplets, aerosols, suspended particles, dry soils, spray lakes, oceans and droplets of moisture on wells, celling floors and foods	Bacteria spores, moulds spores, yeast present in air
Vegetation	
Natural surface of plant flora, outer tissue of unwashed cabbage, exposed plant surface, contamination from soil, water, sewage, air and animal.	Bacteria: *Bacillus*, *Pseudomonas*, *Micrococcus*, coliforms, *Corynebacterium*, *Pectobacterium* Mould: Several genera of moulds
Animal	
Hair, surface flora, respiratory tract flora, gastro intestinal tract, hides, hooves contain microorganisms from soil, manure, feed, water, etc., animal wastes, poultry feather and skin of meat animals.	*Micrococcus*, *Streptococcus*, *Staphylococcus*, *Brucella* sp., *Mycobacterium tuberculosis*, *Clostridium botulinum*, *C. perfringens*, *Salmonella typhi*, etc.
Food equipment and food handlers	
Meat cutting knives, grinders, utensils, containers, machine, equipments. Similarly handlers hand and outer garments or poor personal hygiene practices.	Meat-borne organisms, moulds and yeast.

Major microorganisms spoiling foods are as follows:

- Bacteria
- Moulds
- Yeast

14.1.1 Bacteria

Bacteria are unicellular microorganisms which are classified as prokaryotes, unlike cells of other animals, it do not contain a nucleus. They vary in shape and size. The common shapes are spherical, oval and rod. Bacteria are measured in units called microns (μ). Bacteria commonly range from 1 to 10 μ or more in length and about 0.5 μ in diameter. Under favourable condition (optimum temperature and moisture), bacteria multiply by division of cell or binary fission. Bacteria are of several types. The important group of bacteria and their characteristics are given in Table 14.2.

Table 14.2. Group of bacteria and their characteristic.

Group	Characteristic
Aerobes	Require atmospheric oxygen for growth, e.g., *Acetobacter aceti*
Anaerobes	Do not require oxygen and grow in absence of oxygen
Bacillus	Rod-shaped bacteria, form spores which are more resistant to heat
Coccus	Spherical-shaped bacteria
Coccobacillus	Oval-shaped bacteria
Facultative anaerobes	Grow with or without free oxygen
Facultative thermophiles	Grow over the whole range of temperature covered by mesophylls and obligate thermophiles
Mesophylls	Temperature requirement below 38°C for growth
Obligate anaerobes	Do not grow in atmospheric oxygen
Obligate thermophiles	Grow between 38°C and 82°C
Psychrotroph	Grow fairly well in cold storage or refrigeration temperature and below freezing temperature
Spirillum	Long, coiled threads bacteria
Vibrio	Short, curved rods

14.1.1.1 Bacteria causing food spoilage

The important bacteria causes spoilage of foods are given in Table 14.3.

Table 14.3. Food spoilage bacteria.

Food	Type of spoilage	Bacteria involved
Fruits and vegetables		
Carrot, tomato, potato and fruits	Souring	Saprophytic bacteria
	Acetic acid formation	Acetobacteria
	Soft rot or mushy consistency	*Erwinia carotovora*
	Rotting of potato tubers	*Pseudomonas solanacearum*
Citrus fruits	Scabs and cork like lesions	*Xanthomonas citri*
Refrigerated vegetables	Spoilage- off odour	*Flavobacterium*, *Hafnia*

Refrigerated vegetables products	Acids and gas in most vegetables	*Lactobacillus*
	Red pigmentation in vegetable products	*Serratia* sp.
Pickles	Black pickles	*Bacillus nigricans*
	Soft pickles	*Bacillus* sp.
	Slimy kraut	*Lactobacillus plantarum*
Cereals, flour and dough products such as biscuits, sweet rolls, pizza dough etc.	Acid formation	*Lactobacillus* sp. *Streptococcus* sp. *Leuconostoc* sp.
Fermented bakery products	Ropiness or stringiness of bread or red bread	*B. subtilis* *B. pumillus* *B. licheniformis*
Fermented beverage-Beer	Ropiness	*Gluconobacter*
Wine	Lacting souring	*L. brewis*
Sugar products and honey Syrup and honey	Ropy syrup	*Enterobacter aerogenes*
	Pink syrup	*Micrococcus roseus*
	Green syrup	*Ps. fluorescens*
Dairy products- Raw milk below 37°C temperature	Souring	*Streptococcus lactis* Coliform *Enterococcus* *Lactobacillus* *Micrococcus*
	Proteolysis of milk	*Micrococcus* sp. *Alcaligenes* sp. *Proteus* sp. *Pseudomonas* sp. *Serratia* sp. *Clostridium* sp. *Bacillus* sp.
	Ropiness of milk or string consistency	*Alcaligenes viscolactis* *Enterobacter aerogenes* *En. cloacae* *Es. coli* *L. bulgaricus*
	Blue milk	*Ps. syncyancea*
	Yellow milk	*Ps. synxantha*
	Red milk	*Serratia marcescens*
	Brown milk	*Ps. putrefaciens*
	Gas producers in dairy products	Coliform, *Clostridium* sp. *Bacillus* sp.

	Cheese fermentation	*Propionibacterium*
	Slimy growth on cottage cheese	*Alcaligenes metalcaligenes*
Meat and meat products Fresh meat	Proteolysis and putrefaction	*Bacillus* sp., *Clostridium* sp. *Acinetobacter*, *Pseudomonas* *Alcaligenes*, *Micrococcus*
	Phosphorescence	*Phosphobacterium*
Poultry	Fluorescent pigment	*Pseudomonas* sp.
	Odour and sliminess at the outer surface of carcass or cuts	*Acinetobacter* *Flavobacterium* Enterobacteriaceae *Alcaligenes*
Egg	Green rot	*Ps. fluorescens*
	Black rot	*Pseudomonas* sp. *Proteus* sp.
	Pink rot	*Pseudomonas* sp.
	Red rot	*S. marcescens*
	Colourless rot	*Alcaligenes* sp. *Acinetobacter*
	Bacterial soft rot	*Er. carotovera*
Fish	Discolouration Off flavour	*Pseudomonas* sp. *Flavobacterium* sp. *Proteus* sp. *Serratina* sp. *Es. coli* *Clostridium* sp. *Aeromonas* sp.
	Putrefaction	*Chromobacterium* sp. *Halobacterium* sp.

14.1.1.2 Beneficial/useful bacteria

Some bacteria produce substances of desirable flavour and are cultivated for their beneficial action. Some bacteria are of great importance in the food processing industry. Some of the useful bacteria are as follows:

Lactobacillus sp.: The different organisms of this group of bacteria are also known as lactic acid bacteria. These have different properties but all of them produce lactic acid from carbohydrates. The lactic acid of butter milk, shrikhand, sauerkraut, fermented pickles, cheese and butter are examples of a desirable flavour substance formed by bacterial action. Those bacteria which are used in distilling and brewing industries are facultative thermophiles (heat tolerant) which grow abundantly at 50–55°C and produce much lactic acid. Mesophylls are used in preparation of pickles. *Lactobacillus plantarum* is commonly found in pickles.

Acetobacter sp.: These bacteria, also called vinegar bacteria, are necessary for vinegar production but cause spoilage of wine. The important species are *Ac. aceti*, *Ac. orleansis* and *Ac. schutzenbach* which are very small and generally do not form spores. They are aerobes and in presence of oxygen convert ethylalcohol to acetic acid. These are of two types. One type form a tough shiny film on the surface of wine and growth is known as vinegar mother, while other grows throughout the wine without forming vinegar mother.

Bacteria are very sensitive to acid and their presence can be destroyed in acidic foods at boiling temperature. Most fruits are acidic and can easily sterilized at 100°C. Non-acid or low acid foods with high pH such as vegetables require higher temperature (116°C) than boiling for sterilization or destruction of bacteria. Pressure cooker can be used to obtain higher temperature.

14.1.2 Moulds

Fungi are classified into two groups that are multicellular fungi called moulds and unicellular fungi called yeast. Moulds are eumycetes or true fungi. Moulds are multicellular, filamentous fungi devoid of chlorophyll. They are strict aerobes and require oxygen for growth and multiplication. Moulds are larger than yeast and bacteria and tend to grow slowly than bacteria.

Moulds grow in the form of tangled mass or web-like structure called mycelium and spore. Mycelium is composed of filaments or branches known as hyphae. The group of hyphae is known as mycelium. Mycelium is often white and cottony and penetrates into the attacked food stuffs. Moulds produce spores which germinate under favourable conditions.

Moulds thrive best in closed, damp and dark situations with warm, moist air. Moulds require less moisture than yeast and bacteria. Acid medium favours their growth and grow over a wide range of pH (2.0–8.5). They grow very rapidly at temperature of 20–35°C and in moist atmosphere.

Moulds generally do not thrive in alkaline medium and sensitive to heat. Boiling temperature or below boiling (71–82°C) quickly destroy both moulds and their spores. Low temperature retards their growth but grow in ordinary refrigerator temperature that is 10–15°C.

Major moulds present in food and their characteristic are given in Table 14.4.

Table 14.4. Moulds and their characteristic.

Division	Moulds	Characteristic
Zygomycota	*Rhizopus* sp.	Have non-septate hyphae, asexual reproduction by sporangiospore, sexual reproduction by zygospore and rapid growth as compared to other group

	Mucor sp. (grey mould)	Known as pin mould or bread mould, has non-septate hyphae, asexual reproduction by sporangiospore
Ascomycota	*Aspergillus* sp. (black mould)	Possess septate mycelium, reproduction is by both sexual and asexual manner. Sexual reproduction by formation of ascospores and asexual reproduction by conidiospore. It does not produce off odour and flavour
	Penicillium sp. (blue mould)	Have septate mycelium, sexual reproduction by sexual spore ascospores and asexual reproduction by conidiospore. This produce mouldy odour and flavour
Dueteromycetes	*Alternaria* sp. *Botrytis* sp. *Cladosporium* sp. *Geotrichum* sp. *Trichoderma* sp.	no sexual reproductive stages are known, many of these fungi reproduce asexually by spores.

The important features of mould are hyphae (septate or non-septate), mycelium (dark or clear, coloured or colourless), sexual spores (zygospore, ascospore, oospore, basidiospore) present or not, type of asexual spore (sporangospore, conidiospore, arthrospore, blastospore and chlamydospore), spore head characteristic, sporangio features (colour, size, shape, location, spore head) and conodia features (single, change, budding, mosses, shape and arrangement of sterigma), sexual spore appearance (single or branched, type of branching, size and shape), microscopic appearance of asexual spore/conodia (colour, size, shape, smooth or rough, one or two or many celled) and special structures presence (stolons, rhizoids, foot cell, chlamydospores, sclerotin, etc.).

14.1.2.1 Moulds causing food spoilage

The important moulds cause spoilage of food are given in Table 14.5.

Table 14.5. Food spoilage moulds.

Foods	Type of spoilage	Moulds
Vegetables Onion, garlic, beans, carrot, tomato, peppers, pumpkin, cabbage	Produce grey mycelium	Botrytis cinerea
Onion, garlic, beans, turnip, carrot, radish, lettuce, cauliflower, etc.	Sour rots produces watery soft rots	*Geotrichum candidum*

Sweet potato, beans, melons, tomato, broccoli, cucumber, cauliflower, etc.	Mushi and soft vegetables with cottony growth	*Rhizopus stolonifer*
Tomato	Cottony appearance in initial stage of growth and at latter stage formed spore or conidia	*Penicillium expansum*
Potato	Discolouration, water soaked lesions formation of aerial mycelium and spores and rotting	*Fusarium oxysporum*
Fruits		
Mango	Rotting of fruit surface	*R. arrhizus*
	Black mould rot with brown black spot	*Aspergillus niger*
Banana	Soft rot or fruit rotting	*R. arrhizus*
Apples and pear	Mouldy odour and flavour	*Pe. expansum*
Oranges	Peel becomes watery with blue mycelium	*Pe. digitatum*
Grape	Formation of black spores hence called black mould	*Aspergillus* sp.
Gauva	Development of orange or dark green mycelium	*Macrophoma* sp.
Litchi	Fruit rotting	*Penicillium* sp.
Canned fruit	Disintegration	*Byssochlamys fulva*
Cereals and flour	Mouldy due to mycelial growth and spore	*Rhizopus* sp. *Aspergillus* sp.
Bread	Mouldy	*Rhizopus* sp. *Aspergillus* sp.
	Ropy	*Penicillium* sp.
Pea nuts	Toxin production	*As. flavus*
Sugar syrup	Mouldy	*Aspergillus* sp. *Penicillium* sp.
Butter	Change in colour	*G. candidum*
Eggs	Fungal rotting	*Penicillium* sp. *Cladosporium* sp. *Mucor* sp. *Alternarie* sp.
Cured meat	Mouldy	*Penicillium* sp. *Aspergillus* sp. *Rhizopus* sp.

Majority of the moulds are heat sensitive and are destroyed when heated at 60°C for half an hour. Boiling destroys mould and their spores.

14.1.3 Yeast

Yeasts are unicellular fungi which are widely distributed in nature. Yeast cells are larger than moulds and bacteria. Yeast can be differentiated from bacteria by their larger size, oval elongated spherical cell shape. Yeasts grow luxuriantly at a moderate temperature in a solution of sugar in plenty of water. Under suitable conditions, sugar is converted into alcohol and carbon dioxide gas is evolved.

Yeast + Sugar → Alcohol + Carbon dioxide

This is the reason that carbon dioxide is evolved from food materials spoiled by yeasts and pushes out corks from bottles with great force. Active fermentation can easily be identified by the formation of carbon dioxide bubbles/foam. Yeasts prefer a low concentration of sugar for their growth.

14.1.3.1 Food-borne yeast and their characteristics

Food-borne yeasts are of two types: true yeast and false yeast. True yeast belongs to division Ascomycotina. They produce ascospores and arthrospores. Reproduction takes by fission and budding. These types of yeast are *Saccharomyces*, *Pichia*, *Torulaspora*, *Debaryomyces* and *Zygosaccharomyces*.

False yeast belongs to division *Deuteromycetes*. These are fungi imperfect. Reproduction is by budding. These types of yeast are *Candida*, *Rhodotorula*, *Trichospora* and *Cryptococcus*.

The identification feature of yeast are ascospore production, spore forming yeast characterized with method of ascospore formation that is conjugation of yeast cells or without conjugation of yeast cells, appearance of ascospore (their colour size and shape and ascospore number/ascus, i.e., 1, 2, 4 or 8), vegetative cell appearance and their colour shape and size, asexual reproduction (by budding, binary fission or combined of both or arthrospore), pseudomycelium, mycelium or no mycelium production, growth through the media or film over the surface of liquid, colony colour, physiological characters such as carbon or nitrogen sources, vitamin requirement, oxidative (film yeast) or fermentative (other yeast) lypolysis and production of acid and starchy material.

14.1.3.2 Yeast causing food spoilage

Yeasts causing food spoilage are given in Table 14.6.

Table 14.6. Yeast causing food spoilage.

Yeast	Food spoilage
Brettanomyces	Beers, wines and fruits
Candida	High acid foods, salty foods, butter, fruits, ground beef and poultry
Debaryomyces	Meat, sausages, cheese and brine
Hansenula	Beers
Hanseniaspora	Fruit juices
Pichia	Wines
Rhodotorula	Meat sauerkraut, poultry products, pink kraut
Saccharomyces	Low sugar products such as fruit juices, squashes and honey
Torulopsis	Milk products, poultry products, fruit juices and acid foods
Trichosporon	Chilled beer
Zygosaccharomyces	Honey, syrup, molasses, soya sauce and wines

Yeast prefers low concentration of sugar for their growth and most of them do not develop in media or food containing 66% or more sugar or 0.55 acetic acid. Yeast grow most rapidly at temperature of 20–30°C. Boiling temperature destroys the yeast cells and spores completely.

14.1.3.3 Beneficial effects of yeast

Yeasts play an important role in food industry. The economic importance of yeast is its ability to break down carbohydrate foods into alcohol and carbon dioxide. This process is known as alcoholic fermentation. Yeast fermentation and chemical changes in which enzymes produced are important for production of foods such as bread, vinegar, beer and wines.

14.1.4 Microbial detection technique in food

Food serves as the substrate to initiate the growth of microorganisms. Microorganisms enter into food and grow as contaminants. The quality of food is affected or spoiled by the growth of microorganisms. Consumption of such infected food creates hazardous health effects in human and animal. Microbiological characteristics in the terms of microorganisms (bacteria, mould, yeast) are one of way to assess the quality of food. Therefore, it is important to identify the main types of microorganisms with their characteristic in various foods. The detection of microorganisms mainly examined for the total count of a particular type of microorganisms in particular gram weight of food. The standard microbiological techniques used for the detection of total number of microorganisms in food are as follows:

- Direct microscopic count
- Standard plate counts
- Most probable number
- Microscopic colony count
- Roll tubes
- Dry films
- Agar drop lets
- Dye reduction by methylene blue dye reduction test

14.1.5 Factors affecting microbial spoilage of food

Food is an excellent source of nutrients and microorganisms use food as the substrate for their growth and colonization. Growth of harmful microorganisms particularly bacteria and fungi in food constitutes food spoilage and sometimes cause several diseases on consumption of such food. Under favourable conditions, microorganisms grow rapidly and convert or break down food into sour, foul smell or bad flavour, covered mass of fungus and visible changes in variety of colours.

The factors influence the growth of microorganisms can be divided into two groups that is internal and external factors.

14.1.5.1 Internal factors

The most important internal factors are food or nutrient composition, pH or hydrogen ion concentration, water activity or moisture content, redox potential, inhibitory substances and physical structure of food.

14.1.5.2 Food composition

Food nutrients such as carbohydrate, fats, protein, vitamins and water are the important compounds which influence the growth and function of microorganisms.

Carbohydrates such as cellulose, hemicellulose, starch and pectin are utilized by various microorganisms. Bacterial species of genera *Streptococcus*, *Leuconostoc* and *Micrococcus* are saccharolytic and attack carbohydrates. Carbohydrates are also affected by carbohydrate-fermenting microorganisms such as yeast and moulds that produces acid, alcohol and gases. Proteins are degraded by proteolytic organisms. Bacterial species particularly spore forming gram-negative bacilli (*Pseudomonas*, *Proteus*) and few cocci degrade proteins. Sometimes anaerobic bacteria break down the protein and produce foul smelling amine compounds. The process is known as putrefactions. Spoilage by mould is also common. Protein-rich foods promote more growth of bacteria than moulds and yeasts.

Fats are digested by some microorganisms particularly moulds and some gram-negative bacteria. Fat becomes rancid due to dehydrolytic degradation to malodorous fatty acid.

Food contains different vitamins and minerals which are required by some organisms for their growth. Such microorganisms are known as fastidious organisms.

Water is one of the most important food nutrients which is required for microbial growth and chemical reaction. Foods with higher percentage of moisture deteriorate rapidly.

14.1.5.3 Hydrogen ion concentration (pH)

Influence of pH of food has effect on growth of microorganisms and processing conditions. The pH of most of the foods is generally below 7.0. Foods are classified on the basis of acid and non-acid depending on pH. Foods of acid contents or acid foods promote the growth of acid-loving microorganisms mould and yeast. Yeast can grow at pH of about 4.0–4.5 in acidic foods such as fruits, fruit juices, sauerkraut, pickles and fermented milk. Moulds grow on wider range of acidic pH.

Most of the bacteria preferred neutral or alkaline pH (7.0–7.5) for their growth in non-acid foods such as vegetables, fish, meat and milk. Some bacteria such as fermenters grow in acidic pH, whereas proteolytic bacteria can grow at higher pH. The low pH of acid foods prevents the growth of most bacterial species and such foods are spoiled by yeast and moulds. The neutral or high pH of non-acid foods is subjected to bacterial spoilage.

14.1.5.4 Water activity/moisture content

Water requirement of microorganisms is expressed as available water. Water availability is measured in terms of water activity (a_w). Water activity is defined by the ratio of water vapour pressure of food substrate to the vapour pressure of pure or distilled water at the same temperature. In other words, water activity is the vapour pressure of the solution (water in most food) divided by the vapour pressure of the solvent or pure water. This is expressed as $a_w = P/VP_o$, P is the vapour pressure of solution (water in food) and VP_o is the vapour pressure of solvent or water.

The amount of water required for growth varies with the microorganisms. The water activity of most fresh food is above 0.99. In general, bacteria require more water activity than moulds and yeast.

The lowest or minimum water activity values required for growth of spoilage microorganisms are given in Table 14.7.

Table 14.7. Minimum water activity value for growth of microorganisms.

Microorganisms	Minimum water activity value
Bacteria	0.91
Halophytic bacteria (salt loving)	0.75
Yeast	0.88
Osmophilic yeast (prefer high osmotic pressure)	0.60
Moulds	0.80
Xerophilic mould (dry loving)	0.65

The lowering of water activity below optimum is to reduce or decrease the growth rate of microorganisms.

14.1.5.5 Oxidation-reduction potential

The oxygen concentration in food and type of associated microorganisms contribute to the oxidation-reduction (OR) potential of food which affect the growth of microorganisms. The OR potential of a food expressed the way substrate loses or gains electrons. Microorganisms are classified on the basis of ability to utilize oxygen. These are called aerobes, anaerobes and facultative anaerobes.

Aerobes require free oxygen and anaerobes do not require oxygen and grow in the absence of molecular oxygen. Facultative grow in both aerobic and anaerobic conditions.

Generally mould and yeast are aerobic and bacteria are variables. Some are aerobic, some are anaerobic and some are facultative anaerobes. Aerobes grow better than anaerobes when oxidation potential is high. Anaerobes become dominant when oxygen potential reduced. Highly oxidized substrates have positive OR potential and reduced substrates have negative OR potential. The OR potential is expressed as Eh and measured in millivolts (mV).

Aerobic microorganisms such as *Bacilli*, *Pseudomonas*, *Acinetobacter* and cocci grow at positive Eh (OR) potential and anaerobic microorganisms such as clostridia and bacteriodes require negative Eh (OR potential) for their growth. Most of the fresh plant and animal foods have low redox potential due to their reducing substances such as ascorbic acid and reducing sugar (in fresh fruits and vegetables) and sulfhydryl (in animal tissue). Most of the plant- and animal-based processed food gain positive redox potential and thus promote growth of aerobic organisms.

14.1.5.6 Physical structure of food

The physical protection or natural covering of food helps to protect the inner structure from microbial contamination and spoilage. Protective covering of food such as rind or peel of the fruits and vegetables, shell on nuts, the outer shell and membrane of eggs, layers of fat over meat, skin of poultry and scale of fish prevent the entry of all microorganisms when stored under proper condition of humidity and temperature. Damaged covering of food undergo spoilage very fast.

14.1.5.7 Inhibitory substances

Presence of certain naturally occurring substances in food has antimicrobial activity and affects the stability of food against attack of spoilage organisms. Essential oil of some spices such as eugenol in cloves, cinnamic aldehyde and eugenol in cinnamon and allicin in garlic and allyl isothiocynate in mustard possess antimicrobial activity.

The antimicrobial substances of milk are lactoferrin, conglutinin and lacto peroxidase. Milk casein and fatty acids have also antimicrobial property. Lactoferrin is inhibitory to food-borne bacteria and used as microbial blocking agent on beef carcasses. Lysozyme ovotransferrin and conalbumin content of eggs have also antimicrobial activities.

14.1.5.8 External factors

The external factors which affect the growth of microorganisms are relative humidity, temperature, atmospheric, gasses, light and duration of storage.

14.1.5.9 Relative humidity

Relative humidity is the best known term for expressing the humidity of moist air. It is defined as the ratio of water vapour pressure in the air to the saturated vapour pressure at the same temperature expressed as percentage. Both high and low humidity causes spoilage of foods. In high humidity, foods take more moisture and causes growth of fungus that causes spoilage. High moisture can cause pitting, caking, off flavour, lumping, crystallization and stickyness in food. Similarly foods with low humidity loose moisture and causes shrinkage and weight loss in many foods particularly in fruits and vegetables.

14.1.5.10 Temperature

Microorganisms grow over a wide range of temperature. Microorganisms are classified into three groups on the basis of temperature range. These are given in Table 14.8

Table 14.8. Temperature range of microorganisms.

Microorganisms	Temperature range
Bacteria	
Psychrotrophic	2–30°C

Mesophilic	20–45°C
Thermophilic	55–65°C
Moulds: many moulds	At refrigerator temperature
Yeast	2–45°C

Microorganisms can grow at lowest temperature of –34°C and highest temperature of 100°C and above. The psychrotroph found most commonly on foods belong to the genera *Enterococcus* and *Pseudomonas* which grow well at refrigerator temperature and cause spoilage at 5–7°C in foods. Such as meat, poultry, eggs, fish and other foods at this temperature. Some spore-producing bacteria such as *C. tetani*, *C. perfringens* and *B. stearothermophilus* can grow above 100°C.

Heat and cold both causes spoilage. The rate of reaction doubles for every 10°C rise in temperature. Excessive heat brings protein denaturation, destruction of vitamins, breaking of emulsions and desiccation of food. Food and food products store at room temperature in warm locations spoiled easily by mesophilic and thermophilic organisms.

Sub-freezing temperature of about 7°C does not prevent multiplication of all microorganisms. Refrigerated foods are, therefore, subject to spoilage by mould, some yeast and bacteria.

14.1.5.11 Atmospheric gases

Oxygen and carbon dioxide gases affect the growth of microorganisms. Oxygen is necessary for growth of microorganisms such as moulds. Atmospheric oxygen brings undesirable changes in food such as destruction of colour, flavour and loss of vitamins A and C. Similarly excess of carbon dioxide leads to anaerobic respiration, resulting physiological disorders such as off flavours and discolouration or browning in foods. These atmospheric gases play an important role in control of microorganisms in food. Modified atmospheric packaging of foods is making use of these gases. Ozone (O_3) is another atmospheric gas which has high antimicrobial properties but it has strong oxidizing property hence, not suitable for fat-rich food that causes auto-oxidation.

14.1.5.12 Light

Light cause certain foods to undergo various undesirable changes in chemical composition. Light destroys many food colours and vitamins such as riboflavin, ascorbic acid and vitamin A.

14.1.5.13 Storage conditions and duration

Storage conditions such as temperature, relative humidity, oxygen, light and duration of storage affect microbial growth and food spoilage. Food deterioration is time dependent. The longer the storage time the greater is the deterioration except wine. Therefore, foods should be used or consumed before its quality starts deteriorating.

14.2 Enzymatic spoilage

This is also called biochemical spoilage. Enzymes are organic catalyst produced by living cells. A catalyst is a substance that changes the rate of a reaction without being used in the reaction. Enzymes are found in all fresh foods, plants and animals. Enzymes change constituent of food, for example, convert starch into sugar, protein into amino acids and pectin into pectic acids. The undesirable changes in foods by enzymes are darkening of cut surface, fermentation of soft spots and development of off flavours. Many foods contain natural enzymes such as fruits and vegetables cause enzymatic browning when damaged, peeled or cut surface exposed to air. The enzymes responsible for browning are polyphenol oxidase, phenolase and peroxidase. The action of enzymes can be easily controlled by regulating the temperature and excluding moisture and air. Enzymes can act between 0°C and 60°C and optimum temperature for reaction is 37°C. The rate varies directly with temperature. Boiling temperature destroy enzymes as in the blanching of vegetables before freezing.

14.3 Chemical spoilage

Chemical spoilage is due to the chemical reaction. These reactions are not catalyzed by enzymes in tissues or microorganisms. The example is rancidity of fat due to hydrolytic decomposition to malodourous fatty acids. Certain foods undergo to various undesirable changes in chemical composition due to atmospheric oxygen. Oxidation resulting in production of off flavours is known as non-enzymatic browning or Maillard reaction. Maillard reaction denotes a group of many complex reactions. The degradation reactions of fat, protein and carbohydrates are as follows:

Fat + Lypolytic microorganisms → Fatty acid + Glycerol

Protein + Proteolytic microorganisms → Amino acids + Amines + Ammonia + Hydrogen sulphide

Carbohydrates + Fermenting microorganisms → Acids + Alcohol + Gases

Maillard reaction or Maillard browning is responsible for discolouration of food products such as powdered, egg and powdered milk. The reaction causes loss of essential amino acids. Large number of food items loses its nutritional quality due to Maillard reaction. The factors which influence Maillard reaction are presence of oxygen, types of amino acid and sugar, protein and sugar content of food, high temperature, low water content and high pH.

Browning reaction is also due to caramelization. Sugar in dry condition when heated beyond their melting point decompose and form a brown mass called caramel which has bitter and astringent taste. The process of caramelization occurs at high temperature, whereas Maillard reaction develops brown colour at low temperature.

The reaction of incompatible substances in a food can also lead to chemical spoilage. The examples are the effects of certain metals in brewing coffee and in deep fat frying and effects of iron, copper or other impurities like high alkalinity in water used for carbonated beverages.

Moisture required for chemical reaction also causes spoilage such as lumping, caking, crystallization, pitting and stickiness and deterioration includes off-colour development.

14.4 Physical/mechanical spoilage

The changes caused by drying, burning, freezing, poor packaging material for transportation and storage of food cause spoilage of foods.

Mechanical injury caused particularly in fruits and vegetables during harvesting grading, packing, transportation and storage is the source for entrance of microorganisms that causes spoilage. Improper physical handling can result injuries due to followings factors.

1. *Abrasion*: It can occur during harvesting packing and transport. Rough containers or slackly packed containers permit the individual fruit to rob against each other or against containers surfaces and causes abrasion.
2. *Compression*: Packing more produce into little container or stacking of containers higher than their design strength cause compression damage.
3. *Impact*: Dropping of crates and bags of fruits or vegetables on a concrete floor or careless dumping of produce from containers on to retail display causes impact damage that is bruise or crack.
4. *Punctures*: Punctures are sometime caused by stem or pedicel in brinjal, cucumber, tomato, etc.
5. *Tears*: This is most common in leafy vegetables and tissue exposed lead to rapid dehydration, discolouration and decay.

The important disease which enters through injury and causing spoilage are stem end rot of mango, crown rot of banana, green and blue mould of citrus, pedicel rot of pineapple, *Rhizopus* rot of sweet potato, bacterial soft rot of potato, etc.

Careful handling during harvesting and removal of injured fruits and vegetables during grading, packaging, transport, storage and marketing and chemical protection are useful in preventing spoilage caused by physical damage or mechanical injury.

14.5 Spoilage causing insects, parasites and rodents

Insects such as food flies, borer, buges, weevils, worms, etc., damage foods, reduce nutrient content and render food unfit for human consumption. Injuries caused by insects particularly fruits and vegetables in the field and storage provide source of entry to microorganisms resulting decay. Dry fruits, dehydrated fruits and vegetables are commonly infected by insects during storage.

Insect infestations in grains, dry fruits and spices are generally controlled by fumigation with methyl bromide, ethylene oxide or propylene oxide.

Parasites can spoil foods. A worm belonging to the genus *Anisakis* occurs in some fish and if such fish is eaten raw the worm can infect man. A common parasitic infection of food is *Entamoeba histolytica* responsible for amoebic dysentery. Infected water and poor hygiene also spreads the parasite. Cooking kills most of these parasites.

Rats contribute substantially to destruction of foods in the countries where these are not controlled. A part from consuming large quantity of food they contaminate with their urine and droppings which harbour disease producing bacteria. Rat spreads human diseases such as typhus, plague, typhoid, etc.

15
Food Enzymes

Enzymes are organic biocatalysts which govern, initiate and control biological reactions important for the life process. These are produced by the living organisms and are present in very small amount in various cells. The function of body such as breathing, digestion, synthesis and break down of protein, carbohydrates and fats are catalyzed and controlled by specific enzymes. The substance upon which an enzyme acts is called substrate. The enzyme convert substrate into the product or products. There are thousands of different enzymes found in bacteria, yeast, moulds, plants and animals. Even after harvested food or slaughtered animal, most of the enzymes continue to promote specific chemical reactions and most food contain a greater number of active enzymes.

Enzymes are heat labile, soluble in water, precipitated by protein precipitating reagents (ammonium sulphate or trichloro acetic acid) and contain 16% weight nitrogen. Enzymes have an optimal pH. Broad spectrum of reaction catalyzed by enzymes are hydrolysis, polymerization, oxidation, reduction and dehydration.

15.1 Classification of enzymes

Enzymes are grouped or divided into six major classes. These are given in Table 15.1.

Table 15.1. Major classes of enzymes.

Classes	Function	Examples
Hydrolases	Hydrolysis of esters, either, peptide	Esterase, peptidase, amylase, pepsin, trypsin, chymotrypsin
Oxidoreductase	One compound oxidized and another reduced	Urease , lactic dehydrogenase , catalase , peroxidase, tyrosinase
Transferases	Transfer group containing carbon, nitrogen or sulphur from the substrate to another substrate	Transaminase, hexokinase, transacylase, transaldolase
Lyases	Addition or removal of groups without hydrolysis, oxidation or reduction, producing double bonds at times	Carboxylase, decarboxylase, carbonic anhydrase

Isomerases	Produce optical, geometric or position isomers of substrates by inter molecular rearrangement	Isomerase, epimerase, racemase, etc.
Ligases	Called synthetases and link two substrates together usually with linking of pyrophosphate bond in ATP	Glutamine synthetase and pyruvate carboxylase

15.2 Characteristics and enzyme action

15.2.1 General characteristics

4. All enzymes are protein.
5. Enzymes are true catalyst and affect the rate of reaction but not the equilibrium constant of a chemical reaction.
6. Enzymes are highly specific for their substrate
7. Enzymes form substrate complex as intermediates during their action.
8. Enzymes have enormous power for catalysis.
9. Enzymes regulate rate of metabolic process in living cells precisely so that metabolism may not proceed too fast or too slow.
10. Enzymes lower the activation energy.
11. Enzymes possess active site for interaction with substrate.

15.2.2 Enzyme action mechanisms

The enzyme molecule first combines with a substrate to form an enzyme-substrate complex. Further, dissociates to form product and enzymes back. Enzymes once dissociated from the complex is free to combine with another molecule of substrate. The site at which substrate can meet with enzymes molecule is highly specific and known as active site (catalytic site). The active site is made up of several amino acid residues.

15.3 Enzymes used in food industry

Enzymes are being used in food industry for preservation and processing of a wide variety of foods and beverages. The important industry which utilized the application of enzyme technologies are dairy industry, meat and beer processing, cheese manufacture, beverage industry, chocolate and candies, ice cream industry and soft drink industry. Application of enzymes in various foods is given in Table 15.2.

Table 15.2. Enzymes used in food industry.

Enzymes	Source	Application in food
Amylase	Fungi	Soups and liquefying purees
	Malt, fungi	Bread baking, pre-cooked baby food, breakfast food
	Bacteria, fungi	Syrup production
Takadiastase	Fungi	Bread supplements, syrup production
Invertase	Yeast	Confectionary industry, candies, high test molasses
Pectinase	Fungi	Beverage industry, juice clarification, juice concentration, coffee concentration, coffee bean fermentation, wine filtration
Glucose isomerase	Fungi	Soft drink, high fructose syrup from maize starch
Lactase	Bacteria	Milk industry: milk concentration, ice cream, frozen desserts, low lactate milk, free lactate milk
Catalase	Bacteria	Milk and milk products
Lipase	Bacteria	Cheese flavour dietetic products
Glucose oxidase	Fungi	Glucose removal Oxygen removal in cheese and milk powder
Rennin	Animal, fungi	Cheese production
Proteases: papain	Papaya fruit, Pineapple fruit	Meat industry: Meat tenderization, condensed fish, chill proof beer stabilization
Protease bromelain		

15.4 Factors affecting enzyme activity

15.4.1 Substrate concentration

There is relationship between the rate of an enzyme catalyzed reaction and the substrate concentration. The rate of enzyme catalyzed reaction is directly proportional to the substrate concentration.

15.4.2 Enzyme concentration

The rate of an enzyme catalyzed reaction is the directly proportional to the enzyme concentration. The greater is the enzyme concentration, the faster will be the reaction.

15.4.3 Temperature

Enzyme have an optimal temperature around +50°C where activity is maximum and then false at higher temperature.

15.4.4 pH

The enzyme activity or rate of enzyme catalyzed reactions is maximum or sharp at optimum pH.

15.5 Immobilized enzymes

Immobilized enzymes are defined as enzymes physically confined or localized in a certain defined region of space with retention of their activity and which can be used repeatedly and continuously. The advantages of immobilized enzyme are as follows:

- Increase stability of enzyme
- Recovery and reuse of enzyme
- Product is enzyme free
- Kinetic property of enzyme is enhanced
- Permit continuous operation
- Cost is lower
- Greater control of catalytic power

15.5.1 Immobilization technique

Large number of techniques are available for the immobilization of enzymes on a variety of synthetic and natural supports. These techniques have been classified into four groups: entrapment, covalent binding, cross-linking and adsorption.

- In entrapment techniques, biocatalysts are entrapped in natural polymers such as agar and gelatine or synthetic polymers such as photo cross-linkable resins. The development of hydrogels and thermo reactive water-soluble polymers like albumin poly (ethylene glycol) hydrogel is becoming popular.
- Covalent binding is the covalent attachment or link of enzymes to the insoluble support material (ceramic, metal glass, sephadex) or support containing an alkali amine group through Schiff's base reaction. Enzymes such as peroxidase, glucose oxidase, invertase, etc., have been immobilized using this technique.
- In cross-linking, enzymes have been generally cross-linked in the presence of inert protein, such as gelatine, collagen and albumin.

- Adsorption of enzymes on insoluble matrix by hydrophobic, electrostatic or other non-covalent affinity is the easiest technique of immobilization.

15.5.2 Factors affecting immobilization techniques

The factors which affect the immobilization techniques are as follows:

Matrix stability flow, pressure, temperature and other conditions.

- Enzymes stability during repeated use
- Retention activity of enzymes following immobilization
- Substrate accessibility to the enzymes
- Converting efficiency of substrate to the product
- System compatibility with conversion and recovery of products
- Co-factor needs
- Pure and crude enzyme compatibility for immobilization
- Susceptibility to microbial contamination
- Renewal efficiency and cost

15.5.3 Use of immobilized enzymes in food industry

The important uses of immobilized enzymes in food industry are as follows:

- Conversion of glucose syrup into high fructose syrup by the enzyme glucose isomerase
- Production of aspartic acid by the enzyme aspartase. L-aspartic acid is used in medicines and as food additives
- In dairy industry, used in preparation of lactose-hydrolyzed milk and whey by the enzyme β-galactosidase
- Immobilized enzymes are catalase, super oxide dismutase and glutathione peroxidase
- In pharmaceutical industry used in production of 6-amino penicillanic acid by the deacylation of side chain in penicillin G or V by using penicillin amidase
- Proteolytic enzymes such as subtilin, papain, ficin or bromelain which are immobilized by various techniques used for production of various flavouring compounds
- Immobilized oxidoreductases carry out synthetic transformation
- Immobilized glucose oxidase used in production of gluconic acid, removal of oxygen from beverage and removal of glucose from eggs prior to dehydration

16
Food additives

Food additives are a part and parcel of processed foods. Food additives are defined as a substance or mixture of substances other than the basic food stuff, which is present as a result of any aspects of production, processing, storage and packaging. These are various groups of chemicals added to food generally in small quantities. The substances to be used as food additive should be of good grade and must meet the standard specification. The food additives are non-nutritive substances added intentionally to food generally in small quantities to decrease the risk of contamination by certain microbe, maintain or improve nutritional quality, enhance appearance and flavours, retaining colour, increase shelf life and reduce waste. The additives may be natural or may be synthetics. The principal category of food additives are as follows.

16.1 Preservatives

Substances which are capable of inhibiting, retarding and arresting the growth of microorganism are known as preservatives. Preservatives as additives are important for preserving foods. Natural preservatives such as salt and oils are used for preserving pickles and sugar is used to preserve syrup, jam, jelly marmalade, crystallized and glazed fruit, candy and preserve. Chemical preservatives such as sodium/potassium metabisulphite (sulphur dioxide), sodium benzoate (benzoic acid), sorbic acid and acetic acid are generally used for preserving food products.

16.1.1 Sodium/potassium metabisulphite

These chemical preservatives release sulphur dioxide in the presence of acidic medium and act as antimicrobial agent. This has good preserving action against bacteria, moulds and enzymes. This is most extensively used to preserve fruit pulps, juices, squashes and cordials. Sulphiting or spray and dip prevents enzymatic browning in sliced apples, potato, carrot and minimally processed fruits and vegetables.

1. *Sodium benzoate*: Sodium benzoate is a salt of benzoic acid. Benzoic acid is the most effective agent. This has more effect against yeast than moulds. This is mostly used in coloured juices and squashes such as coloured grapes, phalsa, pomegranate, Indian blackberry,

straw berries, plum, cherries, etc., because it does not bleach the anthocyanin pigments. This is also used in tomato products.

2. *Acetic acid*: It checks aerobic and anaerobic fermentation. Acetic acid acts as a poison for microorganisms. Pickles are preserved by acetic acid.
3. *Sorbic acid*: Inhibits the growth of yeast and moulds. It is used in soft drink, sweets, yoghurt, desserts and frozen pizza.

16.1.2 Antioxidants

Antioxidants prevent oxidation of fat-containing foods and protect from rancidity. These substances should be fat soluble and effective in low concentration (0.01–0.02%). Naturally occurring antioxidants are ascorbic acid (vitamin C), vitamin E, carotene and sulphur. Citric and phosphoric acid increase the action of ascorbic acid which prevents enzymatic browning. Antioxidants generally used in foods are butylated hydroxytoluene, propyl gallate, butylated hydroxyanisole, etc. Antioxidants are used in fat-containing dehydrated fruits and vegetables such as potato chips, nuts, etc.

16.2 Colouring agents

Colour additives are pigments or substances that impart or enhance appearance of the processed, food if added. Colour additives in use are classified into certified and uncertified colours. Certified colours are synthetically manufactured and have to meet strict government regulation. Uncertified colours are generally naturally derived colour substances from fruits, vegetables and flowers sources.

16.2.1 Natural colour agents

The principal natural colours which are mostly in refined form, used as additives or permitted to be added in food products are annatto, anthocyanin, betanin, carmine, caramel, chlorophyll, curcumin, paprika, saffron, etc.

16.2.2 Annato (yellow-orange)

It is water-soluble pigments of yellow to orange colour. It is derived from seeds of the *Bixa orellana* (tropical bush). The pigments in annato are a mixture of bixin (monomethyl ester of a dicarboxylic carotenoid compound) and/or bixin (dicarboxylic derivative of same caroetnoid bixin). It is used in fruit beverage such as syrup, squash, juices and other beverages. It is also used in biscuits, ice-cream, snack food, waffers, sugar confectionary, cakes, sweet, fish and meat products.

16.2.3 Anthocyanins (red purple)

Anthocyanin is water-soluble pigment which gives purple, red and blue colour. Anthocyanin is obtained from variety of flowers, fruits and vegetables such as red/blue grapes, apples strawberry, cherries, raspberries, black currents, *jamun* and red cabbage. It is used in soft drinks and wines. It is also used in preserves, dessert, frozen products, vinegar, confectionery and dairy products.

16.2.4 Betalaines (beetroot red)

Betalaines resemble the anthocyanin and flavonoids in structure but unlike them contain nitrogen. Red violet betacyanins and yellow betaxanthins are water soluble. Betalaines are group of red and yellow pigments. It is obtained from red beetroot (*Beta vulgaris*) and to some extent from cactus fruits, pokeberries and number of flowers particularly *Bougainvillea.* It is used in ice-cream, sugar confectionary and yogurt.

16.2.5 Caramel

It is complex polysaccharides of unidentified chemical structure. It is obtained by heating a food grade carbohydrate such as glucose, fructose or starch in presence of catalyst – acetic sulphurous or citric acid or bases such as ammonium, calcium and sodium hydroxide.

16.2.6 Cochineal (carmine)

Cochineal refers to red colouring matter. Carminic acid is the colourant in cochineal. It is extracted from the dried crushed bodies of female *Dactylopius coccus* just prior to egg laying time. Pigments constitute 22% of their dry weight. Carmine is used in powder form to colour a variety of food.

16.2.7 Chlorophyll

This is fat-soluble pigment responsible for green colour. This is obtained from leafy vegetables such as cabbage, lettuce, spinach, etc.

16.2.8 Carotenoids

Carotenoids are widely distributed in nature. It is fat-soluble orange-yellow pigments. The first carotenoid was isolated from carrot and named carotene.

The most widely distributed carotenoids are lutein, violaxanthin and neoxanthin. Lutein is obtained from extract of marigold. It is mainly used in the fortification of xanthophylls in lemon-flavoured soft drinks and confectionery products. Violaxanthin and neoxanthin are found in green leaves.

The most commercial carotenoid is β-carotene which is also an oil-soluble colour and extracted from various vegetables and fruit sources such as carrot, pumpkin, mango, orange, palm oil, etc. It is mainly used in pharmaceutical and health food industry.

16.2.9 Saffron

Crocetin a dicarboxylic carotenoid found in saffron together with digestion bioside ester crocin. Saffron provides both colour and flavour. Saffron is obtained from stigma of the flowers *Crocus sativus*. It is used in various food products.

16.2.10 Paprica

The orange red colour powder has distinctive flavour. This is obtained from extract of paprika. It is mainly used in meat, sauces and soup.

16.2.11 Curcumin (yellow)

This is yellow pigment obtained from rhizome of turmeric plant (*Curcuma longa*). It contains about 1.5% of curcumin as principle colourant. It is insoluble in water; hence, it is converted into convenient form. It is dissolved in food grade solvents and permitted emulsifiers. Polysorbate 80 is normally used as career for curcumin.

16.2.12 Synthetic colours

Synthetic colour is generally better in colouring power, colour uniformity, colour stability and cost. More over natural colour is difficult to extract. The synthetic colours permitted by act to use in food are red (carmosine, ponceau 4R, erythrosine), yellow (tartrazine, sunset yellow FCF), blue (indigo carmine, brilliant blue FCF) and green (fast green S, green FCF). These colours permitted to use in flavoured milk, ice-cream mix powder, frozen desserts, yogurt, non-alcoholic, carbonated and non-carbonated RTS beverages including syrup, fruit bar, food beverage or drink, synthetic soft drink, concentrate, biscuit waffer, pastries, cakes, confectionery, sweets, papad, canned product of peas, strawberries, cherries which are hermetically sealed containers, preserved candy, jam, jelly, marmalade crystallized, glazed fruits, fruit squash and cordials.

Although colours enhance attractiveness or appearance of food products, it is better to avoid their use as for as possible and educate the consumers to use products not containing colourants. Colour can often be used to cover defects in natural products.

16.3 Flavouring agents

Flavouring agents are responsible for the flavour of foods. These substances are naturally occurring or synthetic. Flavouring agents of natural origin are spices, herbs, root, leaves, stem and flower extracts of plant. These are widely used as flavouring agents. The naturally occurring substances mainly responsible for aroma of food products are volatile compounds which include esters, aldehyde, ketones, hydrocarbons, acetate, alcohol, etc. These substances present in small amount and they are characteristics of each fruits and vegetables. Some of the important volatile compounds are ethyl acetate, contribute aroma to pineapple, pentyl acetate to banana, octy acetate to orange, ethyle-2, methyl butyrate and pentyl valerate to apple, limone to citrus fruit, geraniol and methyl salicylate to grape, methyl and ethyle ester to pear, linalool to papaya, ethyle butyrate to strawberry, benzaldehyde to almond, cherries and peaches, thymol to tangerine cinnamyl acetate to guava, geosmin to beetroot and dry beans, allicin to garlic, 1- octen-3-ol to mushroom, dimethyl sulphide to onion, *S*-methyl cysteine sulphoxide to cabbage and cauliflower and acetaldehyde to butter.

Essential oils and synthetic substances which may or may not occur in nature are used to confectionary, non-alcoholic beverages and other food products. The examples of these are acetyl methyl carbinol, which contribute to flavour of butter, citral to orange, eugenol to clove, vanillin to vanilla and limonene to lemon. Flavouring agents of natural origin such as extracts and essential oil are very costly and sometime difficult to isolate; hence, these substances are being replaced by synthetic ones.

16.3.1 Flavour enhancers

A closely related group of additives to flavouring agents are called flavour enhancers. The function of enhancers is supplement, enhance or modify the original flavour or aroma of a food without contributing flavours of their own. The best known enhancer is mono sodium glutamate (MSG) used in Chinese cookery and beverage. Ajinomoto is a Japanese brand name for MSG. The MSG content of some commonly eaten foods are 50–80 g/kg dehydrated soup powder, 1–3 g/kg canned, 4.5 g/kg processed cheese, 1.3 g/kg ketchup, 2.5 g/kg meat and 1.3 g/kg fish. This is the maximum level of MSG in these foods. MSG is the sodium salt of the amino acid, glutamic acid. It is an extract from Japanese sea weed and Japan has used this for centuries in food.

It is believed to stimulate the taste and enhancing perception of the flavour. Today MSG is made by fermentation process using starch, sugar beets, sugarcane or molasses. It is sold as fine white crystalline substance.

16.3.2 Emulsifiers

These are also known as surface-active agents. These are used for stabilization of oil in water or water in oil and gas in solid or in liquid emulsions. They provide surface wetting and viscosity change. Lecithin is a naturally occurring emulsifier used in chocolate making.

Synthetic emulsifier is a defoaming compound. Monoglycerides, diglycerides, some fatty acids and their derivatives used in ice-cream and confectionery. Acelated monoglyceride is used in pizza.

16.3.3 Stabilizers and thickeners

These substances used in chocolate milk drinks, puddings, baked products and jellies which inhibit crystallization of sugar, stabilize emulsions and foam, reduce stickiness and improve texture of the foods. Some of these are pectin, gelatine, amylose, alginic acid, starch, etc.

16.3.4 Chelating agents

This is also called sequestrants or metal scavengers. Chelating agents are used to suppress the action of some objectionable but practically unavoidable ingredients. For example, in the manufacture of the soft drinks, iron in water reacts with one of the flavouring substances to form an insoluble compound which makes the product cloudy. Citrates form a soluble complex with iron, whereas others give citric acid insoluble. These objectionable ingredients are removed. Chelating agents such as ethylene diamine tetra acetic acid (EDTA), polyphosphates or citric acid, calcium and sodium salts of organic acid, calcium chloride, calcium phosphate and tartaric acid are also examples of chelating agents. The chelating agents are used to remove discolouration, rancidity, turbidity and flavour changes in foods.

16.3.5 Acids and alkalis

Acids and alkali additives are used to adjust pH of the foods. These also affect flavour and texture. Acid in food is a natural constituent in fruits or produced by fermentation. Certain chemicals such as calcium citrate, calcium carbonate, citric acid, acetic acid, lactic acid, malic acid, sodium acetate and tartaric acid are used to adjust pH.

16.3.6 Nutrients

To restoration of losses in processed food and to provide better nutritional value, some nutrients particularly vitamins and minerals are added. The examples of these are vitamin A added to margarine, vitamin B and minerals (iron and calcium) to cereal products, vitamin C to fruit juices, vitamin D to milk and iodine to salt.

16.4 Dietary sweeteners

Various sweetening agents have been used as substitutes for cane sugar (sucrose). Sweeteners may be non-nutritive and nutritive.

16.4.1 Non-nutritive sweeteners

Non-nutritive sweeteners are mostly used in manufacture of soft drinks. They are also added to low caloric liquid foods, canned fruit and frozen desserts. Non-nutritive sweeteners provide less than 2% of caloric value of sucrose per equivalent unit of sweetening capacity when used to sweeten foods. These are aspartame and saccharin synthetic sweetening agents.

Aspartame is a white, odourless, crystalline powder that has sugar-like taste. It has sweetness potency 180–200 times to that of sucrose. It is made by combination of two amino acids aspartic acid and phenylalanine and adding methyl alcohol to form a methyl ester. Aspartame also enhances fruity flavour. It is used in soft drinks. It is allowed daily intake of 40 mg/kg body weight by FAO and WHO.

Saccharin is the first synthetic sweetening agent. It is sodium or calcium salt of orthobenzene sulphonamide which is 300 times sweeter than sucrose. It has bitter and unpleasant after-taste. It has toxic effect and consumption of saccharin has been prohibited by the Government of India.

Acelsulphame-K is synthetic derivative of acetoacetic acid and soluble in water. Acelsulphame-K, the potassium salt of acelsulphame is 200 times sweeter than 3% sucrose solution. The United States approved this compound for use as a table sweetener and in dry beverage mixes, instant coffee and tea.

16.4.2 Nutritive sweeteners

Nutritive sweeteners, provide greater than 2% of the caloric value of sucrose per equivalent unit of sweetening capacity when used to sweeten the foods. Sorbitol, mannitol and polyols are the examples of nutritive sweeteners.

Sorbitol is produced by hydrogenation of glucose sugar. It is low caloric sweeteners. Sorbitol is used in dietetic and diabetic food. Mannitol is used in sugar-free chewing gum. Xylitol is used in drinks. Polyols occur in nature but they are synthesized on industrial scale from carbohydrates such as starch, sucrose, glucose, invert sugar, xylose and lactose. Sugar alcohols such as xylitol, sorbitol, mannitol, lactitol and isomalt are known as polyols which are white crystalline.

16.4.3 Natural non-caloric sweeteners

Non-sugar sweeteners help to control weight and made it possible for diabetic to enjoy food. The natural non-caloric sweeteners are neohesperidin dihydrochalcone, glycyrrhizin, thaumatin, stevia, etc.

Neohesperidin dihydrochalcone isolated from citrus peels. This is about 400–600 times as sweet as sucrose. Glycyrrhizin is obtained from roots of European leguminous plant *Glycyrrhiza glabra* (*licorice*). It is used in beverage and confectioneries. Thaumatin comes from West African fruit plant. It is 2500–3000 times sweeter than sugar. It is used in United Kingdom and Japan.

Stevia comes from sweet herbs botanically known as *Stevia rebaudiana.* It is a native of Paraguay and is widely distributed in the United States, Brazil, Japan, Korea, Taiwan and South East Asia. The plant is a perennial herb growing up to the height of 45 cm. Stevia is a calorie-free bio-sweeteners. The sweet leaf herb is a natural sweetener replacing the chemical sweeteners and even table sugar. Thus sweetening in leaf is due to stevioside and leaf by itself is 20–30 times sweeter than sugar. Stevioside is 100 times sweeter than sucrose. Stevia leaf powder is used for sweetening. About 50 g of stevia leaf powder is equal to 1000 g of cane sugar. The sweetening of stevia is non-fermenting and causes no browning on heating. The beverage industry can blend stevia leafs with tea and coffee. Stevia also possesses antifungal and antibacterial property. Stevia is a potential alternative source for replacing artificial sweeteners like aspartame, saccharin and acelsulphame-K. Stevia is a calorie free and safe and time tasted wonder of nature. Government of India and many other countries support and approved the safety of stevia.

16.5 Other additives

16.5.1 Anticaking agents

These agents prevent food particles from adhering to each other. These substances absorb excess moisture by coating the food particle to act as water repellent as well as diluting the mixture with insoluble particles. Anticaking agents used are calcium silicate, tricalcium phosphate, magnesium carbonate and magnesium silicate. Calcium stearate the salt of calcium and magnesium of fatty acid is used as conditioning agents for dehydrated vegetables.

16.5.2 Bleaching and maturing agents

These are also known as improvers and starch modifiers. Oxidizing agents such as hydrogen peroxide are used to whiten the colour of milk for manufacture of certain kind of cheese. Bromate and iodate are used in bread dough for improving baking quality. Sodium hypochlorite as starch modifiers is used to oxidize starches to increase their water solubility.

16.5.3 Firming and clarifying agents

Firming agents are added to keep the tissues of fruits and vegetables crisp or firm. The examples of the firming agents are calcium chloride and aluminium sulphate.

Clarifying agents are used to remove haziness or sediment produced by oxidative deterioration in fruit juices, wines, beer, etc. Bentonite, gelatine and synthetic resins are the examples of clarifying agents.

16.5.4 Enzymes

Some enzymes such as rennin are used for producing cheese and curd, and papain is used for tenderizing meat and pectinase is use for clarifying beverages.

16.6 Safety aspects of additives

16.6.1 Prohibited additives in food

Brominated vegetable oil, calamus, cobalt salt and their derivatives, coumarin, cyclamate, dulcin, monochloroacetic acid, safrole and thiourea.

16.6.2 Banded colour additives

Acid magenta 11, blue VRS, Brilliant black, red FB and red 6B.

16.6.3 Additives used with caution

Caution is required even in using some of the permitted food additives that causes adverse effects. These additives are as follows:

- Coal tar dyes are used as colourant in vegetable and food products, soft drinks, candy, desserts, pastry, sausage, baked food, ice-cream, hot dogs and burgers. The adverse effects are allergic reaction, cancer and pathological lesions in vital organs.

- Butylated hydroxyl toluene (BHT) is used in potato chips, edible oil, antioxidants in cereals and chewing gum. Possible adverse effects are cancer and allergic reactions.
- Butylated hydroxyanisole is used in potato chips, edible oils, antioxidants in cereals and chewing gum. It is safer than BHT but required more in information.
- Caffeine used as stimulants in soft drinks causes insomnia and other adverse effects at high levels of intake. It is not recommended for children and pregnant mothers.
- Saccharin non-calorie sweetener in food products causes bladder cancer in animals. It is not recommended for normal people (not suffering from diabetes and obesity).
- Sodium nitrite and nitrate used as preservative to prevent growth of *Bacillus*, *Clostridium botulinum* and colourant for bacon, ham, meat, smoked fish. Forms small amount of cancer-producing nitrosamines.
- Artificial flavouring agents used in soft drinks, breakfast cereals, vegetables and food products, ice-cream, custard and alcoholic beverages. Adverse effect is hyperactivity in some children.
- MSG used in soup, poultry meat preparation, sauces and cheese as flavour enhancer. It damage brain cells in infant so not recommended for children. It also causes headache, tightness of head, neck and arms in adults.
- Sulphur dioxide and bisulphate used as preservative for wine, grape juice, dried potato, dry fruits, vegetables and sliced fruits. It destroys vitamin B_1 but safe at prescribed level.
- Phosphoric acid and phosphates used as acidifier, chelating agents, emulsifier, discoloration inhibitor in cheese, cured meat, soft drinks and dried potato. Prolonged use causes osteoporosis or bone thinning.
- Talc and kaolin used in making dry powdery foods, dusting agents for rice, confectionery and chewing gum. It is stored in vital organ and causes cancer.

16.6.4 Situations where food additives should be avoided

- In baby food and invalid food
- Masking spoilage or bad quality of food (deceiving consumer)
- Removing defects in handling and processing
- Making food attractive and appealing at the cost of nutritional quality and safety
- Obtaining desire effects instead of using improved processing technique
- As oxidizing agents that modify the nutrients in food and affect the health of consumer

17

Food preservation

Food preservation is defined as the science that deals with the process of preventing spoilage of food or food products to be stored in a good condition for future consumption. In other words, the measures that can be adopted or used to keep food healthy and normal for longer period of time is called preservation. Foods are preserved for various reasons which are as follows:

- Reducing post-harvest losses by consuming surplus produce for value addition
- Availability of seasonal food throughout the year
- Obtaining stable income
- Adding variety to the diet and meat dietary requirement
- Saving time by reducing preservation time
- Ensuring intensive protection
- Providing employment opportunities
- Establishing agro-based industries

17.1 Principles of preservation

The principles involved in food preservation are as follows.

1. Prevention or delay of microbial decomposition by
   - Hindering microbial growth and activity – chemicals, low temperature, antibiotics, drying, anaerobic conditions
   - Keeping out microorganisms – asepsis
   - Removal of microorganisms – filtration
   - Killing the microorganisms - heat and radiation
2. Prevention or delay of self-decomposition of food by
   - Destruction or inactivation of food enzymes - branching
   - Preventing or delaying of chemical reaction – oxidation by antioxidant

17.2 Methods of food preservation

Methods of food preservation are asepsis, thermal or high heat preservation, low temperature preservation, drying and dehydration, classical methods, food additives, fermentation, carbonation and non-thermal methods.

17.2.1 Asepsis

Absence of infection or preventing the entry of microorganisms is called asepsis. Maintaining general cleaning during handling such as harvesting, grading, packing, processing and transport reduces the number of organisms considerably and increases their keeping quality. Packaging of food widely used application of asepsis. The covering prevents primary contamination during handling and to the hermetically sealed containers of canned foods. This protects the processed contents from contamination by microorganisms.

17.2.2 Thermal or high heat preservation

This is most widely used method of preservation of different products. Most bacteria yeast and moulds grow best in the temperature range of 16–38°C. Most bacteria are killed in the range of 82–93°C but many bacteria in the form of spores are not destroyed even at boiling temperature of water for half an hour. Hence, higher temperature is needed under pressure to destroy bacterial spores. Foods in high acid content increase the killing power of heat. A temperature of 93°C for 15 min may be enough to sterilize food in presence of acid. High temperature used for preservation are generally pasteurization temperature (bellow 100°C) and sterilization temperature (100°C or above).

17.2.2.1 Pasteurization

Pasteurization refers to heat treatment below 100°C to kill part but not all microorganisms present. The primary objectives of pasteurization are to kill pathogenic microorganisms and inactivate enzymes. There are three methods of pasteurization: (i) bottle pasteurization commonly used for preserving fruit juices; (ii) overflow method in which juice is heated to a temperature about 2.5°C higher than the pasteurization temperature; and (iii) flash pasteurization in which juice is heated rapidly to a temperature of about 5.5°C higher than pasteurization temperature and kept at this temperature for about a minute.

The advantages of the technique are enzyme inactivation, destroy microorganisms and simple and efficient operation. Loss of heat-sensitive nutrients and high cost of processing are the disadvantage of the technique.

17.2.2.2 Sterilization

Sterilization refers to heat treatment at or above 100°C to kill or destroy all viable organisms. The time and temperature required for sterilization vary with the type of food. Acid fruit and vegetable products require sterilization at 100°C for 30 min. Non-acidic vegetables such as green peas, beans, okra, etc., require higher temperature (116°C) for 30–90 min to kill the spore forming organisms.

Thermal preservation is applied in various food preservation techniques, including canning, bottling, aseptic packaging, etc.

1. *Canning*

Canning is defined as heating and sealing of food material in a hermetically sealed container. The cans used are known as open top sanitary cans or three peace cans. The cans are made of steel-plate-coated tin. Electrolyte-coated tin cans are generally used for fruit and vegetable preservation such as mango pulp and slices, guava pulp, pineapple slices, orange juice, cherries, apricot, litchi, tomato juice, puree, paste, green peas, beans, mushroom, etc., canning is also used for other products such as meat and fish.

The unit operations of canning fruits and vegetables consist of selection of fruits and vegetables → sorting/grading → washing → peeling/cutting → weighing → blanching (vegetables) → filling into cans → syruping (fruits) or brining (vegetables) → exhausting → sealing → processing (fruits) or sterilizing (vegetables) → cooling → labelling → storage

2. *Bottling*

In bottling, glass bottles are used as containers. Fruit-based beverages, such as fruit juices, ready to serve beverages and nectar prepared from mango, pineapple, litchi, orange, guava, apple, lime, bael, papaya, etc., are most popular bottled products. Beverages are pasteurized, bottled and crown corked. Fruit-based juices and ready to serve beverages are also packed in tetra pack containers using the aseptic process. The consumer packs ranging from 200 mL to 1 L have a place in the market.

3. *Aseptic packaging*

It is high temperature short-time heat processing. The product and packaging materials both are sterilized separately and filled in aseptic atmosphere. The temperature ranges from 90°C to 110°C for acidic products having pH 4.6 or less and 121°C for low acid foods having pH more than 4.6. Aseptic packaging of processed fruit and vegetable products are increasing and it may replace the canning in near future. The aseptic process has many advantages as the heating process is short. The unit operations are also less as compared to canning. The aseptic processing involves sterilization, holding, cooling, sterilizing of packing material, feeling and sealing. Fruits, juices, RTS beverages, pulps, concentrate, wine, etc. are packed using the aseptic technology.

17.2.3 Low temperature preservation

Low temperature can be produced by refrigeration and freezing. Refrigeration or chilling temperature (0–5°C) maintained by means of ice or mechanical refrigeration. The best storage temperature for many foods is slightly above 0°C but varies with the product. Fruits, vegetables and their products can be preserved for few days to many weeks. Refrigeration slow down microbial growth and autolysis of enzymes. This also retains the nutrient of the products.

Freezing is a low temperature preservation process in which product is frozen at –40°C and stored at –20°C. Freezing prevents microbial growth by low temperature and unavailability of water. Frozen products are closer to fresh products and increases shelf life of products for a longer time. It is energy intensive process and causes loss of some B group vitamins and vitamin C during blanching of vegetables prior to freezing. There are various methods of freezing such as plate freezing, blast freezing, quick freezing and dehydro freezing.

In plate freezing, food products are placed in contact with a cold surface. This process is suitable for freezing of packaged products.

Blast freezing refers to vigorous circulation of cold air for freezing the product or cold air is blown a cross the food. The air temperature is about –18°C to –30°C or even lower. This process is cheapest and variety of sizes and shapes can be accommodated.

Individual quick freezing involves the fluidization of the product in the freezing and circulating cold air at –40°C. The advantages of quick freezing are better retention of sensory quality, texture and reconstitution properties due to quick freezing. Large quantity of food can be frozen in a short period of time.

Dehydro freezing consists of drying the food to about 50% of its original weight and volume and then freezing the food to preserve it. The cost in packaging, freezing, storing and shipping is less due to weight and volume saving.

Frozen foods are vegetables, fruits, meat and poultry. Vegetables which can be frozen are peas, beans, carrot, cauliflower, mixed vegetables, minimally processed products, curries, gravies and soups. Fruits which are suitably frozen are mango slices and pulp, guava pieces, orange segments, pineapple rings, etc. Meats, poultry and fishes are also preserved by freezing.

17.2.4 Drying and dehydration

Foods can be preserved successfully by removal of moisture either by sun's heat or by heated air. Sun drying is a removal of moisture from foods by exposure to sun's rays. Dehydration involves moisture removal by artificially produced heat under controlled conditions of temperature, relative humidity and air flow. Fruits are either sun dried or dehydrated. Vegetables are generally dehydrated. Other foods, such as meat, fish, etc., are dried by other methods such as freeze drying. Drying and dehydration reduced the bulk, require less storage space and is usually cheaper than other methods of preservation.

17.2.4.1 Sun drying

Large quantities of fruits are sun dried in tropical and subtropical regions. Fruits suitable for sun drying are raw mango, ripe mango, grape, date, fig, apricot, pears, peaches, prunes, litchi, ber, etc. The process involves in sun drying of fruits are selection of fruits → washing → peeling → preparation or cutting/coring/pitting → traying → sulphuring → drying in drying yard (10-20% moisture) → sweating (dried fruits stacked in boxes to equalize moisture) → packing → storage.

Sun drying has certain limitations such as seasonal variation, exposing to dust insects, loss of some nutrients and require large area for drying.

17.2.4.2 Dehydration

Both fruits and vegetables can be dehydrated. Dehydration is an operation in which both heat transfer and mass transfer take place. Heat is transferred from carrier gas (air) to the product and water in it is vaporized. The water vapour is removed by carrier gas. Commercial drying is carried out by hot air drying with the dryers. The dryers are continuous or batch type where hot air at a pre-set temperature is blown over the material to be dried. The modern drying technologies such as vacuum shelf drying, freeze drying and fluidized drying are used for specific products. Dehydration is much more, faster, done in hygienic condition and products have uniform colour than sun dried.

The major dehydrated fruits and fruit products are apple, apricot, banana, grape, litchi, pineapple, dates, raw mango powder and fruit candies. The process involved in dehydration of fruits of selection is fruits → washing → peeling → cutting → sulphuring → drying → packing → storage at ambient temperature.

The major dehydrated vegetables and their products are green peas, beans, cabbage, cauliflower, bitter gourd, red chilies, okra, leafy vegetables, onions, garlic, ginger, sweet potato, potato, etc.

The process involves in vegetable dehydration are selection of vegetables → washing → peeling or preparation → pre-treatment or blanching → sulphating → traying → drying → packaging. Some vegetables such as tomato, sweet potato, onion and garlic do not require blanching. High quality dehydrated vegetables find wide application in products like soup powder and extruded foods.

Freeze drying involves removal of water by sublimation. Relatively labile foods such as flesh food (meat, chicken, fish and sea foods) and some vegetables and fruits are freeze dried. Freeze dried fruits retain their original shape, texture, flavour and reconstitute quality.

The type of dryers used for drying is governed by the nature of product to be dried, form of finished products, economic and operating conditions. Driers used for various products are given in Table 17.1.

Table 17.1. Driers used for drying various foods.

Foods	Drier
Foods and vegetables	Cabinet, tunnel kiln and continuous belt dryer
Fruit juice, powder, soups and malted beverage	Continuous vacuum belt drier and vacuum shelf drier
Fruit pulp, fruit-based cereals flakes, milk and custard powder	Drum drier
Meat, fish and sea foods	Freeze drier
Egg pulp and milk	Spray drier
Meat products not used as food products	Rotary drier

17.2.5 Classical methods of preservation

Some foods preserved by classical and old procedure. These methods of preservation are with high concentration of sugar, pickling, curing and smoking.

17.2.5.1 High concentration of sugar

Foods such as jam, jellies, marmalade, preserve, candies, crystallized, glazed, syrup and sweetened condensed milk are preserved by high concentration of sugar. The principles involved for preservation is osmosis. Water is withdrawn from microbial cells when they are placed in high concentration or sugar. As a result of this water loss, microbial growth is inhibited.

Jam is a product prepared by boiling fruit pulp with adequate quantity of sugar to a gelatinizing consistency. It should contain not less than 68.5% total soluble solids. Jams can be prepared from mango, pineapple, strawberry, apple, Indian gooseberry, pear, apricot, etc.

Jelly is a product prepared by boiling a clear strained fruit juice with adequate quantity of sugar to a thick consistency. For proper jelly formation, pectin (1%) and acid (3.2 pH) are in important jelly contains 67.5% total soluble solids. Jelly can be prepared from guava, karonda, apple (sour), jamun (gooseberry), wood apple, etc.

Marmalade is a fruit jelly in which peels are suspended. Marmalade has also at least 67% sugar. This is generally prepared from citrus fruit.

Preserve is mature fruit or vegetable pieces impregnated with sugar syrup till it becomes tender and transparent. Sugar syrup should have 68–70% concentration. Suitable fruits for preserve making are Indian gooseberry, bael, karonda, ber, etc. and vegetables such as ash gourd, carrot, etc.

In candy, whole fruits or as pieces impregnated with sugar syrup and subsequently drained and dried. The total sugar content of candy is not less than 70%. Candied fruit can be prepared from Indian gooseberry, ber, karonda, carambola, citrus peels, etc. Candy also can be prepared from ash gourd, carrot and ginger.

Glazed and crystallized fruits have also 70% and above sugar for their preservation. A candied fruit dipped for a moment in boiling sugar syrup to impart a glossy finish, drained and dried is called glazed fruit. The fruits which are suitable for candy are also suitable for making glazed fruits.

Fruit syrup containing 66% are more sugar does not ferment. Suitable fruits for making syrup are lime, lemon, orange, pomegranate, phalsa, etc. Sweeten condensed milk having 70% solids is also preserved by sugar. The product is given slight heat treatment and is not sterilized.

17.2.5.2 Pickling

Pickle is one of the most ancient methods of preserving food. Pickling is a process of preserving fruits and vegetables in common salt or brine. In salt pickle, the percentage of salt varies from 12 to 20. Salt or brine used as curing material improves their texture and flavour and induces translucency. The preservative action of salt is due to high osmotic pressure resulting in the plasmolysis of microbial cells. Pickles are prepared from various fruits such as lime, lemon, mango, Indian gooseberry, karonda, jackfruit, etc. and vegetables such as chilies, cucumber, garlic, ginger and mixed vegetable pickle. Pickles are also preserved by oil and vinegar. In India, mustard, rapeseed and sesame oils are generally used for preserving fruit and vegetables pickles. Oils on surface of pickles, creates anaerobic condition which prevents the growth of microorganism.

17.2.5.3 Curing

Curing is an important method of preserving animal flesh. Meat preservation may be accomplished by dry curing or with pickling solution. The curing agents permitted are sodium chloride, sugar, sodium nitrate, sodium nitrite and vinegar.

17.2.5.4 Smoking

Smoke is commonly obtained by burning the wood preferably of hard wood such as hickory, oak, maple, birch, walnut and mahogany. Smoke contains preservative chemicals such as small amount of formaldehyde, aldehyde, formic acid, acetic acid, etc. These chemicals are unfavourable to the growth of microorganisms. It is also the heat associated with the smoke kills the microorganisms and at the same time dries out the food contributing to preservation. Smoking over a fire is quite effective in preserving foods such as meat and fish. These are smoked after curing.

17.2.6 Preservation with food additives

Food additives are defined as a substance or mixture of substances other than basic food stuffs. It may be chemical preservatives, antibiotics, antioxidant and mould inhibitors.

17.2.6.1 Chemical preservatives

Preservative is defined as any substance which is capable of inhibiting, retarding or arresting the growth of microorganisms. Chemical preservative interfere with cell membrane of the microorganisms and their enzymes. These are added in processed foods. The important chemical preservative permitted in foods are sulphur dioxide and its salt potassium or sodium meta bisulphite, benzoic acid or its salt sodium benzoate, sorbic acid and acetic acid.

Sodium/potassium metabisulphite release sulphur dioxide in presence of acidic medium and act as an antimicrobial agent. This has good preserving action against bacteria, moulds, yeast and enzymes. This is most extensively used to preserve fruit, pulps, juices, ready to serve beverage, squash and cordials. Sulphiting or spray and dip prevent enzymatic browning in pre-sliced apple, potato, carrot and minimally processed fruit and vegetable. Sulphites are not used with anthocyanin pigments, as they discolourize it. Hence, in coloured grape juice, phalsa, jamun, plum, pomegranate sodium or potassium metabisulphite are not used. The permitted level of sulphur dioxide (SO_2) in various fruits is given in Table 17.2.

Table 17.2. Permitted level of SO_2 in foods.

Food production	SO_2 level mg/kg
Fruit pulp, juice, dry fruits, dry ginger, dehydrated vegetables	2000
Fruit juice concentrate and dried soups	1500
Gelatine	1000
Squash, crush, cordials, barley water	350
Ready to serve beverage	70
Cider	200
Alcoholic wines, corn syrup	450
Corn flour/starch, pickles	100

Sodium benzoate is preferred over benzoic acid because of its solubility in water. Sodium benzoate is nearly 170 times soluble as compared to benzoic acid. It is odourless and colourless. This is useful against many spoilage bacteria, mould and yeast. It is most effective against yeast than mould. The mode of action is due to interference with genetic mechanism, affects cell membrane permeability and interferes with enzyme system by inactivating active site. This is mostly used in coloured fruit beverages such as coloured grapes, pomegranate, cherry, jamun, phalsa, plum, strawberries, etc., because it does not bleach the anthocyanin pigment. This is also used in potato products. The permitted level of sodium benzoate in food products is given in Table 17.3.

Table 17.3. Permitted level of benzoic acid in foods.

Foods products	Benzoate (mg/kg)
Fruit squashes with anthocyanin pigments	600
Ready to serve beverage with anthocyanin pigments	120
Pickles and chutney	250
Tomato paste and puree	250
Tomato sauce	750
Jam jelly marmalade and preserve	200

The quantity of sodium benzoate required is dependent on pH. Fruit juices and beverages having pH of 3.5–4.0 can be preserved with 0.06–0.1%. In less acid foods, higher concentration is required. Benzoates in excess of 0.1% may impart a disagreeable peppery or burning taste to the foods particularly to fruit juices.

17.2.6.2 Sorbic acid

It is an organic acid and generally considered non-toxic acid. Sorbic acid and its salt are tasteless and odourless. Sorbate (potassium sorbate) is used for mould and yeast inhibition in a variety of foods. Its reasonable level is less than 0.3% for antimicrobial activity. They provide antimicrobial activity up to pH 6.5. It is used in jam, fruit syrup, soft drink, sweet pickle, sweets, deserts, yoghurt, frozen pizza, etc.

17.2.6.3 Acetic acid

Acetic acid is a general preservative inhibits many species of bacteria, yeast and to some extent of moulds. Acetic acid checks aerobic and anaerobic fermentation and acts as a poison for microorganisms. About 2% acetic acid is enough to prevent the spoilage. The main application of acetic acid is in products such as pickle, sauces, ketchup, cheese, meat, fish, etc. The keeping quality of vinegar depends upon the presence of acetic acid.

17.2.6.4 Antibiotics

Antibiotics are chemical substances produced by microorganisms which have the capacity of inhibiting growth or destroying microorganisms. Application of antibiotics is well-known in medicines. Some antibiotics such as nisin and subtelin are used in preserving foods.

Nisin produced by *Streptococcus lactis* is non-toxic and has no adverse effects on sensory qualities of foods. Nisin suppresses the growth of spoilage organisms particularly gas-producing spore-forming bacteria and toxin-producing bacteria (*Clostridium botulinum*). This is commonly used in canning of mushroom, tomatoes and milk product such as cheese.

Subtelin and antibiotic obtained from strains *Bacillus subtilis.* It is effective against gram-positive bacteria and spore-forming organisms. This is used in canning of asparagus, peas, corn and tomato. Canned peas and tomato containing 10–20 ppm subtelin control the growth of microorganisms.

17.2.6.5 Antioxidant

Antioxidants are generally considered in category of preservative. Antioxidants are phenol compounds and exerts primary anti-oxidative action. Food stuffs particularly fats such as lard, vegetable oils, hydrogenated shortenings and fat-based foods such as fried nuts, potato chips, dry cakes and biscuits may become rancid and produce unpleasant odours. Rancidity may develop as a result of oxidative and hydrolytic degradation of fat. Antioxidants prevent the oxidation of fat-containing foods and protect from rancidity. Antioxidants generally used in foods are butylated hydroxy toluene, propyl gallate, butylated hydroxy anicole, tocopherol, etc. Foods preserved with antioxidant are vegetable oils, cheese, bread, chips, nuts, etc.

17.2.7 Fermentation

The decomposition of carbohydrates by microorganisms or enzymes is called fermentation. This is one of the oldest methods of food preservation. Fermentation encourages the growth of selected microorganisms unlike in other methods of preservation where microbial growth is discouraged. Generally, three types of fermentation are involved in food preservation. These are alcoholic, acetic acid and lactic acid fermentation.

17.2.7.1 Alcoholic fermentation

Carbohydrate-containing fermentable sugar is converted to ethyl alcohol by fermentation of yeast.

$$\text{Carbohydrate} + \text{Yeast} \rightarrow \text{Ethyl alcohol}$$

Wine produced from grape and cider from apple is due to the fermentation by yeast (*Saccharomyces cerevisiae*). About 51.1 g ethyl alcohol can be obtained from 100 g of sugar. About 14% alcohol act as preservative in wines.

17.2.7.2 Acetic acid fermentation

The oxidation of ethyl alcohol by the bacteria such as *Acetobactor aceti* gives acetic acid. Wine, cider or any alcoholic and sugary or starchy products may be converted to vinegar/acetic acid. A total of 67 parts of acetic acid can be obtained from 100 parts of sugar.

17.2.7.3 Lactic acid fermentation

Lactic acid fermentation is very important in food preservation. Lactic acid fermentation is an anaerobic intra molecular oxidation-reduction process. Both hetero fermentative bacteria such as *Leuconostoc* spp. and *Lactobacillus brevis* and homo fermentative bacteria such as *La. plantarum* and *Pediococcus cerevisiae* participate in fermentation.

Sauerkraut is a product obtained by lactic acid fermentation of shredded cabbage called sour or acid cabbage. Pickles of cucumber, tomato, mango and lemon are also due to lactic acid fermentation. 1.8% lactic acid and 2.5% salt act as preservatives in pickles.

17.2.8 Carbonation

Beverage such as fruit based and synthetic or aerated generally bottled with carbon dioxide. Carbon dioxide is a colourless, odourless non-combustible gas. It has acidic flavour. It creates anaerobic condition, removes air and reduces the oxidation of ascorbic acid and prevents browning.

Carbonation is the process of dissolving sufficient carbon dioxide in water or beverage. It gives off the gas as fine bubbles when served. The optimum concentration varies from 20% to 30%. In commercial practice, it is sold as liquid under pressure (58 kg/cm^3) or solidified as dry ice.

Moulds and yeast require oxygen for their growth, become inactive in the presence of carbon dioxide. Carbonated beverage contains sugar much below 66% but the absence of air and presence of carbon dioxide in them help to prevent the growth of moulds and yeast. The aerated or synthetic carbonated beverage are Coke, Pepsi, Thumps-up, Sprite, Dew, Limca, etc.

Fruit juices can be also be carbonated directly or inform of concentrate for subsequent carbonation. The level of carbonation varies with the type of fruit juice and flavour. Generally 1–3 g/L is required. This concentration is lower than that required for complete inhibition (14.6 g/L) of microbial growth. The technique for fruit juice carbonation consists of fruit juice → mixing with strained cooled sugar syrup (sugar + water citric acid) → measuring of total suspended solids → deaerating → cooling (around 8°C) → mixing syrup with water → carbonation (by means of jetting apparatus) → transferring to storage tank → cooling (3–4°C) → bottling → sealing → storage/marketing.

17.2.9 Non-thermal methods of preservation

The non-thermal methods of preservation are new techniques offer promising and wide application in food processing. The major advantage of these methods is in terms of vitamins, essential nutrients and flavour protection, cost efficiency and less energy utilization. Some of the promising non-thermal methods of preservation are membrane processing, high pressure processing, pulsed electric field, minimal processing, hurdle technology and irradiation.

17.2.9.1 Membrane processing

Membrane technology, a separation process which does not involved thermal processing has unlimited potential in food processing industries. Membrane technology simply describes forms of very fine filtration. The membrane filtration is being commercially used in fruit and vegetable juice concentration, clarification of wine and beer, demineralization and purification of water, separation and concentration of enzymes and removal of contaminants. Various types of membranes are used such as ultrafiltration, reverse osmosis, etc.

Ultrafiltration is a molecular filtration where molecules are separated by their size. The ultrafiltration is usually used for clarification of fruit juices (apple, orange, mango, pineapple, guava and pomegranate juices), a part from the use in dairy processing.

Reverse osmosis is the reversal of natural process of osmosis. It is a pressure driven process where pressure is applied to the solution in excess of osmotic pressure of that solution. Juices clarified by ultrafiltration are subsequently concentrated by reverse osmosis. The RO is operative at pressure of 1500 psig. The main advantage of RO in fruit juice industry is retention of flavour with improved quality, low treatment cost and low floor space requirement.

17.2.9.2 High pressure processing

High pressure processing is also known as pascalization. This is a method of preserving and sterilizing food in which a product is processed under very high pressure leading to the inactivation of certain microorganisms and enzymes in food. This inactivates, vegetative microorganisms most commonly related to food-borne diseases and preserve the food with minimal effect on nutritional qualities. The main advantage of this technique is having better sensory and nutritional quality than thermal pasteurization and sterilization. The pressure in range of 100–1000 MPa is used for food. The technique has used in fruit and vegetable industry. The pressure, holding, time and temperature for various food product such as orange juice, grape juice, guava puree and apricot jam and vegetable products such as potato, cubes, chopped tomato, carrot and tomato juices have been standardized. The technique reduces processing time, retains freshness, flavour, texture, appearance and vitamin C.

17.2.9.3 Pulsed electric field

Pulsed electric field (PEF) uses short electric pulses to preserve food. The electric field is applied to food in form of short pulse with pulse duration ranging between microseconds and milliseconds rather than using electricity directly. Minimum heat is generated and process generally remains non-thermal. The technique is a substitute for heat pasteurization. PEF inactivates vegetative microorganisms, including yeast spoilage microorganisms and pathogen. PEF technology is suitable for preserving liquid and semiliquid foods such as orange juice, vegetable soup and dairy products.

17.2.9.4 Minimal processing

Minimal processing refers to lightly processed or partially processed or fresh processed products. Minimally processed products are prepared and handled to maintain freshness while providing convenience to the user. Minimal processed foods are treated very mildly with various treatment (including pH control, antioxidant, chlorinated water dips or combination of these and other treatments) packed in polymeric films and stored at low temperature. Its quality resembles fresh like characters. The colour, texture and flavour are not affected significantly in the minimally processed products. The technique is used for preserving fruit and vegetables, salad vegetables, leafy vegetables, tubers, cucumbers, tomatoes, brinjal, diced fruit chunks and other fruit and vegetables.

The unit operations of minimal processing involve washing → peeling → cutting into required size and shape → pre-treatments → packing in flexible polymeric films→ storing at low temperature.

For safety and greatest quality, these products must be distributed and marketed in cold chain. Many of the minimally processed vegetables are displayed in low temperature cabinet and sold at super markets and other outlets. Minimal processed fruit and vegetables have high quality, convenient and safe. Some pre-cut fruits and vegetables such as cucumbers, brinjal, tomato and tropical fruits have to be handled at high temperature to avoid chilling injury.

The product has sufficient shelf life to make distribution feasible within the region of consumption. The microbiological, sensory and nutritional shelf life of minimally processed fruit and vegetables should be at least 4-7 days but preferably even longer up to 21 days depending on the market, the loss of vitamin C and carotene which are main limiting factors of nutritional quality.

17.2.9.5 Hurdle technology

Hurdle technology involves application of a combination of treatments such as heating, drying, reducing water activity, pH, addition of preservative and other additives. The combination of hurdles used for preserving food products, disturb the homeostasis of the microorganisms there by retarding the growth and resulting microbial stability or safety. Hurdle technology finds the origin in the traditional preservation techniques such as drying, salting and heating. This offers a viable alternative to canning and dehydration. Products prepared with this technique are fruit and vegetable pickles by pH + preservative + salt and dehydration of fruit and vegetables by reducing water activity + heating + preservative. Apricot slices can be preserved by this technique with 50–60% moisture + 0.92–0.95% acidity and heat treatment or pasteurization at 85°C.

17.2.9.6 Irradiation

Food irradiation is a process of food preservation. This is a new technique for pre-treatment of food such as fruits and vegetables by the application of light or radiation. Irradiation involves controlled application of energy of the ionization (gamma rays, X-rays and accelerated electron) in control of sprouting, disinfection, delay in ripening, shelf life extension, destroying harmful bacteria and sterilization. The source of ionization radiation permitted for irradiating foods are as follows:

- Gamma rays from radio isotopes cobalt 60 and caesium 137
- X-rays generated from machine sources at or below energy level of 5 MeV
- Electron generated from machine sources operated at or below 10 MeV

The radiation doses used for perishable are given in Table 17.4.

Table 17.4. Irradiation dose for perishable.

Perishable	Purpose	Dose (kGy)	
		Min.	Max.
Potato	Sprouting	0.06	0.15
Onion	Sprouting	0.03	0.09
Garlic	Sprouting	0.03	0.15
Spices	Microbial decontamination	6.0	14.0
Dried fruits (resin fig, dates)	Insect disinfection	0.25	1.0
Mango	Shelf life extension	0.25	.075
Dried sea foods	Pathogen control	0.25	1.0
Fresh sea food	Pathogen control	1.0	3.0

Frozen fruit	Pathogen control	4.0	6.0
Meat and meat products including chicken	Pathogen control and shelf life extension	2.5	1.0

Unit operations involved in radiation processing are harvesting → pre-cooling → sorting and grading→ short wave energy application → packaging → transportation → marketing/storage.

18
Food quality evaluation

Quality is the measures of excellence or degree of acceptability by the consumers. In other words, quality is the ultimate criteria of the desirability of any food. Food quality can be evaluated by two methods: sensory evaluation and objective methods.

18.1 Sensory evaluation

The ultimate criteria for acceptance or liking and disliking of products to consumer are its eating quality. Therefore, sensory quality is of great importance to both processors and consumers. The quality of food when assessed by means of human sensory organs is called sensory, organoleptic or subjective evaluation.

Sensory quality is a combination of different senses of perception which determines the liking and disliking of the product. People are used as measuring instrument in sensory evaluation.

18.1.1 Sensory properties of food

The principal sensory characteristics which affect the acceptability of food are appearance, texture and flavour.

18.1.1.1 Appearance

This is eye appeal judged by light. Appearance includes size, shape, colour and defects. Size and shape make important contribution to the appearance of fresh produce and processed product. It is a measure interest to the growers and consumers. Grading of produce into various size and shape is one of the first steps in packaging and processing operation. Shape determents the losses during trimming and handling.

Colour is used as an index to the quality of number of products. Surface colour is important for the fresh market and internal colour for processing. Green colour is indicative of insufficient ripeness in fruits but it is desirable attributes in vegetables. Ripeness of various fruits is assessed by the colour. Colour is caused by the spectral distribution of light. Lumps in pudding which is not a desirable characteristic can be judged by the eye. Colour of roast beef is used an index to darkness. Strength of coffee and tea is judged by the colour of beverage.

Defects include deformities, mechanical injury such as damage, bruising, crushing and rupturing, insects and disease injury, specks and sediments.

18.1.1.2 Texture

Texture is also called kinesthetic quality. Texture is one of the most important characteristics of food quality. Texture includes hand and mouth feel judged by sense of touch. Hand feel is a finger feel judged by touch such as firmness in apple, softness in mango and plum, juiciness in citrus fruit, grapes sweet corn, etc., tenderness in vegetables and crispness in potato chips. Mouth feel includes chewiness, fibrousness, grittiness and stickiness. Consistency of custard apple, sauces and soup thin or thick, coarse or fine crystal in ice-cream and crispness of carrot can be judged by mouth feel.

18.1.1.3 Flavour

The flavour of food is a combination of taste, smell and composite of sensation called mouth feel.

18.1.1.4 Taste

Taste is categorized as sweet, salt, sour or bitter. Sugar is the main source of sweetness. Fructose gives most sweet sensation than sucrose, glucose, maltose, galactose and lactose. Sweetness is associated with hydroxyl radicals on the sugar molecules. Sour taste is associated with hydrogen ion provided by acids found in fruits and vegetables or vinegar. Salty taste is due to ions of salt that is sodium chloride.

18.1.1.5 Smell

Smell or odour may be fragrant, acid and burnt. Odour substances are volatile compounds. Volatile compounds are esters, carbonyl compounds, hydroxyl compounds and sulphur compounds. The volatile compounds present in various fruits or vegetables which give flavour or aroma are pentyl acetate in banana, cinamyl acetate in guava, ethyl acetate in pineapple, octyl acetate in orange, pentyl valerate in apple, acetic acid in fruit vinegar, linalool in papaya, cis-3-hexen-1-ol in tomato and raspberry, allicin in garlic, dimethyl sulphide in onion and *s*-methylcystein sulphoxide in cabbage and cauliflower. In eating, pleasant sensation comes more from odour than taste.

18.1.1.6 Composite of sensation

Mixture of substances present in foods gives all four taste sensation. The addition of salt to lime juice or lassi and fruits like guava improve the taste. Acid intensify the saltiness of sodium chloride so it is easier to over salt tart foods.

Sugar reduces the saltiness of sodium chloride, so a little of sugar may improve vegetable soup which have been over salted. Sugar also removes sourness of acid and bitterness of coffee. Hot and cold sensations give to the composite flavour of foods like soup, coffee and ice-cream. Hot coffee is not so bitter as cooled in cup. Iced coffee is not so bitter, as warm but not very hot.

18.1.2 Sensory test

The reasons for testing food quality are to know the consumer preference, to know the effect of variation in processing on quality and to detect the presence of off quality.

Panel of judges are used for sensory test. Member of the panel should be carefully selected and trained to find out difference in specific quality characteristic between different stimuli, direction and intensity of difference.

18.1.2.1 Requirements for an ideal panel member

The requirements of an ideal panel member for sensory test are as follows:

- Member should have good health and do not have habit of chewing supari and pan. Members suffering from cold or sickness cannot judge the food correctly.
- Members should have ability to distinguish differences in taste and odour and discriminate between samples.
- Have experience in particular field.
- Should not be prejudiced, have high personal integrity and ability to evaluate objectively.
- Willingness for sensory evaluation and interest in sensory analysis.
- Have ability to derive right conclusion and willing to periodic test for giving consistent results.

18.1.2.2 Types of panel

Panels are of different types such as trained panel, semi-trained or communicative panel and consumer panel.

Trained panels are carefully trained for specific products and purposes. The number of member varies from 5 to10.

Semi-trained or communicative panels have technical people. They are familiar with the qualities of various foods. The number of members varies from 25 to 30, which are used to find preference or acceptability.

Consumer panels are untrained and selected randomly. The number of members is large and generally not less than 100. The greater the number, the greater is dependability of results.

18.1.2.3 Testing lab

Testing lab should contain three units or rooms. These are reception room, sample preparation room and the test booth are actual place of sensory evaluation. The lab should be air-conditioned, free of extraneous smell and noise, should have facility of colour light (masking the sample colour), stainless steel glass and dishes, cups and plain serving China utensils.

18.1.2.4 Sample preparation

Sample for testing should be prepared by identical methods. The sample should be at same temperature, optimum level and set constant during the test. Use stainless steel spoon and forks for sample tasting. The sample should be presented with code marking and order of presentation should be randomized within each test session.

18.1.2.5 Testing procedure

The testing procedure consists of experimental design smelling technique, testing time and evaluation card. Statistical design is used to measure variables and to establish significance of results. Technique of randomizing is to minimize the error.

Smelling is done with short rapid sequence of sniffs. Tasting of beverages is performed by slurping (liquid is rolled on tongue to rich all parts of tongue). For testing odour of food, a special technique performed to perceive the aroma clearly.

Testing time is considered ideal when panel members are fresh. This is preferably in morning between 10 and 12 h. The number of sample should not be given more than four to five at a time to avoid error.

Evaluation card or score card should be prepared for the test. The card should be a sample and have clear direction. A card with too much detail and too brief should be avoided. No single score card fits all experiments; hence, score card needs to be developed for specific experiment. Score card should contain product, date and name of the judge.

18.1.2.6 Types of test

The different types of sensory tests used for food evaluation are classified into four groups: difference test, rating test, sensitive test and descriptive test.

1. Difference test

The objective of this test is to distinguish minor differences. This is done by obtaining the judgement of experts. The difference test is generally of three types: paired comparison test, triangle test and duo-trio test.

Paired comparison test

The panel members are given two samples or several pairs of samples. These may be different or same samples in each pair; hence, it is known as paired comparison test. Samples are given with code numbers. Members are requested to indicate how they differ in a particular sensory character such as sweetness or bitterness or rancidity or texture. Trained panellists of 5–12 members or untrained panellists of 72–80 members are required to evaluate two samples per test. Evaluation card for paired comparison test consists of name, date, product, code numbers of pairs, difference between the two samples in pairs in sensory characters and signature.

Triangle test

In this test, three samples are presented simultaneously in which two are identical and one is different. The members decide which two of the three samples alike and which is the odd sample. Trained panellists of 5–12 members are required to evaluate three samples (two identical and one different) per test. Evaluation card for triangle test consists of name, date, product, set number (I, II, III), code number of samples, code number of odd sample, comment on odd sample and in last signature of members.

Duo-trio test

In this test, three samples are presented in which two identical and one different. The judge or panel is first given one of pair of identical sample as known reference sample and then the other two samples in random order and asked to match one of these with the first. A positive answer is required. There is 50% chance of a correct answer simply by guessing. Panel members used may be trained or untrained. Trained panellists of 5–12 members are required to evaluate three (two identical and one different) samples per test. Evaluation card for duo-trio test consists of name, date, product, reference sample, set number (I, II, III, IV), code number of pairs and decide sample same as reference. In the last, there is signature of panel member. Generally paired comparison test and triangle test are more useful than duo-trio test.

2. Rating test/ preference test

The objective is to indicate preference for a particular sample. This is done by the public and called market test. Rating test gives more quantitative data than difference test. This can be used for the analysis of more than two samples at a time. Rating tests are of various types such as ranking, monadic, two-sample different test, multiple sample different test, hedonic rating test, numerical scoring test and composite scoring test.

Ranking test

Several samples are presented at a time. These are ranked or determined the differences in several samples by the members on the basis of intensity of single sensory characteristic. This test is useful for evaluation of large number of samples at a time. Members are asked to rank the coded sample according to their preference in consumer analysis. Trained panellists of 5–12 members or semi-trained panellists of 10–25 members are required to evaluate 2–7 samples per test.

The evaluation card for ranking test consists of name, date, product, intensity/preference, sample code and signature.

Monadic test

This is also known as single sample test. The members are asked to indicate the presence or absence or intensity of a particular quality characteristic. The complete analysis of two or more samples evaluated at different time is compared with the trained members or panellists. Trained panellists of 6–25 members or untrained panellists of 72–80 members are required to evaluate one sample per test.

The evaluation card for monadic test consists of name, date, product and ranking of sample. Yes or no, if there is any off flavour and signature.

Two-sample difference test

This test measures the amount of difference or variation of the paired comparison. Each pair consists of an identical reference and coded test sample. In two pairs, the test sample is a duplicate of the reference sample. The members asked to decide each pair independently for the degree of difference between the test sample and standard on scale of 0 (*no difference*) to 3 (*extreme difference*). Trained panellists of 6–25 members are required to evaluate four pairs on unknown and control sample per test. The evaluation card for two-sample difference test consists of name, date, product, degree (no difference – 0, very slight difference – 1, moderate difference – 2 and large difference – 3) and direction (inferior to standard – I, equal to standard – E and superior to standard – S) and signature.

Multiple sample difference test

More than one test variables is evaluated in this test. Each member of panel is presented three to six samples, depending upon the number of test variables. One sample is known as standard. The panel members compare each coded sample with known standard. One coded sample is the duplicate of the standard. The score of blind standard assigned by the members is subtracted from the score assigned to the test variables. Trained panellists of 6-25 members or semi-trained panellists of 10-25 members are required to evaluate three to six samples, including control per test. Evaluation card for multiple sample difference test consists of name, date, product, degree of difference (rating 0, 1, 2, 3 and difference are standard – none, slight, moderate and large, respectively), direction of the quality (equal to inferior and superior) and signature.

Numerical scoring test

Each panellist is given one or more sample in random order or according to statistical design. Each sample is evaluated by panellists on a specific scale for particular sensory characteristic corresponding to the agreed quality description. Trained panellists with 5–12 members are required to evaluate 1–6 or 5–10 samples and untrained panellists with 72–80 members are required to evaluate 1–4 samples per test. The evaluation card for numerical scoring test consists of name, date, product, score such as 60, 70, 80 and 90 and quality description such as poor, fair, good and excellent corresponding to score, comments and signature.

Composite scoring test

Specific characteristics of a product are rated separately; hence, rating scale is defined. The definition of rating scale is weighed so that the most important characteristic will account for a large part of the total score. Scores obtained are compounded for any one panellist to rich or arrive a composite score. Method is useful for grading products and comparing quality components. This method, provide more information than the numerical scoring test. Trained panellists with 5–10 members are required to evaluate one to four samples per test. The evaluation card for composite scoring test consists of name, date, product, quality (such as colour consistency, flavour, absence of defects and total score), possible score (corresponding to quality component, respectively, are 20, 20, 40, 20 and total 100) and sample, score and signature.

Hedonic rating test

Hedonic rating test relates to pleasant or unpleasant experiences. This test is used to measure the consumer acceptability of food products. In this test, panellists to rate the acceptability to provide on a scale genomally of nine points ranging from like extremely to dislike extremely. The results are analyzed for preference with data from large untrained or small semi-trained panels. Semi-trained panellists of 10–25 members are required for sensory test of 5–10 samples per test.

The evaluation card for hedonic rating test consists of name, date, product, hedonic scale (like extremely, like very much, like moderately, slightly, neither like nor dislike, dislike slightly, dislike moderately, dislike very much and dislike extremely), sample code (A, B, C), reason and signature.

3. Sensitive tests

Sensitivity tests are performed to assess the ability of individual to detect different tests such as odour and feel the specific characteristic like hotness or astringency in food products. In this test, trained panel members are selected to evaluate the quality of products such as spices, salt and sugar in tomato sauce. Sensitivity test are of two types: sensitivity-threshold test and dilution test.

Sensitivity-threshold test

Threshold is defined as a statistically determent point on the stimulus scale at which a transition in a series of sensation or judgement occur. Threshold test is of three types:

- Stimulus detection threshold: This is a magnitude of stimulus at which transition occurs from no sensation to sensation.
- Recognition, identification threshold: It is minimum concentration at which stimulus is correctly identified.
- Terminal saturation threshold: It is the magnitude of a stimulus above which there is no increase in perceived intensity of the stimulus.

Threshold value is given as a more number that is the denominator of the dilution where flavour or odour is recognized. These tests are also used for detecting the minimum difference of an additive. In this test, untrained panellists evaluate the test of 5–10 samples per test.

Dilution test

This test is designed to establish the smallest amount of an unknown substances or material developed as a substitute for a standard product which can be detected when it is mixed with the standard product. Examples are mixing of synthetic orange flavour ingredients in natural flavour, dried whole milk in fresh milk, margarine in butter, etc. The quality of the test material is represented by the dilution number which is the percent of the test material in mixture of standard products. The bitterness is the quality of test material with bigger number of dilution. Trained panellists of 12–24 members are required to sensory test of 5–10 samples per test.

The evaluation card for sensitivity threshold test consists of name, date, product, set number (1, 2, 3, 4, 5), description of test, feeling factors and signature.

4. Descriptive flavour profile method

This method describes both quantitative and qualitative characters for flavour analysis in products containing different tastes and odour. For example, the flavour profile analysis of tomato sauce consists of aroma (spices, taste sour, sweet, salty), mouth feel (chilies) and texture (smoothness). In this test, trained panellists of three to six members required to evaluate one to five samples per test.

Limitation of sensory evaluation

- Results are highly variable.
- People suffering with cold or other health problems loose their maximum effectiveness.
- Individual ability may be influenced by emotional burdens.

18.2 Objective evaluation

Objective methods of evaluating food quality depend on measure other than human senses are generally known as objective evaluation. Objective evaluation involves analysis and lab instruments. Objective methods of food quality evaluation have certain advantages which are as follows:

- Accurate results and minute differences can be observed.
- Human sensitivity is not involved as compared with sensory method.
- It is less subjected to errors and provides permanent records; hence, comparison can be made over a period of time.
- Overcome the limitation of emotional burden and individual ability and confidence can be gained as they are reproducible.

Various methods or test used for objective evaluation of food quality are

1. Physical methods
2. Chemical methods
3. Physicochemical methods
4. Microscopic examination

18.2.1 Physical methods

Physical methods include size and weight, volume, specific gravity, moisture, colour, texture and odour.

18.2.1.1 Size and weight

Size makes important contribution to the appearance of fresh produce. It is major interest to the growers, consumers and processors. The instruments used for measuring size and shape are vernier calliper, micrometers, and planimeters. Weight indicates the quality in various fruit such as avocado, apple, orange and egg. Weight is taken or measured by weighing machine.

18.2.1.2 Volume

Liquid volumes can be measured by using measuring cups.

Specific gravity is a measure of the relative density of a substance in relation to that of water. To obtain specific gravity, the weight of sample in air is divided by its weight in water. This method in used in measuring the quality of potato. Potato with low specific gravity has good cooking quality and with higher specific gravity has good processing quality. Specific gravity is very useful technique for measuring the maturity standard or harvest in dices in various fruits and vegetables.

18.2.1.3 Moisture

Fresh fluids or juice contents indicate the quality of various fruits such as the minimum juice content in oranges should be 35% and in limes and lemons 25%. Moisture content can be obtained by drying technique that is the weight of the original sample is determined and then it is dried at 60°C for 6 h or longer until it gives constant weight. Moisture content (%) is calculated as initial weight minus dried weight upon initial weight into hundred.

18.2.1.4 Colour

Colour is caused by the spectral distribution of light. Colour is the most important quality attributes in food. Surface colour is important for the fresh market and internal colour for the processing. Green colour is indicative of insufficient ripeness in fruit but it is desirable attribute in vegetables. Chlorophylls, carotenoids and anthocyanins are reasonable for colour of fruits and vegetables. The measurement of surface colour presents many problems. When the unit size is large such as mango, papaya, apple, melons, etc., individual units have to be measured. When the unit size is small such as karonda, strawberry, grape berries, phalsa, etc., a representative sample can be measured.

The instruments used for colour measurement in food are Hunter colour-difference meter, spectronic-20 (reflectance measurement) and spectrophotometer.

18.2.1.5 Texture evaluation

Instruments are used to measure the texture of liquids, semi-solid and solid. The instrument used for measuring textural quality of liquids and semi-solids are jelmeter (determines viscosity in foods such as jelly), viscometer (measures viscosity or consistency), consistency meter (measuring the consistency of tomato ketchup), synchrolectric viscometer (measures consistency of custard, tomato products, dairy products, etc.) and penetrometer (measures tenderness in gels and baked products).

The instruments used for measuring the texture of solids are A-ender-meter (measures compression and shearing such as suitability of peas for canning), succulometer (measures the maturity of corn and storage quality of apples), fibrometer (differentiate fibrousness between mature and tender vegetables such as beans, okra), shortometer (measures the breaking strength of cookies, idli, pastries etc.), chrystal texurometer (measures the texture of meat), shear press (measures textural characteristics of some fruits and vegetables) and universal testing machine (hardness, springiness, gumminess, chewingness, cohesiveness and adhesiveness).

18.2.1.6 Flavouring substances

Odour substances are volatile compounds. Volatile compounds are esters, carbonyl compounds, hydroxyl compounds and sulphur compounds. Gas chromatographic technique a sensitive procedure has been developed to detect and estimate volatile flavouring compounds of foods.

18.2.2 Chemical methods

Chemicals are estimated in adulterated food such as presence of metanil yellow in turmeric powder, starch in milk, vanaspati in ghee or butter, invert sugar in honey, minerals in soft drink and some chemical is also estimated in food spoilage like peroxidase in fats and nutrient losses during cooking such as vitamin, minerals, fibres, etc.

18.2.3 Physicochemical methods

Instrument used for measuring chemical are pH meter for pH or hydrogen ion concentration. Digital salto meter used for salt percentage in pickle, sauce, etc. Brix refracto meter is used for measuring total soluble solids in various fruits. Brix hydro meter measures direct sugar percentage in syrups and polarioscope used for quantitative analysis of sugar. Butyro meter finds butter content in milk.

18.2.4 Microscopic examination

Microscopic examination is used for spoilage of various foods caused by microorganisms such as bacteria, fungi or yeast. Some properties of foods such as size of crystal in sugar relating to smoothness of products, types of organism in fermented products, starch cells identification and number and size of air cells in batters can be obtained by microscopic examination.

Limitations of objective evaluation

- It is expensive methods
- It is time consuming
- Required technical knowledge
- Non availability of instrument some time
- Some aspects of food quality cannot be evaluated by objective method

19

Food packaging

Packing makes a bridge between production and marketing. Packaging is defined as a techno-economic means for minimizing cost of delivery and maximizing the sales. In other words, it is a means of ensuring safe delivery to the consumers in safe and sound condition at an affordable cost. Packaging has gained importance in recent years. Packaging industry has made excellent strides to develop more and more varieties of packaging material and packaging machinery. This is mainly due to growth of consumer awareness and increase of willingness to pay for value and hygienic product, growth of export market and growth of innovations in fresh and processed foods. Packaging has great role and contribution that how best fresh and processed products could be delivered to the consumer in right quantity with a right quality. Packaging provides three basic functions:

1. Preservation: Packaging does not improve the quality but it retains quality.
2. Protection: Packaging protects from mechanical and environmental hazards.
3. Presentation: Adds value and assists sale.

The principles of packaging should be cheap, strong, smooth surface and ventilated. The requirements for designing packaging containers of food products are as follows:

- Sanitary protection
- Gas and odour protection
- Moisture protection
- Light protection
- Compatible with specific fruit and vegetable product
- Non-toxic
- Low cost
- Resistance to breakage
- Ease of opening and disposal
- Size, weight and shape consideration
- appearance and printability

19.1 Packaging containers for fresh produce

Packaging containers for fresh produce particularly for fruits and vegetables are classified into two groups: bulk packaging and consumers packaging.

19.1.1 Bulk packaging containers

The containers used for bulk packaging are (i) baskets, (ii) wooden boxes, (iii) rigid plastic creates, (iv) corrugated fibre board boxes, (v) plastic corrugated boxes and (vi) sacks. Merits and demerits of these packaging containers are as follows.

19.1.1.1 Baskets

Baskets are made up of various local materials such as bamboo and pigeon pea, mulberry and phalsa sticks, etc. These are of various capacity, shapes and sizes. These are cheap but have low strength and inadequate stackability; hence, these are not suitable for transport of fresh fruits and vegetables to distant markets.

19.1.1.2 Wooden box

Wooden boxes provide better impact and compression strength than basket; hence, it has good stackability during transport, handling and storage. However, the use of wooden containers is discouraged due to occupying large space in storage and problem of deforestation.

19.1.1.3 Plastic crates

Plastic crates available in various sizes, shapes and colour are made up of high-density polyethylene. These are strong, rigid and reusable and can be cleaned easily. The normal capacity varies from 20 to 40 kg. These have advantages of easy handling, reducing the storage space and transport cost of empty crates. This is most suitable in handling of fresh produce.

19.1.1.4 Corrugated fibre board box

Corrugated fibre board boxes which have higher stacking strength, smooth and non-abrasive surface, reusable and recyclable are widely used particularly for export of fresh produce. In such boxes, ventilation can be provided easily and can be laminated with plastic film as per need.

19.1.1.5 Bags

Bags of different materials such as jute, light weight fibre cotton and plastic particularly low-density polyethylene are very useful for packing of fruits and vegetables due to low cost, high tensile strength and reusability. However, these materials have problems of impact injuries, puncture and poor stackability for fresh produce. It is suitable for serials, dry fruits, potato, onion, etc.

19.1.1.6 Plastic corrugated box

Plastic corrugated box made up of polypropylene and high-density polyethylene are better than corrugated fibre board boxes due to their high degree of moisture resistance, reusability and low weight. However, it is very expensive and has low compression strength and cushioning property.

19.1.2 Pre-packaging containers

Pre-packaging means packaging in consumer size container before sale. Packages can be designed to suit specific individual fresh fruits and vegetables and handling device to carry. Pre-packaging reduces spoilage, increases shelf life both under normal and cold storage conditions and offers hygienic method of distribution and storage. These types of packaging are preferred by the buyers in supermarkets and departmental stores. The materials of pre-packaging are of various types: plastic net bags, trays with over wrap, plastic crate of light weight, shrink wrap, etc.

19.1.2.1 Plastic net bags

Plastic net bags are of different size, shapes and colour. These may be extruded or woven and made of high-density polyethylene or nylon this is most suitable for packing of small size fruit such as ber, date, gooseberry, apricot, etc.

19.1.2.2 Trays with over wrap

Trays with over wrap materials are to hold individual fruits. These are made up of waste paper or thermo formed trays made of polyvinyl chloride or polypropylene with cavities. The film made of low-density polyethylene or polyvinyl chloride used to cover the trays as over wrap. This is suitable for packing for mango, apple, kiwi fruits and eggs.

19.1.2.3 Plastic crate of light weight

Plastic crates of light weight are made of high-density polyethylene which has high compression strength. The crates have perforation for ventilation.

19.1.2.4 Shrink wrap

Shrink wrap of individual produce is one of the recent trends in fresh fruits and vegetables packaging. These are made of low-density polyethylene and have ability to reduce transpiration rate, control moisture loss and maintain firmness.

19.1.2.5 Modified atmosphere packaging

The development of modified atmospheric packaging system (MAP) is important to reduce oxygen concentration and increase carbon dioxide. The technique utilizes polymeric film with selective permeability for O_2, CO_2 and H_2O vapour. This creates modified atmosphere around the packed produce due to respiration of the products and selective permeability of packaging material. Polyethylene and polyvinyl chloride film which have CO_2, O_2 ratio of 2 to 5.9 and 3.6 to 6.9, respectively, are very useful for packaging of fresh produce. The MAP technology does not require high investment and can be also adopted where refrigeration facilities are not available.

The map technology is very popular in packaging of apple, apricot and kiwi fruits. By using MAP at ambient conditions, storage life of banana, tomato, capsicum and green chilies are 15, 15, 13 and 8 days, respectively. The storage life of banana, tomato, capsicum and chilies by using MAP at optimum low temperature is 42, 30, 21 and 28 days, respectively. There is about 50% increase in shelf life of these crops both at ambient and optimum low temperature by using MAP. Biodegradable laminate of chitosan, cellulose and polycaprolactone as film for MAP is used for fresh produce such as shredded cabbage, lettuce, tomato, sweet corn and blue berries.

19.2 Active packaging

This is interactive or smart packaging. The potential technologies for active packaging are oxygen scavenging, antimicrobial packaging, ethylene control packaging, moisture control packaging and gas permeability control packaging.

19.2.1 Oxygen scavenging

In this packaging, oxygen is removed by using absorption and scavenging. Containers are so designed that they absorb oxygen of the packed produce. This retard respiration and increase the shelf life. This is suitable for fresh produce.

19.2.2 Antimicrobial packaging

Antimicrobial agents are incorporated in plastic film/sheet surface coatings and into absorbent pads for fresh produce. For example, sodium/potassium metabisulphite is used in sawdust mixture in pads inside the box or carton to release sulphur dioxide to control fungal spoilage in grapes.

19.2.3 Ethylene control packaging

Ethylene accelerates ripening of various fruits; hence, the removal of ethylene retards ripening and promotes longer shelf life. Active packaging permit, containers that control ethylene. Ethylene absorbents used in packaging are potassium per magnet, activated carbon, tetrazine film and methylcyclopropene which binds ethylene receptor. This is most suitable for packing of climacteric fruits which generate ethylene during transport and storage.

19.2.4 Moisture control packaging

Moisture control gives protection to produce during handling, transport and storage of fresh food. Metabolism of fats and carbohydrates produces water condensation or sweating is a problem in packed fruits. Use of humectants between two highly permeable layers of plastic film to buffer the humidity inside the package.

19.2.5 Gas permeability control packaging

High oxygen permeable packaging materials have been developed which help in extending shelf life. A mixture of iron powder and hydrated lime is used in sachet to scavenge both O_2 and CO_2 in package.

19.3 Packaging containers for processed food

Various types of containers depending upon the type of processed products are used for sale. Considerable shift is being experienced towards modern packaging of processed food due to growing consumer awareness for health and hygiene, consumer convenience, increased purchasing capacities, product branding and export thrust. Containers used for packaging of food products are given in Table 19.1

Table 19.1. Packing containers for processed food products.

Packaging containers	Processed food products
(A) Glass bottles	Beverages (RTS, squash, syrup, cordial, wine, cider, vinegar), jam, jellies, pickles, chutney, ketchup, etc.
(B) Cans	
Plain can	Canned products of mango, guava, litchi, apricot, banana, papaya, etc.

AR lacquer can (R-enamel) Acidic product	Canned product of strawberry, plum, coloured grapes, etc.
SR lacquered can (C-enamel) Non-acidic product	Canned product of pea, asparagus, beans, mushroom, corn and some sea foods
Citrus enamel	Citrus products and concentrates
Sea food enamel	Fish products, and meat and meat products
Milk enamel	Milk, eggs and other dairy products
Beer can enamel	Beer and carbonated beverages
Midget can (picnic pack)	Mango juice, coconut water, etc.
(C) Plastic packaging	
Pouches (made of laminates and multi layer film)	Fruit juice concentrates, fruit juice based beverages, wine and country liquor. Edible oils, processed and convenience food, snack food, spices, tea, coffee, malted milk products, pan masala, betel nut powder
Metalized laminates	Dry fruits such as pecan nuts, cashew nuts, etc.
Polythene bag	Frozen fruits and vegetables
Thermo formed cups and tubes	Jelly, portion packs: pickle, chutney, ketchup, jams, yogurt, ice-cream, shrikhand, fruit salad and butter
Thermo form film meat trays	Processed meat
Tetra packs	Non-carbonated beverages
Stretched blow moulded bottle of polyethylene terephthalate and olyvinyl chloride film	Non-alcoholic and alcoholic beverages, vinegar and ketchup
Printed wrappers of laminates	Fruit bar and cheese
Expanded polyesterine	Fresh meat, poultry meat
Low-density polyethylene (LDPE) over wrap films	Sausage
Heat sealed plastic film (linear LDPE)	Frozen meat

Packaging industry has made excellent strides to develop more and more varieties of packaging material and packaging machinery due to growth of export markets and innovation in processed foods. It is essential to select right type of packaging material and technique to provide and optimum shelf life of the product at optimum cost.

19.4 References

1. Anthikad, J. 2014. Enzymylogy. In: *Nutrition and Biochemistry for Nurses*. Jaypee Brothers Medical Publishers (P) Ltd., New Delhi, pp. 112-126.
2. Babu, S. and Bhat, R.V. 1997. Know your food additives. *Nutrition* 31, 4.
3. Barmore, C.R. 1987. Packaging technology of fresh and minimally processed fruit and vegetables. *J Food Quality* 10, 207.
4. Bhat, R.V. and Mathur, P. 1998. Changing scenario of food colors in India. *Curr Sci*, 74, 198-202.
5. Dash, S.K. and Chandra, P. 2001. Evaporative cooling system for storage of fruits and vegetables. *Indian Food Packer*55, 79-87.
6. Das, Madhusweta. 2003. Safety of Using Monosodium Glutamate in Processed Foods. Processed Food Industry.
7. D'Mellow, J.P.F. 2003. *Food Safety: Contamination and Toxin*. CABI Publishing Wallingford, Oxon, UK.
8. Frazier, W.C. 1988. *Food Microbiology*. Tata McGraw, Hill Pub. Co. Pvt. Ltd., New Delhi.
9. Jood, S. and Khetarpaul, N. 2002. *Food Preservation*. Geeta Souraz Agrotec Publishing Academy, Udaipur.
10. Kader, A.A. 2004. Controlled atmosphere storage. In *Commercial Storage of Fruits and Vegetables and Florist and Nursery Stocks*. Agriculture Hand Book No. 66, USDA.
11. Ladaniya, M.S. and Singh, S. 1999. *Post Harvest Technology and Processing of Citrus, Fruits in India*. National Research Center for Citrus, Nagpur.
12. Mitra, S. 2001. *Post Harvest Physiology and Storage of Tropical and Subtropical Fruits*. CAB International, UK, pp. 167-189.
13. Mudambi, S.R. and Raja Gopal, M.V. 2009. Fundamentals of Foods, Nutrition and Diet Therapy, 5th edn. New Age International (P) Ltd. Publishers, New Delhi.
14. Parekh, J.V. 2005. Screening tests for detecting adulteration in food. Food and Pack.
15. Pandey, U.B. 2004. Onion and garlic storage: status, constraints and challenges. Souvanir. First Indian Horticulture Congress, New Delhi.
16. Parker, R.O. 2001. *Introduction to Food Science*. Thomson Delmar Learing, Albany, NY, USA.
17. Potter, N.N. and Birch, G.G. 1986. *Food Science*. AVI Publishing, Westport CT, USA.
18. Salunkhe, D.K. and Kadam, S.S. 1995. *Hand Book of Fruit Science and Technology: Production, Composition, Storage and Processing*. Marcel Dekker Inc., New York, USA.
19. Skariyachan, S. and Abilash, M. 2012. Food spoilage and food borne diseases. In *Introduction to Food Biotechnology*. CBS Publishers and Distributors Pvt. Ltd., New Delhi, pp. 123-143.

20. Shrilakshmi, B. 2013. *Food Science*, 5th edn. New Age International (P) Ltd. Publishers, New Delhi.

21. Sucheta, B. 2000. Development in Packaging of Processed Food. Processed Food Industry.

22. Thompson, A.K. 2003. *Fruits and Vegetables Harvesting, Handling and Storage*. Blackwell Publishing Ltd., Oxford.

23. Varnam, A.H. 1994. *Milk and Milk Products: Technology, Chemistry and Microbiology*. Chapman and Hall, London.

24. Zagory, D. and Kader, A.A. 1988. Modified atmospheric packaging of fresh produce. *Food Technol.* 7(2), 70-77.

PART III
Food Technology

20

Cereal food products and processing technique

Cereals are major source of calories and protein in the diet of Indian population. Cereal processing particularly grain processing is the biggest component in the food sectors. The principal cereals are wheat, rice, maize, jwar, bajra, ragi and barley. Wheat and rice have been used as staple food. Earlier wheat has been used as wheat flour. Now, refined wheat flour/maida finds greater application in the preparation of bakery foods such as breads, biscuit, cakes, etc. Traditionally rice has been used as whole cooked grain, but now several products are processed. A gradual change in processing and utilization of cereals has taken place in the country. The common cereals and their products are given in the following sections.

20.1 Wheat

Three species of wheat namely *Triticum aestivum* (common hard wheat), *T. durum* (durum wheat) and *T. dicoccum* (soft white wheat) are cultivated in India. Wheat is naked caryopsis. The wheat grain consists of germ or embryo rich in protein and oil, endosperm rich in starch and various outer coverings such as pericarp, seed coat or testa, hyaline layer and aleurone cell layer rich in fibre.

Wheat varieties suitable for processing of various products such as chapaties are C 306, Raj 3765, HD 2285, K8027, K9107, Sujata, HI 1500, HW 2204, HD 2833, for making breads are HS 240, BL 738, HD 2285, HD 2733, PBW 396, HS 277, GW 120, GW 173, HI 977, HD 2189, for making biscuits are Sonalika, HS 490, UP 2425 and for making pasta are PDW 233, WH 896, HI 8498, HD 4632, Raj 1555 and MACS 2846.

Wheat is popularly consumed in the form of chapaties, puries, paratha, daliaa, etc. Wheat is rich in protein, carbohydrates, iron and nicotinic acid.

20.1.1 Products

The important product of wheat are flour, refined flour and processed food products like bread (brown, plain, sweet, milk bread, fruit bread, high fibre bread), biscuit (salted, sweet, cardamom flavour, wheat germ, sugar-free bread), cakes and pastries, flakes, starch, gluten, instant food (noodles, macaroni), etc. The techniques for preparation of wheat-based products are as follows.

20.1.1.1 Whole-wheat flour (Atta)

The whole-wheat flour contains finely ground bran, germ and endosperm of whole kernel. It has distinctive flavour and coarse texture but has poor keeping quality. The technique for preparation of wheat flour is as follows:

Wheat grain → Cleaning (stones and other foreign matter) → Grading for bold size, free from broken, immature and shrivelled grain → Milling (burr mills/mini grain mill/roller mills) → Collection → Packing in bags of 5–10 kg capacity

20.1.1.2 Refined flour (maida/white flour)

The bran and germ are separated in making white flour. The technique used for preparation is as follows:

Wheat → Cleaning → Grading → Milling (roller mills) with 13% bran and 3% germs as by products → Packing

Milling operation consists of breaking, sifting, purifying, reduction, scratching, entroleter and air classification.

20.1.1.3 Fortified wheat flour

Wheat flour can be fortified with 10% defatted soya flour (poustic atta). This improves quality of protein and functional characteristics such as moisture retention and less oil absorption.

20.1.1.4 Bread

Ingredients

Flour 100 g, compressed yeast 2.5 g, sugar 5 g, salt 2 g, shortening 3 g, potassium bromate 15 ppm, 10 mL water optimum for desirable consistency can be calculated by water absorption method.

100 g of flour is weighed and transferred to the mixing container → Remaining ingredients which are dissolved in solution form are added to flour in the mixing container → Kneading for 1 min and 40 s → Fermentation for 1 h 40 min at 33°C → Remixing 25 s at room temperature → Recovery (ferment) for 25 min at 33°C → Proofing for 55 min at 33°C → Baking for 25 min at 230°C → Cooling for 25 min at room temperature

Other method

Wheat flour/maida → Sieving through 60 mesh to remove foreign material → Mixing of ingredients sugar, vegetable oil, yeast, salt and chemicals thoroughly until dough is formed → Fermentation volume of dough increases due to carbon dioxide released by the yeast → Punching/knock-back by folding the ends and the sides of the dough from one side to other → Intermediary first proofing (short resting period of 15 min) → Dividing of dough (450 g pieces) → Rounding to provide a skin around the dough → Moulding mechanically → Panning → Baking at 205°C for 25–30 min in the oven → Depanning and cooling about 60–90 min → Slicing through mechanical slicer → Packaging

20.1.1.5 Biscuit

Ingredients

Flour 75 g, ghee 25 g, sugar powdered 50 g, egg $^1/_2$, sodium bicarbonate 0.5 g and baking powder 0.5 g.

Sieving (flour, sodium bicarbonate + baking powder) → Creaming (ghee + sugar) → Mixing (flour mix + beaten egg + creamed mixture) → Dough making → Dough chilling (1 h) → Shaping → Baking (160°C for 15-20 min) → Natural cooling → Stocking → Packaging

20.1.1.6 Cakes and pastries

Ingredients

Wheat flour, beaten eggs, yeast, baking powder, cream, sugar and ghee/vanaspati. The technique for preparation of cakes and pastries is as follows:

Mixing of wheat flour, baking powder, cream, sugar and ghee till it becomes fluffy → Addition of beaten eggs with caramel colour and chopped fruits → Baking for about 30–40 min → Placing of butter cream, jam, etc., between the layers of cake → Chilling of layered cake → Cutting with salt knife an required shape and size → Icing of sides of the pieces with butter cream → Topping with finally ground cake crumbs/ pieces of fruits or chocolate strips → Decorated with proper design. Pastries are made in various shapes such as square, rectangular, from thick cake seeds.

20.1.1.7 Wheat flakes

This is a breakfast wheat product. The product can be sugar coated. The technique of processing consists of tempered wheat → Bumping rolls → Agitating pressure cooker (123.7°C for 90 min) → Conditioning over (moisture 20%) → Smooth flaking rolls → Toasting over (final moisture 3%) → Vitamin, mineral spray → Packing.

20.1.1.8 Wheat popcorn

This is a snack food. Texture is positively correlated with popping volume. The expansion volume is the critical quality factor for popcorn. The commercial popcorn has 30–40 fold expansion. Popping occurs at 177°C which is equivalent to a steam pressure of 2.5 ton/cm^2 inside the kernel.

20.1.1.9 Instant noodles (ready to cook and snack food)

Ingredients

Wheat powder containing ash content of 0.3–0.4%, carbonic salt, water, common salt, soft water, refined vegetable, cooking oils.

Mixing of raw materials → Making of dough sheet → Cutting (strip cutting) → Measuring → Steaming → Casing → Frying → Cooling → Inspection → Packing → Storage/marketing

20.1.1.10 Macaroni (gold finger): ready to eat food

Ingredients

Wheat maida, tapioca starch and soda bicarbonate. The technique used for preparation is as follows:

Mixing of maida, tapioca starch and sodium bicarbonate in a vertical mixer → Addition of boiled water → Preparation of dough in dough mixer for 15 min → Kneaded dough taken to macaroni making machine → Extrusion (desired shape and length is obtained by using appropriate die) → Collection of product in wooden trays (moisture content is around 30%) → Semi-drying by exposing the product to indirect sun rays (shade) → Exposing the product to steam for about 10 min → Drying up to moisture content of 10% → Packing → Storage/marketing

20.1.1.11 Energy food

Ingredients

Wheat flour 60%, gram dal 10%, edible ground nut cake 10%, jaggery 15%, Calcium carbonate and vitamins can also be added. The technique for preparation is as follows:

Wheat → Cleaning → Roasting into golden brown colour → Grinding (hammer mill) → Gram dal and edible ground nut cake are also roasted and ground → Mixing of jaggery with calcium carbonate and wheat flour and processed in multi-mill to obtain coarse flour → Finally mixing of all ingredients thoroughly → Packing → Storage/marketing

20.1.1.12 Wheat starch and gluten

Wheat starch has market for paper and textile industry. Wheat gluten is needed in confectionery industry as well as food processing industry. The technique for preparation of the wheat starch and gluten is as follows:

Wheat flour → Conversion into dough → Washing using water → Separation of wheat starch in the form of thick slurry → Thickening of slurry (using series of centrifuges) → Separation of light weight wheat germs and wheat gluten using conical hydroclones → Processing of wet germs for extraction of germ oil and germs containing gluten (protein) is dried into powder (wheat gluten). Wheat starch is also dried using rotary dryers and converted into powder form.

20.1.1.13 *Malted wheat*

Malted cereal flour is inexpensive and can be prepared at home and commercially. Malt is used in brewing and in preparation of malt extract for pharmaceutical purpose and in making of malted milk powder. The process of malting consists of steeping of good quality grain in cold water for 36 h with two changes of water → Speeding of steeped grain on wire mesh tray of 5–7.5 cm thickness → Germination is allowed to proceed for 3 days → Slow drying of germinated grain at low temperature → Drying of malt to moisture content of 13%.

20.1.2 Fermented wheat products

A variety of cereal-based fermented foods are prepared in India and most of them are used as staple food. Wheat-based products are bhatura, kulcha, naan, jalebi, etc.

20.1.2.1 *Bhatura*

Bhatura is leavened deep fried bread prepared from white wheat flour. It is consumed as breakfast food and snack food. The technique for preparation is as follows:

Making dough by mixing white wheat flour with water → Kneading for 20 min at room temperature → Supplementing dough with 1% common salt and inoculated with portion of previous batch ripe batter → Keep in open to proceed fermentation for 2–14 h → Dough is made or converted into balls → Flatten ball by hand using vegetable oil (12–18 cm diameter) before deep frying in oil

20.1.2.2 *Kulcha*

It is also used as staple food. The technique for preparation of kulcha is as follows:

Dough preparation by mixing white wheat flour, sugar, portion of dough from previous fermented batch and water in ratio of 100:1:10:50 at room temperature → Kneading by hand and proceed to fermentation overnight in earthen pots (gram flour can be added at 20% level) → Dough is prepared into balls after fermentation → Keep on smooth surface lightly sprinkled with flour→ Flattened by hand into 15-20 cm diameter → Transfer smoothly flattened dough on to a metallic baking tray → Baking for 30 min to obtained final product.

20.1.2.3 Naan

Naan is leavened flat bread generally consumed as a staple food. The technique for preparation of naan is as follows:

Dough preparation by mixing white wheat flour (1 kg), water (500 mL), yeast (20 g) or sour dough from previous batch (350 g) → Kneading the mixture vigorously for 15 min using vegetable oil for softening→ Divide dough into balls and left for fermentation at 25–32°C for 22–2.5 h → Mechanically kneading back → Flattened into discs (5–7 mL thickness) → Dusting with flour → Covered → Proceed to ferment at 25–32°C for 30–36 min. Naan is baked rapidly in hot oven at 230–260°C either on metal dry for 5–10 min or directly in contact with hot oven wall at 460–500°C for 2–3 min

20.1.2.4 Jalebi

This is a popular product prepared from soft smooth fermented wheat flour, deep fried and crisp, 5–7 cm in diameter and soaked in sugar syrup. This is eaten as snack and very popular at festive occasion. This is prepared from fine wheat flour (1 kg), curd (200 g) and water (650 mL). It is mixed together to form a thick batter and fermented overnight. Saffron can be added for better colour. Fermented batter is squeezed through cloth with a hole of about 4 mm diameter and deposited as continuous spirals into heated oil or ghee (160–180°C). In about a minute, these spirals become light brown and are removed from the frying pan. Drained away the excess fat and jalebi is immediately immersed into sugar syrup of honey consistency for 2 min and then removed for use.

20.2 Rice

Rice is extensively grown in India and forms staple article of diet of a majority of people. Rice is rich in carbohydrates in the form of starch which provides energy in the body. It has also fair amount of protein. Rice is also rich in vitamin B_1.

Rice is a covered caryopsis. The rice kernel consists of hull or husk, seed coat or bran, embryo or germ and endosperm. Milling of rice removes the hull (indigestible) and additional portion of bran to obtain unbroken endosperm. Rice is obtained through rice milling which is the largest agro processing industry of the country. The technique used for processing of paddy into rice is as follows:

Paddy → Cleaning of stones, chaff, dust, etc. → Parboiling → Dehulling/dehusking → Brown rice → Whitening or rice polishing → White rice → Milled or polished

20.2.1 Parboiling

Parboiling involves soaking of paddy in water for a short period followed by heating once or twice in steam and drying before milling. Parboiled rice is harder than raw rice, resist of breaking, has greater resistance to fungus and insects, losses of nutrients is less, improves digestibility, easy dehusking and stabilizes the oil content of bran. However, it has some disadvantage like dark colour, unpleasant smell, prolonged cooking, loss of antioxidants due to heat treatment. The process involved in parboiling is given in flow sheet.

Paddy → Stipping in water at 54.4–65.6°C for 9–12 h → Steaming at 110–118 for 8–20 min → Drying at 11–30% moisture → Milling → Parboiled or converted rice.

20.2.2 Rice products

Rice can be processed into various food products such as flaked rice, puffed rice, popped rice, rice papad, extruded food and fermented products.

20.2.2.1 *Flaked rice*

Flaked rice is prepared from parboiled rice. It is a breakfast food. It can be fried with spices and popularly known as poha. The technique for preparation of flaked rice is by traditional and improved methods.

Traditional process

Paddy → Soaking in warm water overnight or up to 30% moisture → Draining of water → Roasting of paddy with vigorous stirring in batch of 2 kg with sand in iron pan, over direct fire for about a minute → Removal of sand by sieving → Flattening of paddy either by pounding in mortar and pestle or by edge runner → Removal of husk → Flaked rice → Packing in polythene bag → Storage/marketing

Improved process

Paddy → Soaking in hot water overnight → Roasting of soaked paddy in sand → Passing successively through dehusker → Aspirator polisher and roller faster → Finely drying → Flaked rice → Packing → Storage/marketing. Recovery is more, no breakage and flakes are free from any husk bran specs and sand particles. Pure bran and husk can also be obtained with this process.

20.2.2.2 *Puffed rice*

This is popular snack product obtained by puffing milled parboiled rice. The traditional process consists of rice → Gently heated on furnace without sand (for reducing moisture content) → Mixing with salt solution → Roasting again on furnace in small batches with sand on fire for few seconds → Rice (expanded about eight times → Packing → Storage.

Better puffing can be obtained with dry heat parboiled rice than steam parboiled rice. Still better puffing can be obtained with pressure parboiled rice. Puffing can also be done with the method of over puffing.

20.2.2.3 Popped rice

This product is obtained by puffing the paddy directly. The process consists of Paddy → Pre-drying to 9% moisture → Raising moisture up to 14% → Resting → Puffing.

20.2.2.4 Extruded food

Extruded foods are ready to eat food manufactured from rice grits. The technique for preparation is as follows:

Rice grits → Feeding into homogenizer mixer → Transferring to semi-finished product forming machine → Formation of raw product → Giving desired shape (through compression, generation of heat and extrusion expansion) → Raw flips transported to raw flips silo → Exposed to counter current dryer (dries the semi-finished product to <1% moisture) → Processing via preparation system to the drum → Coating → Packing → Storage/marketing

20.2.2.5 Rice papad

Ingredients

Rice 1 kg, salt 50 g, red chillies 30 g, cumin seeds 20 g, lemon juice 2 tea spoons, water 1.5 L. The technique used for preparation of papad is as follows:

Rice → Washing → Drying → Grinding into powder → Adding of boiling water → Cooking 10-15 min → Mixing all the ingredients together → Kneading well → Rolling into balls → Taking each ball in a piece of polythene paper → Rolling into thin layer → Drying → Packing the bundles of papad in polythene bags → Sealing → Storage/marketing.

20.2.3 Fermented rice-based products

Fermented rice-based products are idili, dosa, dhokla, etc.

20.2.3.1 Idili

Idili is a small white acid-leavened steamed cake made by fermentation of a thick batter of washed and soaked rice and black gram. These are spongy and soft with a desirable sour flavour. This is eaten with coconut chutney, pickles and lentil curry.

The traditional method of idili preparation consists of washing and soaking rice and black gram in a ratio of 2:1 for 2–4 h at ambient temperature → Grinding them separately (rice is coarsely ground and black gram finely ground) → Mixing together with water to form uniform batter → Ferment the batter for 18–30 h by inoculating with fermented batter of previous batch after adding 1% salt → Pour fermented batter with a ladle on to greased metal plates or round shapes moulds → Steam cooking for 10–20 min → Idili with fine texture for use.

20.2.3.2 Dosa

Dosa is a thin, crisp, fried, breakfast or snack food becoming popular throughout India. The technique for preparation consists of soaking rice (1–3 parts) and black gram (1 part) at ambient temperature → Grinding to a fine paste by adding 2–3 parts of water → Mixing the two to form running batter → Allow the batter mixture to ferment overnight for 12–24 h after adding of 1% salt and inoculating with fermented batter of previous batch → Pour 60–80 mL of batter on a hot greasy griddle for few minutes → Formation of crisp pan cake → Rolling of dosa and serving with coconut chutney.

20.2.3.3 Dhokla

Dhokla is a fermented food prepared from a batter made of coarsely ground rice and Bengal gram. The preparation technique consists of preparation of batter from ground rice and Bengal gram powder in a ratio of 3:1 → Mixing 1 part of curd with adequate water → Ferment overnight as room temperature → Addition of salt and green chillies → Pouring of batter on greased plates → Steaming in a suitable pan for 20 min → Cooling of dhokla → Cutting into square → Seasoned with coriander leaves and green chillies for serving.

20.3 Maize (corn)

Maize is also an important staple food crop of India. Maize is rich in carbohydrates, fibre, minerals and protein. Maize grains are white yellow and reddish. Its kernel consists of hull or bran coat with high fibre content, embryo rich in oil and endosperm rich in starch which is predominant carbohydrate. The principal types of maize are sweet corn, flint corn, dent corn, pop corn, flour corn and waxy corn based on distribution of starch in the endosperm.

20.3.1 Maize shelling

Grains are separated from maize cobs by machine called maize sheller. Maize sheller may be hand operated or power operated. In hand operated corn sheller, the cobs are fed one by one and shelling takes place in between the long, bevel wheel and shelling disc.

20.3.2 Milling

The major process utilized for milling is by dry and wet. In both processes, germ is separated from the grain to recover oil. In dry milling, the object is to recover maximum quantity of grits with minimum amount of flour or meal. Grinding of whole grain produces these products. Grits are used for production of corn flakes. Dry milled germ can be pressed or solvent extracted to recover valuable oil. Flour is consumed shortly after processing because presence of crushed germ in the flour produced rancid odour and flavour. Maize dry milling has lower capital cost than wet milling. Wet milling process consists of steeping stage and disintegration of endosperm to recover starch and protein. Wet milling products are high fructose corn syrup and ethanol.

20.3.3 Products

Maize is processed into various products such as flakes, popcorn, extruded food, flour, degerminated flour, starch, corn germ oil, liquid glucose, dextrose monohydrates, etc.

20.3.3.1 Flakes

A maize flake is a product accepted as health food. Deep fried flakes are used extensively. Dry roasted maize flakes are consumed along with sugar and milk. The technique of preparation of flakes is as follows:

Maize nuts → Cleaning to remove dust and stones → Grading → Soaking in hot water → Draining → Drying → Roasting → Fed to flaker polisher → Flakes → Sieving to remove bran and broken maize → Packing in polythene bag → Storage/marketing

20.3.3.2 Popcorn

Maize popcorn is very popular. It is very tasty, easy to carry and eat. It is low-cost snack, nutritious and is consumed regularly. The technique for preparation of popcorn is as follows:

Maize grains → Washing → Drying → Feeding to automatic popping machines → Roasting and popped → Mixing with salt and black pepper → Packing in polythene bag → Storage/marketing

20.3.3.3 *Extruded food*

The technique for preparation of extruded food is as follows:

Corn grits → Feeding into homogenizer mixer → Transferring to semi-finished product forming machine → Formation of raw product → Giving desired shape (flips stars stick or plasticised) through compression → Transporting of raw flips to raw flips silo → Drying with counter current dryer to <1% moisture → Processing → Coating → Packing → Storage/ marketing

20.3.3.4 *Maize flour*

The technique for preparation of maize flour is as follows:

Maize grain → Cleaning → Conditioning → Removal of germ and husk mechanically → Processing of maize grits into fine flour

20.3.3.5 Degerminated flour

This flour is mostly consists of endosperm. It has low content of B vitamins. This flour is utilized by brewers as a starch source for the action of barley malt making of wort for production of beer.

20.3.3.6 Starch

Maize starch has many uses. It is used in domestic as food in soup, pudding and gravy thickness, as preferential water absorber in baking powder and in manufacture of confectionery. The technique for preparation of starch is as follows:

Maize grains → Cleaning → Steeping in hot water (52°C) → Draining → Discharging by screw conveyors to the degerminating mill → Flowing of maize slurry into containers → Pumping to refiner mill → Delivering to extraction section for coarse fibre washing → Correction of starch milk → Dewatering of husk, shells and coarse fibre mechanically → Pumping of crude starch milk to the extraction section for fine washing → Flowing of starch milk to the containers → Filtering and gluten is separated from the starch milk → Washing of milk again in second and third separator → Gluten is separated and concentrated → Collection of gluten water in a container → Pumping to the concentrator → Flowing of concentrated gluten into container be mixed with the pre dewatered fine fibres coming from extraction section → Pumping of collected starch milk in the starch milk container to centrifuge → Transporting of scraped starch to the starch dryer to reduce water content → Collection of dried starch in a cyclone → Sacking off product (starch) → Packing → Storage.

20.3.3.7 Corn germ oil

Germ oil can be extracted by solvent extraction. Maize oil is valuable vegetable oil due to high content of linolenic fatty acid and its pleasant flavour.

The fat content is low about 3.6% and oil can be refined to obtain high quality vegetable oil for cooking.

20.3.3.8 Liquid glucose

Liquid glucose can be obtained from starch conversion. Starch is converted into acid or enzyme hydrolysis which gives liquid glucose and dextrose.

20.3.3.9 Dextrose monohydrate

Assimilates with blood instantly and work as an energy agent. It is also used in ice-cream, soft drinks, bakery products and ready to eat food.

20.3.3.10 Dextrose anhydrous

Used in manufacture of baby foods, frozen dairy products and manufacture of beer.

20.3.3.11 Malto dextrose

It is used in manufacture of baby food, frozen dairy products and beer.

20.4 Sorghum (jowar)

Sorghum is popularly known as jowar. Jowar is a very popular food grain and it is cheaper than the wheat and paddy. It is the most important food and fodder crop of dry land agriculture. Starch is the major carbohydrate of the grain. Sorghum is richer in protein than rice and maize. Riboflavin and pyridoxine content of sorghum is similar to maize.

Sorghum grain is small, rounded and varies in colour such as off-white, shades of red and yellow or brown. Sorghum grain consists of an embryo, scutellum and endosperm enclosed in seed coat called testa and fruit coat called pericarp fused together. Pigment layer is found in outer layer of pericarp or beneath the pericarp.

20.4.1 Dehulling

Dehulling of sorghum is done by mechanical dehuller. Mechanical dehulling improves appearance and functional properties. Dehulling removes the colour of all sorghum verities. Mechanical dehulling converts millets into convenient ready to cook grain and improves the flour quality. Mechanical dehulling process consists of following steps:

Clean sorghum → Drying of grain (8–10 h) → Grading → Filling of grain (5 kg) in dehuller → Running of dehuller for 6–8 min → Removal of dehulled grain → Winnowing → Separation of husk and dehulled sorghum grain

20.4.2 Sorghum products

The sorghum grain is used as human food in various forms such as chapaties and cooked as rice. Sorghum can be processed into flour, semolina, flakes and popping.

20.4.2.1 Flour and semolina

The fine quality sorghum flour can be substituted in place of wheat flour or semolina. Bengal gram flour and semolina can be used for preparation of various products such as instant food mixes, infant and weaning foods, dehydrated foods (papad), breakfast food, snack food (deep fried food) and baked food (biscuits).

The process used for sorghum flour and semolina is as follows:

Sorghum (dehulled) → Milling → Cooling → Sieving (24 mesh) → Coarse semolina and fine semolina with flour → Sieving (40 mesh) → Flour and fine semolina

20.4.2.2 *Instant food mixes*

Idili and dosa mixes ready to cook can be prepared from sorghum flour. Idili contains dehulled sorghum rawa 60%, black gram flour 30.5%, salt 3%, sodium bicarbonate 2%, citric acid 2.5% and sodium acetate 0.65%.

Dosa mix contains the ingredients sorghum flour 30%, rice flour 30%, black gram flour 30%, salt 3.2%, citric acid 3.8% and calcium carbonate 1.9%.

20.4.2.3 Infant mix

Infant mix formulation such as sorghum and pigeon pea flour in ratio of 80:20 or sorghum and soya bean flour with sugar in ratio of 70:10:20 can be used for preparation of infant mix foods.

20.4.2.4 Papad

Papad can be prepared from dehulled sorghum flour. Steps involved in preparation of sorghum papad are as follows:

Dehulled sorghum flour (500 g) → Addition of chilli powder (15 g), salt (25 g), cumin seed (10 g) → Mixing well → Addition of lemon juice (2 spoon) → Addition of mixture to boiling water (1 L) → Cooking for 15 min → Removal from fire → Kneading thoroughly → Making into round ball → Rolling into papads → Drying → Packing in polythene bags → Storage/ marketing

20.4.2.5 Flakes

The technique for preparation of flakes is as follows:

Jowar grains → Cleaning → Soaking in hot water for 10 h → Draining → Roasting → Resting to obtain wrinkle-free flakes → Polishing → Flaking → Drying → Packing in printed polythene bag → Storage/marketing.

20.5 Pearl millet (Bajra)

Bajra is the predominant crop among millets in India. It is used as food. It is also used as animal feed and green plant serve as excellent fodder. The coarse grain contain 10% husk. The carbohydrate consists mostly starch. It is rich in protein, mineral such as calcium, phosphorus and iron. The grains are rich in thiamine, riboflavin and niacin.

Pearling improves appearance and taste of the products. Wet millings have developed. In pearling, most of the germ is intact and nutritive value is not much affected.

20.5.1 Products

Bajra is usually processed into flour, bread, chapaties and porridge. The grain can be parched and product is like popcorn. The grain is also used for malting.

20.6 Finger millet (ragi)

The grains of finger millet is very small and its colour vary from deep brown to sheds of red to almost black. Several verities have been developed which have higher production. The nutritive value of ragi is better than wheat and rice. Prolamins and glutelins are the major proteins and are adequate in all essential amino acids. It is very rich in calcium mineral and fibre.

20.6.1 Milling

Milling is done by wet conditioning. After steaming, milling is done in a hammer/plate mill or roller flour mill.

20.6.2 Products

Ragi is used as chapaties, dosa, porridge, gruel and dumpling. Ragi is most suitable for malting (malted ragi). The malted ragi flour can be used with milk and in combination of germinated green gram flour to form weaning food of high calorie. Ragi is also roasted and used as snack food.

Fermented product ambali can be prepared from ragi millet flour. The technique of preparation consists of Ragi flour → Combine with water → Formation of thick batter → Fermentation for 14–16 h → Addition of partially cooked rice to batter with continuous stirring and cooking → Addition of curd when cooked → Ambali is ready to use.

20.7 Barley

Barley is an important cereal of North Indian plains. The major portion of the grain produced is consumed as flour. Barley flour is easily digestible and is used for preparation of chapaties either alone or mixed with gram or wheat flour. It is rich in carbohydrates, fibre and minerals. Barley is the source of fermentable carbohydrate. It is an important raw material for the distilling and brewing industry.

20.7.1 Milling

Barley is milled to make shelled barley, pearl barley, barley grits, barley flakes and barley flour. Barley grains have fused husk and pearling involves to stage that is dehusking and then bran abrasion. Pearl barley used in soup and infant food.

20.7.2 Barley products

Barley can be processed into flour, and parched grains to make sattu. It is used to prepare malt for production of beer and whisky and other products such as industrial alcohol and vinegar. The techniques for preparation of some of these products are as follows.

20.7.2.1 Beer

It is the fermented product of and extract of malt cereal preferably barley. In addition, hopes are added to the mesh to provide pleasant bitterness flavour and increase the shelf life of beer. The technique for preparation of beer is as follows:

Barley → Steeping → Germinating (green malt) → Milling → Mashing (sweet wort) → Boiling (hopped wort) → Addition of yeast → Fermentation → Aging (maturing) → Packaging/bottling → Storing/marketing

20.7.2.2 Whisky

The technique used for preparation of whisky from barley is as follows:

Barley → Steeping → Germinating → Milling → Mashing → Fermentation → Distillation (double continuous distillation system) → Maturation (2–3 years) → Blending for consistent flavour → Bottling of blended whisky

The types of units which have come up in cereal processing are flour, refined flour, bakeries food, bread, biscuit, cakes, etc. Starch, glucose, cereals flakes (corn, wheat, rice and millets), malted food, whole cooked grain (rice, papad, beer, grain-based alcohol and instant food). Recent development in cereal processing are shift from stone milling to roller milling in wheat flour mill, development of fast foods based on refined wheat flour, development of extruded cereal products which have greater demand and production, production of high fibre bread, development of health foods such as diabetic food and low calorie food, development of ready to eat or instant food, recovery of rice bran during milling of rice, parboiling of rice in minimum time and branding and packaging of cereal and cereal-based food. Breakfast cereal, based on wheat, corn, rice and millets, instant food, malted food and bakery products have great potential for export.

21

Pulse products and processing technique

Various types of pulses are cultivated throughout the country. Most of the pulses produced are milled into dal. Use of pulses is very common in Indian diet. Pulses are used in different forms such as whole, split with skin and without skin, germinated or fermented, etc. Pulses are rich in protein and B vitamins. Pulses improve the quality of cereal protein. Pulses provide safety due to high protein and fibre content. They are also rich in carbohydrates and minerals. The important pulses are pigeon pea, Bengal gram, black gram, peas, cow peas, green gram and lentil. The common pulses and their products are discussed in the following sections.

21.1 Pigeon pea (red gram)

Red gram is the most important pulse of India. It is extensively used for dal. Pigeon pea is rich in protein.

21.1.1 Products

Pigeon pea grain is mainly processed into dal. Nutritionally 5–10% husk in dal is considered desirable but the consumer preference is for husk-free dal.

21.1.2 Dal milling

Mini dal mills have been developed which are suited for small scale operation. The technique for preparation of dal is as follows:

Pigeon pea → Cleaning to remove dust, stones, chaff, etc. → Soaking in water → Seasoning (kept in shed for around 8–10 h) → Milling → Dehusking and splitting → Grading → Packing → Storage/marketing

21.2 Bengal gram (chana)

This is the most important crop of pulses in India. It is rich in fibre, minerals such as calcium and iron and vitamin particularly niacin. Beside its food value, it has medicinal importance as the germinated gram seeds recommended to cure scurvy.

21.2.1 Products

Bengal gram can be processed into dal, besan (flour), sattu, crushed or whole gram, boiled or parched, roasted or cooked, salted and is also used in sweet preparations.

21.2.1.1 Dal

The technique for preparation of dal is as follows:

Bengal gram grains → Cleaning for broken grains and other impurities → Conditioning → Sun drying up to 12–14% moisture → Milling (splitting) → Grading → Packing → Storage/marketing

21.2.1.2 Flour/besan

The technique for preparation of Bengal gram flour is as follows:

Gram → Cleaning → Conditioning (removal of coloured gram shell) → Drying → Milling (breaking, scalping and purification) → Reduction and dressing → Finishing into excellent flour/besan → Packing → Storage/marketing

21.2.1.3 Sattu

Steps involved in the preparation of Bengal gram sattu are as follows:

Bengal gram → Cleaning with pulse cleaning machine → Roasting with electrically operated roaster → Grinding to obtain finer mesh size → Sieving to remove coarse powder and foreign material → Packing → Storage/marketing

21.2.1.4 Parching

Bengal gram is parched to give highly acceptable product. Parched Bengal gram is used in the treatment of protein-calorie mal nutrition in children. The traditional method of parching consists of the following steps:

Sprinkling of grains with little water → Mixing with preheated sand in a frying pan → Keeping on open fire at temperature 200–250°C for 2 min → Sieving parched Bengal gram → Packing/marketing

21.3 Black gram (Urad)

Black gram is known as urad/mash. It is one of the important pulse crops and is highly prized pulse. It is very rich in phosphoric acid. Its use is similar to green gram (mung).

21.3.1 Products

Black gram is processed into dal (whole or split). Dal is processed into papad and bari (spiced ball of ground dal).

21.3.1.1 Papad

Papad is a dry product, which adds variety to the diet. It is nutritious and quite popular.

Ingredients
Dal 1 kg, water 0.5 L, salt 50 g, cinnamon powder 10 g, cumin seeds 20 g, black pepper powder 20 g, sodium bicarbonate 50 g.

The technique for preparation of black gram papad is as follows:

Black gram dal (urad) → Washing → Drying → Grinding into fine powder → Addition of boiling water with sodium bicarbonate salt → Cooking for 15–20 min → Mixing of all the spices → Kneading well with hot water and beating with grinding stone → Stretching it with hands (plasticizing) → Rolling into balls → Take each ball in piece of polythene paper → Rolling out into very thin layer → Drying → Packing in polythene bag → Sealing → Storage/marketing

21.3.1.2 Bari

Ingredients
Black gram dal 1 kg, fenugreek leaves 1 kg, salt 100 g, black pepper 30 g, red chillies 40 g, cumin seeds 20 g, cloves 5 g, cinnamon 5 g, asafoetida 0.5 g, ginger 125 g.

The technique for preparation of bari is as follows:

Black gram → Dehulling → Washing → Soaking overnight in water → Grinding into paste (dough) → Spicing with all spices → Moulding into balls of 5–8 cm in diameter → Fermentation → Drying in open air about a week → Packing → Storage/marketing.

21.4 Green gram

Green gram or mung is spread all over the country. Green gram is rich in minerals particularly in iron. It is also rich in nicotinic acid.

21.4.1 Products

The grains are used as pulse (whole or split). It is also processed into vadian and flour. Grains are eaten whole after germination, parched and salted. Bari can also be prepared from green gram like black gram bari.

21.4.1.1 Vadian

The ingredients used and the technique used for the preparation of vadian are as follows.

Ingredients
Mung dal 1 kg, fenugreek leaves 1 kg, salt 100 g, black pepper 30 g, red chillies 40 g, cumin seeds 20 g, cloves 5 g, cinnamon 5 g.

Green gram dal (mung dal) → Cleaning → Soaking in water (overnight) → Washing, cleaning and chopping of fenugreek leaves → Grinding of mung dal to make dough → Keep it overnight for fermentation → Mixing of dal, chopped fenugreek leaves and all spices together → Divide the mass into small balls and place them in sun (spread out muslin sheet or greased polythene sheet in sun and putting the balls on it) → Drying vadian completely in the sunlight → Packing the vadian in polythene bags → Sealing airtight → Storage/marketing

21.5 Soya bean

Soya beans have higher content of protein than any other legumes. It provides a high quality of protein and low saturated fat. It has good source of minerals such as calcium, iron, phosphorus and zinc and vitamins such as B complex and E. Soya beans contain all three macro nutrients needed for good health. It is also an excellent source of dietary fibre. Soya bean protein provides all the essential acids in good amount as required for human health. It has also higher percentage of oil and quality fatty acid profile. Soya beans are extensively used in many food items. Soya products are becoming popular with health conscious people.

21.5.1 Products

Soya beans are processed into number of products such as soya milk, paneer, flour, curd, sauce, roasted nuts, nuggets, soya flakes, soya papad, etc. The techniques for preparation of these products are as follows.

21.5.1.1 Soya milk

Soya milk is extracted from soya beans. It is rich in proteins, vitamins and minerals. Soya milk is lactose free, cholesterol free and low in saturated fat. Soya milk can be used as such or cold and hot beverage such as shakes, coffee or tea and ice-cream. It is also used for the preparation of curd and ice-cream.

Ingredients
Soya bean 1 kg, baking soda 15 g, sugar 150 g, salt 10 g, calcium sulphate 30 g or citric acid 5 g.

The technique for the preparation of soya milk is as follows:

Soya bean → Cleaning → Sorting or removal of cracked, damaged and discoloured soya beans → Addition of soya bean in boiling water and blanching for 5 min → Draining and rinsing with hot water → Addition of rinsed soya bean in vigorous boiling water containing 5 g baking soda → Blanching for 5 min → Draining and rinsing with hot water → Grinding blanched soya bean with 6 L of very hot water (boiling) for 3 min by using blender at high speed → Filtering of soya milk through cheese cloth and extracting as much of the soya milk as possible → Addition of salt and sugar → Simmering (cook near boiling) for 20 min → Addition of flavours according to preference (vanilla, chocolate, etc.) → Stirring frequently to avoid burning → Serving hot or cold

21.5.1.2 Soya paneer

The technique for preparation of soya paneer is as follows:

Soya bean → Cleaning→ Soaking in water for 4 h → Washing with warm water → Grinding in water (7–8 times more water than beans) for 25 min → Slurry → Cooking in grinder cum cooker (for 3 min at 120°C) → Filtering → Soya milk → Addition of citric acid → Coagulation of material → Pressing with mechanical press for half an hour to remove water → Paneer → Marketing

21.5.1.3 Soya flour

The technique for preparation of soya flour is as follows:

Soya bean → Cleaning → Drying → Dehulling and separation of hulls from cotyledons → Preconditioning (boiling/cooking) for denaturing of hydrolytic enzymes which causes rancidity → Extrusion (enzymes and anti nutritional factors are inactivated) → Drying → Cooling → Milling/grinding → Flour → Packing → Storage/marketing

21.5.1.4 Soya sauce

Ingredients

Defatted soya flour, salt, baking soda, vinegar and preservatives.

The technique for the preparation of soya sauce is as follows:

Soya flour → Processing (hydrolysis process) → Mixing with all ingredients homogenously → Formation of semi-liquid/paste type mixture → Filtering through filter sieves to remove impurities → Mixture is taken to SS nutrilization tanks → Keeping for 2 h → Packing → Storage/marketing

21.5.1.5 Roasted nut

Soya nuts are whole soya beans soaked in water and then baked until browned. Soya nuts have less fat and more protein as compared to pea nuts or other nuts. It is also less expensive than pea nuts. The technique for preparation of roasted nut is as follows:

Soya beans → Cleaning → Sorting → Soaking for 8 h → Draining of beans → Spreading into a single layer → Baking at 175°C → Stirring after 15 min and again stirring after 5 min until it becomes golden brown and crunchy (total time takes about 25 min) → Packing → Storage/marketing

21.5.1.6 Nuggets (bari)

It is prepared from defatted soya flour. It has about 50% protein and <1% fat. Nuggets are healthy alternate to meat.

21.5.1.7 Soya flakes

Soya flakes are a popular dietary product. This can be prepared with soya bean flaking machine. The steps involved in preparation are as follows:

Soya bean → Cleaning → Dehulling → Blanching of dehulled soya bean in boiling water (60 min) → Drying of bean in sunlight up to 25–305 moisture → Flaking of beans in soya bean flaker → Drying of flakes up to 8% moisture → Packing

21.5.1.8 Soya papad

Papad is another traditional food product of India. Soya papad can be prepared by blending soya flour with 30–40% of black gram flour. This is soya-fortified papad. Fortification of soya flour with black gram flour increases the protein content of papad.

21.5.1.9 Instant soya wheat meal

This is a pre-cooked product of defatted soya flour and wheat flour. This product is convenient alternate to dalia called breakfast cereal.

21.5.1.10 Noodles and vermicelli

Noodles are of two types: wet noodles and fried noodles. Mixing of 10–12% defatted soya flour to wheat flour provides a product with increased moisture retention called wet noodles, whereas in case of fried noodles, it saves oils during frying.

21.5.1.11 Extruded snacks

Extruded snack prepared are defatted soya flour and combination of rice, wheat and corn flour. Extruded soya snacks have very little fat and more than double protein, compared to regular snacks.

21.5.1.12 Soya protein isolates

Protein isolates contain about 90% protein from soya bean. Protein isolate can be used in production of toned milk, infant food, protein rich biscuits and bread. It is used as meat substitute. The technique for preparation of soya bean protein isolate is as follows:

Defatted soya bean → Dispersion at pH 9.0 → Sieving of coarse material → Centrifugation (fine material) → Precipitation at pH 4.5 by addition of HCL → Curd → Vacuum filtration → Drying → Soya bean protein

22

Nuts and oil seed products and processing technique

India occupies a prominent position in oil seeds. Oil seeds are considerably higher in protein than cereal grains. It is also higher in fat. Oil seeds contain 20–40% protein and 20–50% fat. The important oil seeds crops grown are groundnut, rapeseed, mustard, sesame and sunflower.

22.1 Groundnut (peanut)

Groundnut is the most important oil seed crop grown in India. Groundnut is rich in protein and vitamins A and B.

22.1.1 Products

Groundnut is processed into edible oil, blanched and roasted peanut, groundnut flour, hand-picked and selected (HPS) groundnut and peanut butter.

22.1.1.1 Blanched and roasted peanut

The techniques for preparation of these products are as follows:

Groundnut → Cleaning → Decortication (separation of kernels) → Grading (according to size) → Sorting (through colour sorting machine, removal of infected/unwanted kernels) → Roasting (in roaster at 60–70°C) → Blanching (removal of outer red skin with mild pressure) → Packing (polythene bag) → Storage/marketing

22.1.1.2 Peanut butter

It is an ideal substitute for milk butter. It has low calorie and high protein product. The technique for preparation is as follows:

Groundnut → Cleaning → Shelling → Grading → Roasting and blanching → Grinding in peanut butter mill to obtain fine and creamy butter → Cooling → Packing in pet jar/metal drum → Deaeration for removal of air in vacuum → Storage/marketing

22.1.1.3 HPS groundnuts

Groundnut pods → Decortication (shells are broken and kernels are separated) → Sieving (through mechanical shaker sieves for removal of dirt and stones, splits and shrivelled peanuts) → Grading (different sizes) → Packing (gunny bags) → Storage/marketing.

22.1.1.4 Groundnut flour

Groundnuts → Passing through bucket elevators to destoner and decoraticator → Groundnut kernels separated → Feeding to viabratory grader to remove immature kernels → Mild roasting to facilitate removal of red skin → Passing through blancher → Skin and germs are separated → Inspecting of blanched kernels → Feeding to a screw type expeller → Oil and cake are obtained → Cooling of cake → Grinding in a hammer mill → Flour → Packing → Storage/marketing

Oil is filtered through pressure filter and packed in tins/barrels.

22.1.1.5 Chikkies

Groundnut kernels → Roasting to remove the outer red skin → Splitting through splitting machine → Boiling of jaggery in water till thick syrup is formed and filtered → Mixing of hot syrup with groundnut splits → Pouring of the mixture in trays → Cooling → Cutting of small square-shaped pieces → Packing of pieces in plastic wrappers → Storage/marketing.

22.1.1.6 Peanut milk

Peanut milk can be used as supplement to the diet of children. The technique for preparation of peanut milk is as follows:

Peanut kernel → Cleaning → Light roasting for red skin removal → Decuticling → Removal of germ and spoiled seed → Grinding to smooth paste (seven times the weight of paste) → Mixing with addition of calcium hydroxide solution to pH of 6.8 → Addition of a mixture of disodium phosphate and acid potassium phosphate having pH 7.0 to stabilize milk → Filtration → Fortification (vitamin A, D, riboflavin, folic acid, vitamin B_{12} and mineral calcium and iron salt) → Addition of cane sugar (7%) → Homogenization → Steamed → Bottling → Storage (under refrigerator) → Distribution

22.1.1.7 Protein isolate

Protein isolate is blend, cream coloured and has 90% protein. Groundnut protein is used in baby foods, milton, biscuits, coffee and tea whiteners and confectionery. The technique used for preparation of protein isolate is as follows:

Groundnut flour → Solubilization in aqueous alkaline medium → Separation of insoluble carbohydrates by filtration or centrifugation → Precipitation of protein isolate

22.2 Mustard and rapeseed

Mustard is an important oil crop of the country. The oil obtained is the main cooking medium in North India. The seed and oil are used as condiment in the preparation of pickles and for flavouring curries.

22.2.1 Products

Major portion of the seeds is utilized for extraction of edible oil. Mustard powder is also prepared and used as condiment in pickles particularly stuffed green and red chillies. The technique for the preparation of powder is as follows:

22.2.1.1 Powder

Mustard seeds → Cleaning → Grading → Conditioning (to loosen the husk) → Drying of seeds → Subjecting to splitting and dehiscing → Mixture of husk and cotyledons → Screening → Classification into individuals fractions → Grinding of cotyledons to desired fineness to obtain mustard powder on triple roller mill → Mustard powder → Packing → Storage/marketing

22.3 Sesame (gingelly seed)

Sesame seeds are oil seeds but their oil is not commonly used in India as it is expensive. Sesame seeds have medicinal values and they control the ageing process.

22.3.1 Products

Sesame is processed for seeds, hulled seeds, oil, chikkies, etc.

22.3.1.1 Hulled seeds

Sesame seeds have thin shell/husk which needs to be removed and removing process is called hulling. The technique used for hulling seed is as follows:

Sesame seeds → Soaking in water for 5–6 h (to facilitate hulling and minimizing breakages) → Putting in concrete pits → Hammering with help of mechanized wooden hammers → Washing thoroughly in water (to remove skin, dirt, etc.) → Sun drying of deskinned sesame seeds → Packing in gunny bag → Storage/marketing

22.3.1.2 Chikkies

The technique for preparation of chikkies is as follows:

Sesame seeds → Roasting→ Boiling of jaggery in water till thick syrup is formed and filtered → Mixing of hot syrup with sesame seeds → Pouring of the mixture in trays → Cooling → Cutting into small square-shaped pieces → Packing of pieces in plastic wrappers → Storage/marketing

Oil can also be extracted from sesame.

22.4 Sunflower seed

Sunflower is grown mainly for its oil. The oil is used for culinary purposes and it is recommended for heart patients. Seeds contain 35–50% oil and 17–25% protein.

22.4.1 Products

22.4.1.1 Dehulling of seeds

The technique for dehulling of seeds preparation is as follows:

Seeds of sunflower are coated with dry brittle hull. Dehulled sunflower seeds have major application in extracting high quality edible oil. The technique for dehulling of sunflower seeds is as follows:

Sunflower seeds → Cleaning → Grading with the help of vibrating sieve → Dehulling with the help of sheller → Sieving for separation of kernels, broken, fines and hulls → Packing → Storage/marketing

Dehulled sunflower seeds are used for extraction of oil, preparation of snacks confectionery and chikkies. Edible quality of cake is also produced.

22.5 Soya bean

Soya bean is also used as oil seeds. The good quality oil can be obtained from soya bean seeds. The oil is good source of tocopherols and as poly unsaturated fat intake is increased, the need for dietary vitamin E in cases. The oil is also find use in emulsions for parenteral nutrition due to its high n-3 linolenic content.

23
Fats and oil processing

Fats have high melting point and are solid at room temperature. Oils have lower melting point and are liquid at room temperature. Fats and oils do not occur free in nature. They occur in animal tissue and in seeds and fruits from which they are isolated, refined and processed for specific use. Fats and oils are good source of energy, excellent source of fats soluble vitamins A, D, E and K and provide essential fatty acids which are component of membrane of living cells. In addition to their nutritional value, fats and oil play an important role as medium of cooking improving texture of food, improving palatability of food, influence flavour and one of the essential constituents in food emulsions.

23.1 Animal-based fat

The animal-based fats and oils used are lard, tallow, fish oil and butter.

23.1.1 Lard

Lard is a fat of pork or hogs. It is low cost fat and popular in western countries for frying and baking. The technique used for extraction of fat from animal tissue is by rendering are heat. The process involved is as follows:

Mincing or division of fatty tissue of animal into fine particle size → Flash heating for 15 s → Pulverization → Centrifugation → Blended and stable fat → Packing

23.1.2 Tallow

Tallow is a animal fat from beef. This is also extracted by rendering process.

Meat scraps or mincing of fatty tissue of animal → Heating for melting of fat → Rising of melted fat and settling of water and remaining tissue → Separation of melted fat by skimming or centrifugation

23.1.3 Fish oil

Fish oil is of two types that is fish body oil and fish liver oil.

23.1.3.1 *Fish body oil*

Fish body oil can be obtained from fishes such as whale, sardine, salmon and herring which are good source of oil. Fish body oil can also be obtained by rendering process. The process is as follows:

Fish tissues → Heating in kettle for melting of fat → Rising of melted fat → Separation of melted fat by centrifugation → Packing

23.1.3.2 *Fish liver oil*

It is a natural source of vitamin A and to some extent vitamin D. Shark, cod and halibut are good source of fish liver oil. The method used for obtaining fish liver oil is as follows:

Minced fish liver → Cooking at 85–95°C → Resulting disintegration of liver cells and freeing of oil → Oil flooding on the stream condensate → Skimmed off by centrifugation → Packing

23.1.4 Butter

Butter is fat concentrate obtained by agitation or churning of cream, milk and curd. Butter may be table butter or white butter. Table butter is prepared from sour cream which has more pronounced flavour. Table butter contains 80% fat, 1.5% curd and 3% salt. White butter contains 76% fat not more than 1.5% curd and no salt and colour. The technique for preparation of table butter is as follows:

Reception or separation of cream → Neutralization of cream or partial reduction in acidity of sour cream → Standard digestion of cream or adjustment of fat level in cream 30–35% → Pasteurization of cream by HTST method at 95–100°C for 15 s → Cooling at 5–10°C → Ripening of cream or fermentation of cream with the help of desirable starter culture → Ageing at least 4 h → Churning and addition of colour and salt → Butter with 80% fat and 16% moisture → Packing for bulk or retail → Storage at –23°C to –29°C or marketing

23.1.5 Margarine

Margarine is made from one or more optional fat ingredients churned with cultured pasteurized skim milk or whey. Vitamins A and D are added to margarine for improving nutritive value.

23.2 Vegetable-based fats and oil

The techniques for oil extraction from oil seeds are pressing and solvent extraction by pressing is by the use of high pressure expellers or power ghanis which as now replaced non-power units. The process involves oil bearing seeds or material, cleaning, tempering, dehulling, crushing or flakening and passing through expeller for oil separation. Deoiled cake is used as cattle feed. This is most common and about 80% oil is extracted by this method. However, this method is not very efficient as cakes contain considerable amount of oil. Hence, solvent extraction or combination of both pressing and solvent extraction is becoming popular. Solvent extraction is especially more useful for removing oil with the materials have low content of oil. Among various solvent used, the hexane is very common solvent. Solvent is removed from the oil after extraction of oil. The residue is used for processing of edible flour.

Oil extracted by this method is crude and contains many other undesirable constituents. Therefore, refining is done to remove the suspended particles by filtration or centrifugation. The process of refining oil consists of oil seeds/nuts, cooked in steam, screw pressing, addition of food grade hexane, oil is extracted and solvent is removed, degumming, addition of alkali (formation of soap with free fatty acid), removal by centrifugal filtration, refined heated oil in vaccum, removal of plant pigment by bleaching and finally deodourized to obtain refined oil.

The source of vegetable-based fat and oils are mustard and rape seed oil, groundnut oil, soya bean oil, sesame oil, sunflower oil, rice bran oil, olive oil, coconut oil, palm oil and mahua oil.

23.2.1 Mustard and rape seed oil

Mustard and rape seed are the important oil crops of India. The oil content of seeds ranges from 30% to 48%. Its oleic and linolic acids have higher nutritive value. Rape seeds oil is also known as canola oil. Mustard and rape seed oils are used in cookery and pickles in North India. The process involved in extraction or production of mustard/rape seed oil consists of following steps:

Dry mustard/rape seed → Cleaning of impurities → Screw pressing or power ghani (expeller) →Filtering of liquid oils → Packing in tin/jar/plastic pouches → Storage/marketing.

23.2.2 Groundnut oil

Groundnut oil is extensively used in cooking, and in salad, it is also used for preserving fish such as tinned sardines. It is one of the most important fats used for making margarine. The processes for oil extraction of groundnut consist of following steps:

Good quality groundnut kernels → Cleaning of all impurities → Roasting of kernels for 5–10 min → Remove of red cuticle (decuticling) by rubbing → Separation of germs → Oil is extracted by screw pressing (power expeller) → Packing

The resulting cake is powdered into hammer mill and these can be extracted by food grade hexane to get fat-free flour.

23.2.3 Peanut butter

It is an ideal substitute for milk butter. It is low calories and high protein product. The technique for preparation is as follows:

Peanut kernel → Cleaning of all impurities → Moderate roasting → Removal of red skin (testa) through blanching machine → Separation of germ by sieving and spoilt kernel by hand picking → Grinding of kernels is grinding machine → Addition of hydrogenated fat at 5% to prevent separation of oil → Addition of sodium chloride at 2% → Mixture is grounded to smooth paste → Packing

Peanut butter can be fortified with calcium, salt and essential vitamins for supplementing the diets of children.

23.2.4 Soya bean oil

This is a leading vegetable oil in the world in terms of both production and consumption. Soya bean oil has both n-6 and n-3 fatty acids and good source of vitamin E. The oil is used in vanaspati, cooking oil, sandwich spreads, baby food and making non-dairy butters. The process for extraction of oil is as follows:

Soya bean (raw bean) → Cleaning of impurities → Passing through huller to remove hulls → Dehulled seed → Splitting → Soaking in water for an hour → Draining of water → Wet material → Heated in steam for 30 min at 6.34 kg pressure to inactivate trypsin and growth inhibitors → Drying of steamed seed under sun or tunnel drier → Removal of oil from died seed in screw pressing or by solvent extraction

23.2.5 Sesame (gingelly oil)

Sesame oil contains antioxidant, linoleic acid, α-linoleic acid and lecithin. Seeds contain about 25% oil. Sesame oil has medicinal value. It is used in pickle for its flavour and has preservative property. The oil extraction technique is as follows:

Sun-dried sesame seeds → Cleaning of impurities → Dehulling of seeds by soaking the seeds in water or in diluted alkali and removing the skin by rubbing → Drying of dehulled seed in tunnel drier → Pressing of dehulled dried seed in screw press expeller or solvent extraction to get oil → Filtering of oil → Packing → Marketing

The resulting cake is powdered in hammer milk.

23.2.6 Sunflower seed oil

Sunflower seeds contain 35–50% oil. The oil is used for culinary purpose and is useful for heart patients. The processing technique for extraction of sunflower seed oil is as follows:

Sunflower seeds → Cleaning of impurities → Decortications in decorticator → Kernels or decorticated seed pressing in screw press or power expeller to obtain oil.

The residual cake contains 10–15% oil and can be further extracted by solvent using food grade hexane.

23.2.7 Rice bran oil

Rice bran oil is rich in vitamin E and possesses antioxidant activity. The oil also has higher cholesterol lowering effect than other oils. Rice bran oil is used in cooking and it has less absorption in fried food. Rice bran oil can be extracted through solvent extraction technique.

23.2.8 Olive oil

Olive oil contains mono unsaturated fatty acid, poly unsaturated fatty acid and antioxidant such as vitamin E, A and phenols. The oil is beneficial in combating coronary heart diseases. It is used in cooking, seasoning and salad dressing. The technique used for extraction of highest grade olive oil (virgin oil) is as follows:

Olive fruits → Crushing → Resulting mass → Putting the mass in press → Oil and water is forced out → Oil is separated → Filtered (no refining) → Left to settling for little time → Filtering again → Bottling/marketing.

Pure olive oil can be obtained by further pressing (cold pressed) of extra virgin oil. Refined olive oil can be produced by using the technique of refining to remove the oil which remains in olive mass after the pressing.

23.2.9 Coconut oil

Coconut oil is produced from dried coconut meal or copra. Coconut oil is poor source of unsaturated acids. It is used in confectionery, cookery and manufacture of vanaspati, margarine, pharmaceuticals preparations and soap. The process for obtaining edible oil from coconut is as follows:

Coconut meat → Cutting into small pieces → Drying in tunnel drier → Screw pressing or solvent extraction with food grade hexane to get oil → Filtering → Packing

23.2.10 Palm oil

Palm oil contains both saturated and unsaturated fatty acids in equal proportion. It has also vitamin E content. Palm oil is used in cooking, preparation of margarines and shortening and various food products. It is also useful in extending the shelf life of products. Various types of oils are produced from palm. These are palm kernel oil, palm oil, palm olein and palm stearin.

Palm kernel oil contains 50% oil. Palm kernel oil is used in making ice-cream, in baking and confectionery. The oil is extracted from seed kernel through screw pressing or solvent extraction.

Palm oil is derived from flesh pericarp of palm fruit which contains about 49% of palm oil. It consists of olein (liquid fraction) and stearin (solid fraction). The palm oil is extracted from fleshy pericarp through pressing and solvent extraction.

Palm olien is purely a liquid in warm climate; hence, it differs from palm oil. The oil has ability to blend with any seed oil. It is a popular cooking oil. The oil can be refined, bleached and decolourized.

Red palm oil is unrefined unbleached crude palm oil and has edible grade quality. It is rich in β-carotene. It is good source of vitamin E. It is used in cake, halwa, upma, etc.

Palm stearin is a co-product of palm olein which is the solid fraction of palm oil. It is natural shortening for pastries.

23.2.11 Mahua oil

Mahua kernel has 48% oil which is higher than many oil seed crops. It is used for vanaspati manufacture and extensively used in cooking in growing reasons. The major unsaturated fatty acid found in mahua oil is linoleic which has therapeutic use in reducing the cholesterol content in blood serum, thus renders oil useful for heart patients. The technique for extraction of oil is as follows:

Mahua seed → Removal of brown cell or seed coat → Kernel drying up to 5% moisture → Oil extraction through pressing and solvent extraction → Refining → Packaging → Marketing

24

Fruit products and processing technique

Fruits have special significance to human beings as protective food. They are rich source of mineral and vitamins in diet. Fruit are available only for a limited period during the season; hence, they need to be processed and preserved for consumption during off season. India produces a variety of fruits such as mango, banana, citrus, grape, guava, litchi, papaya, pineapple, pomegranate, aonla, jackfruit, ber, bael, jamun, karonda, apple, pear plum, apricot, strawberry, etc. The products from various fruits and their preparation technique are given in the following sections.

24.1 Mango

Fruit is very rich source of vitamin A. It is also good source of vitamin C, carbohydrate, fibre and minerals (potassium and iron). Ripe mango is very useful in constipation and helps to prevent blindness. It is also highly invigorating, flattening, laxative and diuretic. Raw mango drink (*Panna*) is useful in heat stroke during hot summer. The kernel of the stone is rich in calcium, fat and carbohydrates, which can be used as food, soap industry and also as substitute for cocoa in confectionary.

24.1.1 Products

24.1.1.1 Raw mango products

Raw mango fruits are processed into various products such as slices, pickles, chutney and amchoor. The techniques for preparation of these products are given in the following sections.

24.1.1.2 Slices

Preparation technique

Mature raw mango fruit → Washing → Removing of stem → Slicing → Cutting into small pieces through dicer → Storing of pieces in cemented tank under brine of 15% salt containing citric acid (2%) and acetic acid (2%) → Maintaining the salt percentage by adding more salt with time of storage and covering the slices completely under the brine. Slices are the base product for pickles, chutneys and amchoor

Other technique
Raw mango fruit → Washing → Removing of stem → Slicing/cutting of either peeled or unpeeled fruit of desired thickness → Dipping of slices in potassium metabisulphite (KMS) solution (300 ppm or 0.7 g/L of water) for 5 min → Draining of slices and air dried → Mixing with powdered salt properly → Filling into flexible pouches/container → Storage for about 3–4 months or used for making desired products

24.1.1.3 Pickles

Pickles can be prepared in various ways such as with salt, with oil and sweet pickle.

Pickle with salt
Recipe
Mango slices 1 kg, salt 200 g, chillies (powder) 10 g, fenugreek 10 g, black pepper 10 g, cardamom 5 g, cumin 10 g, asafoetida 5 g and clove (head less six in number).

Preparation technique
Raw mango fruit → Washing → Peeling with the help of peeler to remove outer green skin → Cutting into four quarters either by machine or manually → Removing stones → Curing mango pieces with salt under the sun for 2–3 days → Mixing with all spices → Storage

Pickle with oil
Recipe
Mango pieces 1 kg, salt 120 g, garlic chopped 100 g, ginger chopped 50 g, fenugreek powder 25 g, turmeric powder 25 g, red chillies 25 g, black pepper 30 g, nigella seed 15 g, aniseed powder 25 g, asafoetida 2 g, mustard oil 350 mL and glacial acetic acid 10 mL.

Preparation technique
Raw mango fruit → Washing → Peeling with the help of peeler to remove outer green skin → Cutting into four quarters either by machine or manually → Removing kernal → Curing mango pieces with salt under the sun for 2-3 days → Heating oil and cooling → Mixing spices in little oil → Mixing with mango pieces → Little heating → Addition of glacial acetic acid → Filling into container → Addition of remaining oil → Capping → Storage

Sweet pickle
Recipe
Sliced mango 1 kg, salt 120 g, red chillies, cumin, cardamom (large), aniseed, black pepper, coriander powder 10 g each, clove six in number and sugar/jaggery 500 g.

Preparation technique
Raw mature mango → Washing → Removal of stem → Peeling with the help of peeler → Slicing → Removal of kernel → Mixing slices with salt → Mixing with spices → Mixing with sugar → Packing in clean sterilized bottles → Capping → Storage

24.1.1.4 Chutney

There are two types of mango chutney, that is, sweet and hot.

Sweet chutney
Recipe
Raw mango grated slices 1 kg, sugar 1 kg, salt powder 50 g, onion chopped 50 g, garlic chopped 15 g, ginger shreds 10 g, spices (red chillies, cardamom, cumin, cinnamon, black pepper and aniseed powder 10 g each) and vinegar 180 mL.

Preparation technique
Mature raw mango → Washing → Removal of stem → Peeling of green skin → Grating into fine slices → Cooking slices in little water for softening → Mixing with sugar and salt → Allow to sweat for an hour (so that sugar and salt dissolve) → Heating/cooking slowly → Tying all the ingredients except vinegar in cloth bags → Putting in mixture while cooking → Pressing the spices bag occasionally during cooking → Cooking up to jam consistency → Removing spices bag after squeezing the extract in the mixture → Addition of vinegar → Cooling slightly → Packing into clean sterilized bottles → Cooling → Capping/sealing → Storage in cool and dry place

Hot chutney
Recipe
Raw mango grated slices 1 kg, sugar 0.5 kg, salt powder 50 g, ginger shred 50 g, onion chopped 75 g, garlic chopped 20 g, red chillies powder 15 g, black pepper 10 g, cumin 10 g, cardamom 10 g, cinnamon 10 g and vinegar 180 mL.

Preparation technique
Method of preparing hot chutney is precisely the same as that for sweet mango chutney. Only proportions of some of the ingredients are more and sugar is less as compared to sweet chutney.

24.1.1.5 Dehydrated raw mango (Amchoor)

Preparation technique
Raw green mango → Washing → Peeling → Slicing (12mm thickness) → Deeping in KMS solution (1.5%) for 5 min → Draining → Drying in sun or

Dehydration at 45–50°C for 2 h (up to 4% moisture) → Grinding into powder (amchoor) → Packing → Storage.

24.1.1.6 *Ripe mango products*

Ripe mangoes can be processed into several products such as mango slices in syrup, mango, pulp, beverages, jam, fruit bar, mango leather, cereal flakes, strained baby food, sweetened mango powder and frozen products.

Canned mango slices in syrup

Preparation technique

Firm ripe mangoes of suitable variety → Sorting and grading → Washing → Peeling → Cutting (2–4 longitudinal slices of approximately equal size) → Weighing → Filling into plain A2 or A2^1/2 tin can (550 g/can) → Syruping (hot syrup of 35–40% total soluble solid strength 666 g sugar/L of water containing 0.25% citric acid) leaving head space 0.3–0.5 cm → Exhausting (at 100°C for 7–10 min or temperature in the centre of the can reaches at least about 75°C) → Sealing → Processing in boiling water at 100°C for 25 min of A2 size of can and 30 min for A2^1/2 size can → Cooling (at 37°C) → Wiping → Labelling → Storing

Canned pulp

Preparation technique

Pulpy variety of ripe mango → Washing → Peeling → Extracting pulp with the help of pulper → Homogenizing (blender or homogenizer) → Heating (80°C) → Filling hot into sterilized cans (A2^1/2 size) → Sealing → Processing in boiling water for 30 min → Cooling (37°C) → Labelling → Storing/marketing

Canned juice

Recipe

Pulp content 45%, total soluble solids 15% and acidity 0.3%.

Preparation technique

Suitable variety of fully ripe mangoes → Washing → Peeling → Cutting → Pulping/juice extraction → Mixing with syrup solution (sugar + water + citric acid, heating just to dissolve the sugar and filtering clear syrup) → Heating 80–85°C → Filling hot into sterilized cans (A2^1/2 size) → Processing in boiling water for 25 min → Cooling (37°C) → Labelling → Storing/marketing

RTS beverage

Recipe

Mango juice 10%, total soluble solids 12–15%, acidity 0.3% and sodium metabisulphite 70 ppm.

Preparation technique

Suitable varieties of ripe mango → Washing → Peeling and cutting → Passing through pulping machine → Pulp → Mixing with syrup solution (sugar + water + citric acid, heating just to dissolve the sugar straining and filtering clear syrup) → Addition of preservative → Bottling → Crown corking → Pasteurization at 75°C for 30 min → Air cooling → Storing/marketing

Nectar

Recipe

Pulp content 20%, total soluble solids 15% and acidity 0.3%.

Preparation technique

Suitable varieties of ripe mango → Washing → Peeling and cutting → Passing through pulping machine → Pulp → Mixing with syrup solution (sugar + water + citric acid, heating just to dissolve the sugar straining and filtering clear syrup) → Addition of preservative → Bottling → Crown corking → Pasteurization at 80–85°C for 30 min → Air cooling → Storing

Squash

Recipe

Pulp 25%, total soluble solids 45%, acidity 1.2% and sodium metabisulphite 350 ppm.

Preparation technique

Ripe fruit → Washing → Peeling → Passing through pulping machine → Pulp → Mixing with syrup solution (sugar + water + citric acid) → Addition of preservative → Bottling → Capping → Labelling → Storing/marketing

Jam

Recipe

Pulp 1 kg, sugar 0.75 kg, citric acid 2 g and water 100 mL.

Preparation technique

Ripe fruit → Washing → Peeling → Cutting/grating → Seed removal → Pulp → Addition of sugar and water → Cooking up to desired consistency → Addition of citric acid → Judging of end point [temperature 105°C or total suspended solids (TSS) 68–70%] → Filling hot into clean and sterilized bottles → Cooling → Capping/sealing → Storing/marketing

Toffee

Recipe

Mango pulp 1 kg, sugar 0.65 kg, glucose 0.85 kg, skim milk powder 170 g and hydrogenated fat 100 g.

Preparation technique
Mango pulp → Concentrating (steam jacketed kettle) to about one-third of its original volume → Mixing with other ingredients → Cooking continue to a desired consistency → Transferring cooked mass in tray having smooth surface and smeared lightly with fat → Spreading of product into a thin sheet about 0.5 cm thick → Cooling to set → Cutting of solid sheet into shape of toffees → Wrapping in tissue paper → Packing in air tight container (jar/tins) → Storing/marketing

Fruit bar
Recipe
Mango pulp 1 kg, sugar 150 g, citric acid 1 g and KMS 1 g.

Preparation technique
Pulpy variety of ripe mangoes → Washing → Peeling → Pulping → Mixing with sugar, citric acid and KMS → Spreading on trays → Drying in cross-flow air dryer → Cutting into small bars → Wrapping in cellophane paper → Packing in polythene pouches/suitable containers → Storing/marketing.

Leather (Amawat)
Recipe
Mango pulp 1 kg, citric acid 3 g and sodium metabisulphite 0.5 g.

Preparation technique
Mango pulp → Washing → Peeling → Extraction of pulp → Homogenization (in blender) → Addition of citric acid and sodium metabisulphite by dissolving separately in small quantity of water to the pulp → Mixing thoroughly → Pouring of pulp to 1 cm thickness in trays smeared with butter → Drying in a dryer → After drying another layer of 1 cm thickness of the pulp may be poured on it → Drying again up to 5–8% moisture → Cutting of leather into small/suitable pieces → Packing in polythene pouches → Storing in a cool and dry place

Cereal flakes
Recipe
Mango pulp 1 kg, wheat flour (maida) 100 g, sugar 60 g, glucose 60 g, calcium carbonate 1 g, sodium bicarbonate 1 g and pectin 0.06 g.

Preparation technique
Ripe mango fruits → Washing → Peeling → Extraction of pulp → Heating to 80–85°C and pH adjusted to 5.0 → Mixing with wheat flour paste (prepared by cooking with three times its weight of water at a temperature of 75–80°C for 2 min) → Heating of mixture to a temperature of 80–85°C → Addition of other ingredients (sugar, glucose, calcium carbonate and sodium bicarbonate) → Mixing thoroughly → Cooking → Addition of pectin in the form of 2%

solution in water → Drying in a double drum dryer → Flakes → Secondary drying (in cabinet dryer) → Packing in hermetically sealed closed tin or glass container → Storing

Custard powder (strained baby food)

Recipe

Mango pulp 10 kg, sugar 500 g, skim milk powder 500 g, cornstarch 250 g and sodium bicarbonate to reduce the pH of the pulp 5.6.

Preparation technique

Ripe mangoes → Washing → Peeling → Pulp extraction → Sieving pulp → Mixing with sugar and skim milk powder → Addition of gelatinized starch (by cooking the corn starch with water, four times the weight of corn starch) → Mixing thoroughly → Passing mixed mass through the homogeniser to make it fine → Drum drying (double drum dryer) → Further drying in cabinet dryer (about 1–1.5% mass) → Powdering → Packing in tagger-top tins → Storing

Frozen slices

Preparation technique

Firm ripe fruits → Washing → Peeling → Slicing → Filling into polythene bag → Covering with 40° brix sugar syrup solution containing 0.3% citric acid and 0.5% ascorbic acid/vitamin C → Sealing of polythene bag → Placing in waxed cartons → Freezing at –40°C → Storing at –20°C

Frozen pulp

Preparation technique

Ripe mangoes → Washing → Peeling → Pulping → Pulp → Adjusting brix to 20% and acidity 0.5% → Heating to 85°C → Cooling at room temperature → Filling into polythene bag → Sealing → placing bag in waxed carton → Frozen at –40°C → Storing at –20°C

24.2 Banana

Banana is the most nourishing fruit prized for its nutritive value and desert qualities. It is available in large quantity throughout the year. Fruit is good source of energy. Fruit is very rich in carbohydrates, minerals such as calcium and vitamin B particularly riboflavin. Fruit is helpfully reducing depression and blood pressure.

24.2.1 Products

Ripe banana can be processed into pulp, juice, squash, brandy, fig, toffee, food bar, canned banana and powder. Unripe fruits used for preparation of chips and flour.

24.2.1.1 Banana pulp

Preparation technique

Fully ripe fruit → Washing → Peeling→ Extraction of pulp in a screw type pulper → Homogenization of pulp → Deaerating with centrifugal deaerator → Heating of pulp aseptically in heat exchanger → Cooling → Packing aseptically into containers (A-0 can/drums)

24.2.1.2 Clarified juice

Preparation technique

Ripe banana preferably Cavendish → Washing → Peeling → Pulping in a pulper (with stainless steel sieves) → Addition of SO_2 → Treating with pectic enzyme (at 40°C) till the clear juice is separated from pomace → Pressing mass through cheese cloth → Filtering with the filter aid → Blending of filtered juice with sugar and acid if required → Pasteurizing → Filling hot into sterilized bottles → Sealing → Cooling → Storage

24.2.1.3 Squash

Recipe

Banana juice 1 kg, sugar 1.5 kg, water 500 mL, citric acid 5 g and SO_2 350 ppm.

Preparation technique

Ripe banana → Washing → Peeling → Cutting into pieces → Heating with little water to soften → Pulping → Mixing with sugar syrup (sugar + water + citric acid, heating just to dissolve the sugar) → Addition of SO_2 350 ppm or 0.7 g/L of finished product → Filling into clean sterilized bottle → Capping → Storage

24.2.1.4 Brandy

Preparation technique

Fully ripe banana/over ripe → Washing → Peeling → Pulping → Treating with pectin enzyme → Clarified juice → Fermentation by inoculating suitable yeast in a fermenter (complete fermentation within 4–5 days) → Distillation of fermentated liquor brandy having ethanol content of 35–40%

24.2.1.5 Fig

Preparation technique

Ripe fruits → Washing → Peeling → Cutting into halves length wise → Spreading on wooden trays → Sulphuring for an hour (3.6 kg sulphur/tones of fruit) → Drying of slices (60°C) in a cabinet drier till it becomes soft and non sticky → Packing cardboard cartons (lined with polythene film) Storing

24.2.1.6 Toffee

Recipe

Banana pulp 1 kg, sugar 750 g, glucose 100 g, skimmed milk powder 150 g and butter or ghee 70 g.

Preparation technique

Ripe banana → Washing → Peeling → Pulping → Sieving (30 mesh sieve) → Concentrating pulp (steam jacketed kettle) to one-third of its original volume → Addition of all ingredients (sugar, glucose, skimmed milk powder, butter) → Mixing → Cooking continue to final weight (one-fifth of the fruit pulp taken) → Transferring cooked mass to smooth surface tray smeared with fat (flavoring matter is added at this stage) → Spreading into thin (0.5–0.75 cm) sheet → Allow to cool and set (2 h) → Solid sheet cut into pieces of toffee size → Drying at 50–55°C to a final moisture of 5–6% → Wrapping in butter paper → Filling in jars or tins → Sealing → Storage

24.2.1.7 Fruit bar

Recipe

Banana pulp 1 kg, sugar 100 g, citric acid 2 g and KMS 1 g.

Preparation technique

Ripe fruit → Washing → Peeling → Pulping → Pulp → Heating (83°C for 10 min) → Mixing with sugar, citric acid and KMS → Spreading on tray → Drying in cross-flow drier at 60°C until can be taken out in the form of sheet → Cutting of sheets into small bars → Wrapping in cellophane paper → Packing in polythene pouches → Storing

24.2.1.8 Canned banana

Preparation technique

Firm ripe banana (Cavendish or other suitable varieties) → Washing → Peeling → Cutting into thin slices (1.25–2 cm thickness) → Filling into cans → Covering with boiling hot sugar syrup of 30° brix containing 0.3% citric acid → Exhausting (till the centre of the can reaches 80°C) → Sealing → Processing for 15 min at 5 psig → Cooling → Storing

24.2.1.9 Powder

Preparation technique

Fully riped fruit → Washing → Peeling → Pulping → Addition of milk solids at 10% → Drying (spray drying) → Packing → Storing

24.2.1.10 Chips

Preparation technique

Unripe, firm fruits of suitable variety (Cavendish, Nendran) → Washing → Peeling → Trimming → Slicing/cutting (2 mm thickness) → Washing in boil water → Drying → Deep frying in hydrogenated fat at 160°C → Seasoning (salt and spices) → Packing in HDP bags and keeping in sealed tin → Storing

24.3 Citrus fruits

Citrus fruit have a place of pride in Indian fruit industry. Commercially grown citrus fruits in India are mandarin oranges, sweet oranges, lime and lemons. Citrus fruit is very well known for its vitamin C content which protects from scurvy a disease causing body sores and bleeding gum.

24.3.1 Mandarin orange products

Mandarin oranges can be processed into quality beverages such as concentrate ready to serve (RTS), squash and crush. Marmalade can be prepared from mandarin oranges.

24.3.1.1 Juice concentrate

Preparation technique

Fruits → Washing → Cut into halves/hand peeling → Fed to citrus juice extractor with lower and upper cup projectors → Screening of juice to remove seed, sacs, etc. → Flash pasteurization of juice to temp of about 180–190°F → Concentrated in vacuum evaporators to 60° brix → Transferring to refrigerated closed tank for blending with dearated fresh juice to reduce concentrate to 42° brix → Addition of peel oil → Packing in tin cans and HDPC containers → Storage at 15°C (when preserved with SO_2 1500 ppm) for 9 months or at 0°C (without SO_2) for 6 months

24.3.1.2 RTS beverage

Recipe

Mandarin orange juice 10%, acidity 0.3% and total soluble solid 12%. This can also be prepared by using the ingredients orange juice 1 kg, sugar 1.5 kg, citric acid 18 g, water 7.5 L and orange essence 5 mL.

Preparation technique

Fully riped mandarin orange (Nagpur santgtra/Kinnow mandarin) → Washing → Removal of peel and separate the segments → Extraction of juice → Straining of juice → Mixing with sugar syrup (sugar + citric acid + water, heating just to dissolve the sugar and filtered) → Addition of orange essence

→ Bottling → Crown corking → Pasteurization in boiling water for 20 min → Cooling → Storing

24.3.1.3 Squash

Recipe

Mandarin orange juice 25%, sugar 50%, acid 1.2%, sodium metabisulphite 350 ppm. Ingredients calculated for 1 L of juice for preparation of squash are: sugar 1.75 kg, water 1 L, citric acid 20 g and preservative (SMS 2.25 g).

Preparation technique

Fully riped mandarin fruit → Washing → Peeling → Juice extraction → Filtering/Straining → Mixing with sugar syrup solution (sugar + citric acid + water, heating just to dissolve the sugar and filtered) → Addition of preservative (by dissolving in little quantity of squash) → Filling into clean and sterilized bottle → Capping → Storing

24.3.1.4 Crush

Recipe

Mandarin orange juice 25%, total soluble solids 55%, citric acid 1%, sodium metabisulphite 350 ppm or 0.6 g/L of finished product.

Preparation technique

Fully ripe fruit → Washing → Peeling → Juice extraction → Straining → Determination of total soluble solids and acidity → Calculation of their require quantity → Mixing with sugar syrup solution (sugar + water + citric acid, heating just to dissolve the sugar and filtered) → Addition of preservative → Mixing/homogenization → Filling into sterilized bottles → Capping → Storing

24.3.1.5 Marmalade

Recipe

Mandarin orange and khatta in ratio of 2:1, juice extract 1 L, sugar 0.75 kg and shredded peel 60 g.

Preparation technique

Ripe fruit → Washing → Peeling outer portion (Flavedo) → Cutting peel into fine shreds (2 cm long and 0.1 cm thick) → Cutting of peeled fruit about 0.4 cm thickness → Addition of water in ratio of 2:1 → Boiling for 40–50 min → Straining the extract → Testing for pectin content (alcohol test) → Addition of sugar → Cooking to 105°C → Addition of prepared shred (peel boiled for 15 min for 3–4 times by changing the water for softening and removing bitterness) → Boiling till jellying point → Testing for end point (drop/sheet/temperature test) → Cooling with stirring → Addition of flavor (orange oil)

→ Filling into sterilized bottles → Capping/sealing → Storage in cool and dry place

24.3.2 Sweet orange products

24.3.2.1 Freeze dried powder

Preparation technique
Fruit → Washing → Juice extraction → Addition of sugar (100/kg of juice) → Pasteurize (85°C for 2 min) → Freezing (–20°C) → Cutting into small Blocks → Freezing (–30°C) → Freeze drying → Powder → Packed in N_2

24.3.3 Lime and lemons products

Lime and lemon can be processed into various products such as squash, syrup, cordials, barley water and pickles.

24.3.3.1 Squash

Recipe
Lime/lemon, juice 1 L, sugar 2 kg, water 1 L, sodium metabisulphite 2.5 g or 0.7 g/L of finished product.

Preparation technique
Lime/lemon fruit → Washing → Cutting into halves → Juice extraction → Straining → Measuring → Mixing with strained sugar syrup solution (sugar + water, heating, just to dissolve the sugar and straining) → Addition of preservative by dissolving in small quantity of squash → Mixing thoroughly → Filling into clean sterilized bottles → Capping → Storage

24.3.3.2 Crush

Recipe
Lime/lemon juice 25%, total soluble solids 55%, citric acid 1.0%, sodium metabisulphite 0.6 g/L of finished product.

Preparation technique
Lime/lemon fruit → Washing → Cutting into halves → Juice extraction → Straining of juice → Mixing with strained syrup solution → Addition of preservative → Mixing thoroughly → Filling into clean and sterilized bottle → Capping → Storage

24.3.3.3 Syrup

Recipe
Lime/lemon juice 1 L, sugar 2.25 kg and water 0.5 L.

Preparation technique
Lime/lemon fruit → Washing → Cutting into halves → Juice extraction → Straining of juice → Mixing with syrup solution → Filling into clean sterilized bottles → Capping → Storage

24.3.3.4 Cordials

Recipe
Lime/lemon juice 1 L, sugar 1.25 kg, water 1 L and sodium metabisulphite 0.7 g/L of finished product.

Preparation technique
Lime/lemon fruit → Washing → Cutting into halves → Juice extraction → Straining of juice → Addition of sodium metabisulphite (1 g/L of juice) → Storing in glass containers for 7 days at room temperature for setting of suspended material → Siphoning/filtration of supernatant clear juice → Straining and measuring → Mixing with strained sugar syrup → Addition of preservative (0.6 g SMS/L of finished product) → Bottling → Capping → Storage

24.3.3.5 Barley water

Recipe
Lime/lemon juice 1 L, barley extract 1 L, barley flour (15 g + 1 L water), Water 0.8 L, sugar 1.2 kg and sodium metabisulphite 2.4 g.

Preparation technique
Lime/lemon fruit → Washing → Cutting into halves → Juice extraction → Straining of juice → Mixing with barley extract (barley flour + little water making thin paste + remaining water to make 1 L and heating, cooking and straining) → Addition of preservative (0.6 g/L of finished product) → Addition of essence if desired (8 mL) → Mixing → Filling into clean sterilized bottle (leaving 2.5 cm space on top) → Capping → Storage

24.3.3.6 Pickles

Pickle with salt

Recipe
Lime/lemon 1 kg, salt 200 g, red chillies powder 15 g, cumin, cardamom, cinnamon and black pepper10 g each and clove (headless five in number).

Preparation technique
Lime/lemon fruit → Washing → Cutting into four pieces of lime/small pieces of lemon → Squeezing juice about one-fourth → Mixing all spices and salt → Mixing with lime pieces → Filling in jar → Covering with lid → Keeping in sun (4–5 days) → Ready to use/storing

Pickle with oil

Recipe

Lime 1 kg, salt 150 g, red chillies powder 25 g, black pepper, turmeric powder, cumin, aniseed, rye powdered 10 g each, asafoetida 2 g and mustard oil 400 mL.

Preparation technique

Lime fruit (yellow colour) → Washing → Cutting into four pieces → Squeezing out juice partially → Mixing all spices and salt with juice → Mixing with lime pieces → Filling in jar → Keeping in sun for 5 days → Addition of oil after heating and cooling → Sealing of container → Storage

24.4 Guava

This is an ideal fruit for the nutritional security. Fruit is rich source of vitamin C and pectin. It has also fair amount of calcium and iron. Guava juice is an excellent substitute for orange juice in feeding babies. Fruit is very useful in digestion, scurvy and cough. Guava juice is an excellent substitute for orange juice in feeding babies. Excellent flavour, nutritive value and medicinal properties of guava fruits show great potentiality for processing into valuable products

24.4.1 Guava products

Guava can be processed into various quality products such as RTS beverage, squash, cider, canning, jelly, toffee and cheese.

24.4.1.1 RTS beverage

Recipe

Pulp 10%, total soluble solid 11%, acidity 0.25% and SO_2 70 ppm.

Preparation technique

Ripe/overripe fruit → Washing → Cutting → Mixing with water in ratio of 1:1 → Passing through pulper → Pulp → Determination of TSS and acidity and calculation for required quantity of sugar and citric acid → Mixing of strained pulp with strained syrup solution (sugar + water + acid heating just to dissolve the sugar and straining) → Addition of SO_2 → Mixing → Bottling → Crown corking → Pasteurization in boiling water for 20 min → Air cooling → Storage

24.4.1.2 Carbonated beverages

Preparation technique

Guava pulp/juice → Addition of sugar and citric acid (adjusted at 60° brix TSS and 2% acidity) → Addition of preservative (500 ppm sodium benzoate) →

Syrup filled in pre-sterilize bottles (200 mL capacity) → Carbonation at 60 or 80 psi with the help of carbonation machine → Crown capping → Carbonated guava beverage → Pasteurization (at 60°C for 30 min) → Labelling → Storage

24.4.1.3 Squash

Recipe

Pulp 25%, total soluble solid 45%, acidity 1% and SO_2 350 ppm.

Preparation technique

Pulp (extraction as mentioned above) → Mixing with syrup solution → Addition of SO_2 → Mixing → Bottling → Capping → Labelling → Storage

24.4.1.4 Cider (fermented beverage)

Preparation technique

Fully ripe fruits → Washing → Cutting into pieces → Addition of water (1:1) → Passing through pulper → Pulp → Adjusting to total soluble solids 22% and acidity 0.5% → Addition of KMS (SO^2) 100 ppm → Keeping for half an hour → Inoculate with 4% *Saccharomyces cerevisiae* yeast → Fermentation → Addition of pectic enzyme → Filtration and removal of pomace → Siphoning clear juice and filling into container → Addition of 50 ppm SO_2 → Storage (maturation) under sealed container for 6 months → Bottling of clear fermented juice → Crown cooking → Pasteurization at 60°C for 20 min → Cooling → Storage

24.4.1.5 Jelly

Recipe

Guava juice 1 kg, sugar 0.75 kg and citric acid 2–3 g.

Preparation technique

Firm ripe fruit → Washing → Cutting into slices → Boiling with water for 20–30 min (water and fruit ratio 1.5:1) → Addition of citric acid during boiling 2 g/kg of fruit → Straining of extract → Testing of pectin for addition of sugar (alcoholic or jel meter test) → Addition of sugar → Boiling → Judging of end point (temperature 105°C or TSS 65%) → Removal of scum (foam) → Addition of remaining citric acid → Filling hot into clean and sterilized bottle → Sealing/capping → Storage

24.4.1.6 Cheese

Recipe

Guava pulp 1 kg, sugar 1.25 kg, citric acid 3 g, butter 100 g and salt 2 g.

Preparation technique

Firm ripe fruit → Washing → Cutting into slices → Boiling with water (in ratio 1:1) till it becomes soft → Addition of citric acid during boiling →

Screening/sieving pulp and removal of seeds and skin → Addition of sugar → Cooking/concentrating till desired consistency (mass starts leaving the pan) → Addition of salt and mixing → Transferring the mass in tray smeared with butter → Spreading hot cheese (layer of 0.6 cm thickness) → Cooling and allow to set overnight → Cutting into suitable pieces/size → Wrapping in butter or cellophane paper → Packing in jar → Capping/sealing → Storage

24.4.1.7 Toffee

Recipe

Guava pulp 1 kg, sugar 0.75 g, butter 100 g, glucose 100 g and skimmed milk powder 150 g.

Preparation technique

Firm ripe fruit → Washing → Cutting onto pieces → Boiling with water (1:1 ratio) → Sieving (removal of seeds) → Pulp → Heating/cooking to one-third volume → Mixing with sugar and glucose and heating → Addition of butter → Cooking till sufficient solid → Addition of milk powder (by dissolving in little water) → Addition of colour and essence → Mixing → Transferring the mass in tray smeared with butter → Spread mass uniformly (0.5–0.75 cm thick layer) → Cooling (4–5 h) → Cutting into pieces of suitable size → Wrapping in butter or moisture proof paper → Packing in jars → Capping/sealing → Storage

24.4.1.8 Canning

Preparation technique

Selection of variety → Firm ripe fruit → Grading → Washing → Peeling [Lye peeling, i.e., 2% boiling lye (20 g NaOH/L of water) till the surface becomes black] → Washing with water (several changes with slight rubbing to remove the black skin) → Dipping in 0.5% citric acid solution to neutralize the residue of NaOH → Transfer in 1% sodium chloride solution/brine (10 g/L of water) to prevent browning → Cutting into halves or into quarters → Scooping the seed cavity → Washing with plain water → Filling into plain cans (500 g for A2½ cans) → Syruping [Hot syrup of 40% total soluble solids strength, i.e., 1 kg sugar in 1.5 L of water with 0.1% citric acid and 0.1% ascorbic acid (1 g citric acid and 1 g ascorbic acid per kg sugar solution)] → Exhausting (at 100°C for 6 min) → Sealing → Processing (in boiling water for 20 min for both A2 and A2½ tin cans) → Cooling (up to 37°C) → Labelling → Storage

24.5 Grape

Grape is one of the most delicious and nourishing fruit. It is very sweet and juicy. It contains and abundance of sugar, vitamins B and C and minerals specially calcium, phosphorus and iron. Besides its value as a food, it has various medicinal uses. Grape juice is nourishing, thirst quencher, stimulant to the kidneys and laxative.

24.5.1 Products

An excellent quality of juice, raisin and alcoholic beverage can be prepared from grapes. Canning can also be done.

24.5.1.1 Juice

Preparation technique

Fully ripe grape → Washing → Stalk removal → Juice extraction by crushing the berries with basket press → Filtration → Clarification (setting of cream of tartar by low temperature storage for 90 days) → Filtration of clear juice → Bottling → Crown corking → Pasteurization → Cooling → Storage

24.5.1.2 Sun dried Raisin

Preparation technique

Ripe clusters → Shade drying till development of greenish/light amber ting Colour of berries → Separating dried berries from cluster → Packaging → Storage

24.5.1.3 Dehydrated raisin

Preparation technique

Selection of suitable variety (Thompson seedless or Pusa seedless for raisins and seeded variety for Monucca) → Ripe clusters → Washing → Removal of stem → Dip in boiling lye solution (0.5% for 20 s) → Rinsing → Sulphuring for about 30 min (To prevent browning) → Drying at 66–82°C for 20–30 h or up to the moisture content of 15–20% (yield varies from 21–27%) → Packing → Storage

24.5.1.4 Alcoholic beverage

Grape is an ideal fruit for making wines because of high content of fermentable sugar and natural association of fermenting yeasts with the grape berry. The quality of wine depends upon the grape variety, fermentation technique and by the processing and aging of the wine. The wines prepared from grape are often named after the variety. Examples are Muscat (prepared from Muscat variety), Tokay (prepared from Tokay variety), etc. The suitable varieties for making wine in India are Beauty seedless, Arka Shyam, Pusa Navrang, Banglore Blue, etc.

Preparation technique

Fully ripe cluster of grape → Destalking (removal of stems from the berries) → Crushing (to produce the juice) → Must (crushed material) → Transfer must in jar (should not be filled more than three-fourth) → Addition of sugar (70 g/kg grapes) to raise total soluble solids to 20–24% (if the grapes are sour) → Adjusting pH or acid content of juice to 0.6–0.8% (If the pH of juice is too low, it should be diluted with water to raise the pH of desired level and extra amount of sugar has to be added to raise the sugar percentage to desired level. If the pH is high, tartaric acid has to be added to bring down the pH of desirable level) → Addition of preservative (sodium metabisulphite at 1.5 g/10 kg of grapes) → Mix and allow to stand for 2–4 h (This serves inhibitor for wild yeast and other spoilage organism) → Addition of wine yeast inoculums (4 mL thick yeast suspension/kg of grapes) → Fermentation for 2 days in a cool place (20–25°C) by covering the mouth of jar with cloth → Filtration (On third day through a thin muslin cloth) → Fermentation (allow to ferment in a cool place for another 10 days without disturbance) → Racking (siphoning of fermented wine to separate the yeast cells and other solids deposits from wine is known as racking) → Fining (new wine is sometime not clear and requires fining hence suitable fining agent such as bentonite is added to settle down the colloidal matter) → Filtration (the clear wine is siphoned off or filtered) → Filling (clear wine is filled into bottles or barrels completely and sealed airtight) → Maturation (allow the wine to mature for 6–8 months at room temperature preferable in cool place the process is known as aging) → Pasteurization (83–87°C for 2 min) → Bottling → Crown corking → Pasteurization (87°C for 20 min) → Cooling → Storage

24.5.1.5 Canning

Preparation technique

Firm ripe berries of seedless varieties (white) → Removal of stem → Washing → Filling into plain cans (white varieties) or lacquered (colour varieties) of A2 or A2½ → Syruping (hot syrup of 40% TSS) → Exhausting for 10 min → Sealing → Processing and boiling water (100°C) for 10 and 12 min A2 and A2½ can, respectively → Cooling → Labelling → Storage

24.6 Pineapple

The fruits develop from entire inflorescence at the apex of stem with centre of plant. The fruit is a good source of vitamins A, B_1, B_2 and C and minerals such as calcium, iron, phosphorus, magnesium and potassium. It is also a source of bromelin a protein digestive enzyme. Bromelin is commonly used in food production and in pharmaceutical industries.

24.6.1 Products

A number of processed products are made from pineapple. These are slices, juice, RTS beverage, squash, juice concentrate, powder, jam, etc. The Kew and Giant Kew are the most suitable variety for canning of pineapple slices, and Queen and Mauritius varieties are good for beverage.

24.6.1.1 Canned slices

Preparation technique

Select fully ripe, cylindrical-shaped uniform-sized fruit of suitable variety (Giant Kew) → Washing thoroughly → Removing crown → Peeling eyes and removing core with corer → Slicing (Transversely) either mechanically are manually (1 cm thick) → Punching of slices to get uniform rings → Rinsing of slices in water and dried → Feeling into plain cans (8–10 rings in A_2 or $A2^1/2$ size cans) → Feeling of cans with hot syrup of 40% total soluble solid strength with 0.2% citric acid → Exhausting (At 100°C for 7–12 min or till temperature at the center of can reaches 75–80°C) → Sealing of cans → Processing in boiling water for 20–25 min → Cooling → Wiping dry → Labelling → Storing in cool and dry place

24.6.1.2 Pineapple titbits

Undersized and broken slices are used for preparing titbits. The technique of preparation is same as that of slices.

24.6.1.3 Juice

Preparation technique

Removal/cutting of crown → Peeling → Slicing → Crushing → Juice extraction → Straining → Heating at 85°C → Filling hot into plain cans → Sealing → Processing at 100°C for 15 min → Cooling in water → wiping → Labelling → Storage/marketing

24.6.1.4 Canned pulp

Preparation technique

Fruits of 90% maturity/broken slices → Crushing in a fruit mill → Crushed mass sweetened and acidify by adding hot syrup and citric acid → Heating to 85–90°C → Filling in cans → Processing of cans at 100°C for 45–50 min → Cooling → Labelling → Storage

24.6.1.5 RTS Beverage

Recipe

Pulp 10% , total soluble solids 12% , acidity 0.3% and SO_2 70 ppm.

Preparation technique

Ripe fruit → Washing → Removal of crown and stem → Peeling → Cutting/slicing → Passing through pulper → Pulp → Straining → Mixing with syrup solution → Addition of preservative → Mixing/homogenization → Bottling → Crown corking → Pasteurization (100°C for 15 min) → Cooling → Storage

24.6.1.6 Squash

Recipe

Juice 25%, sugar 50%, acid 1.2% and SO_2 350 ppm or juice 1 L, sugar 1.5 kg, water 1 L, acid 20 g and sodium metabisulphite 2 g.

Preparation technique

Ripe pineapple fruits of suitable variety (Queen) → Washing thoroughly → Removing crown with sharp twisting → Peeling with stainless steel knife and removing eyes with V-shaped steel knife → Cutting the fruit into small pieces → Crushing/passing through pulped → Juice extraction → Mixing with syrup solution (sugar + water + citric acid, heating just to dissolve the sugar) → Addition of preservative and mixing → Bottling → Capping → Wiping dry → Labelling → Storing/dispatch

24.6.1.7 Juice concentrate

Preparation technique

Pineapple juice → Pasteurization (to inactivate enzyme) → Centrifuge to remove excess pulp → Partial evaporation (stripped juice) → Concentrate to 60° brix → Cut back with small quantity of fresh juice and volatile flavour → Concentrate (47° brix) → Cooling (1.6°C) → Filling into cans → Frozen at –8°C → Storage at –18°C

24.6.1.8 Juice powder

Preparation technique

Ripe pineapple fruit of suitable variety → Washing → Removing crown → Removing eyes and core → Cutting into small pieces → Extracting juice by passing the slices through mechanical juice extractor → Pasteurization of juice at 85°C for 10 min → Cooling → Packing in HDPE bags → Storing at –20°C → Blending of thawed juice with 121.5% egg albumen for 10 min with blender for foaming → Spreading of foam on a tray (uniform layer of 3 mm thickness) → Drying up to 6% moisture → Grinding with addition of 1% magnesium stearate → Passing through sieve (0.5 mm size) → Vacuum packing (300 gauge HDPE bags) → Storing at ambient temperature

24.6.1.9 Jam

Recipe

Pulp 1 kg, sugar 0.75 kg, citric acid 2 g and water 150 mL.

Preparation technique

Ripe fruit → Washing → Removing crown → Peeling → Removing eyes → Cutting into small pieces → Crushing the pieces to obtain uniform mass → Addition of sugar and citric acid → Cooking slowly with stirring till desired consistency → Testing end point (Temperature 105°C or TSS of 68%) → Filling into sterilized bottle → Cooling → Capping → Storing in a cool and dry place

24.6.1.10 Nata-de-Pina

This is value added product of pineapple. It is developed through bioprocessing of pineapple into pineapple gel. The product is rich in fibre and low in calories.

The bacterium *Acetobacter xylinum* strain grows fast in the dilute pineapple juice and curdles into a thick translucent, gelatinous in soluble layer. The jelly layer formed on the top of the liquid by the bacterium is removed and cut into pieces of desired shapes and sizes, boiled in light sugar syrup and bottled or canned. It is delicious chewy and no stickiness. The product can also be blended with fruit salad, ice-cream and kheer. The product can also be prepared from the peels and pulp waste of pineapple.

24.7 Papaya

The fruit has high nutritive and medicinal value. It is very rich in vitamin A and fairly rich in vitamin C. It is also rich in minerals such as calcium, phosphorus and iron. Medicinal property of papaya is very well known. It improves digestion and is said to cure chronic constipation, piles dyspepsia of liver and spleen and digestive disorders. Papain prepared from dry latex of raw papaya is a proteolytic enzyme used for meat tenderization, manufacture of chewing gum, cosmetics and pharmaceutical industries. Bothraw and ripe papaya can be processed into number of quality products.

24.7.1 Raw papaya products

24.7.1.1 Papain

Preparation technique

Raw papaya → Making incision longitudinal (four sides) → Collection of latex (milk) → Filtration → Addition of 1000 ppm SO_2 → Mixing thoroughly → Sun dying up to 5% moisture → Powdering → Blending → Packing → Storage

24.7.1.2 Jelly

Recipe

Mature but unripe papaya 1 kg, ripe papaya 1 kg, citric acid 5 g and sugar (as/ pectin test) 1 kg.

Preparation technique

Mature unripe papaya → Washing → Peeling → Cutting into pieces → Removal of seeds → Addition of water 2.5 L/kg of fruit → Addition of ripe papaya after peeling and seed removal and citric acid → Heating the mixture for 35 min → Cooling of extract and settling of mixture about 2 h → Decanting/filtering the extract → Testing for pectin → Addition of sugar according to pectin test → Cooking up to desired consistency → Testing of end point (temperature/sheet/drop test) → Filling into clean sterilized jar → Capping/ sealing → Storing

24.7.1.3 Chutney

Recipe

Raw papaya 1 kg, sugar 750 g, onion 100 g (chopped), garlic 10 g (chopped), ginger 60 g (chopped), red chillies powder 20 g, cumin seed 5 g, cinnamon powder 5 g, black paper powder 5 g and salt 40 g.

Preparation technique

Raw papaya fruit → Washing → peeling → Grating → Mixing with onion, garlic, ginger, chillies and salt → Cooking with stirring till smooth → Addition of sugar → Cooking till desired consistency (jam like) → Mixing powder spices → Filling into a clean sterilized bottle/jar → Capping → Storing

24.7.1.4 Pickle

Recipe

Raw sliced papaya 1 kg, salt 15 g, mustard powder 10 g, turmeric powder 10 g and vinegar to cover the slices.

Preparation technique

Raw papaya → Washing → Peeling → Slicing→ Cover with boiling water for 3 min → Straining of water → Sprinkling of salt on blanched slices → Drying the slices little → Filling the slices in jar → Covering with vinegar → Addition of mustard and turmeric powder → Capping/sealing → Curing about 2 weeks → Storing

24.7.1.5 Preserve and candy

Preparation technique

Mature but unripe papaya → Washing → Peeling → Cutting into halves → Removal of seeds → Cutting into pieces of 7.5 cm cubes → Pricking →

Immersing the pieces in lime solution for 3–4 h (15 g of lime/L of water) → Blanching till softening → Steeping in syrup of 40° brix → Keeping overnight → Steeping in 50° brix syrup → Keeping overnight → Steeping in 60° brix syrup → Keeping overnight → Steeping in syrup of 65° brix → Addition of citric acid (0.5%) → Steeping in syrup of 70° brix → Filling into sterilized wide mouth bottle or tin cans → Pouring of syrup to fill interspaces → Sealing → Storing

In case of candy, pieces from syrup of preserve are drained, shade dried, packed and stored.

24.7.1.6 Sweet (Burfi)

Recipe

Papaya 1 kg, sugar 750 g, cardamom (small) powder 10 g and coconut shreds 20 g.

Preparation technique

Mature but unripe papaya → Washing → Peeling → Cutting into halves → Removal of seeds → Grating into shreds → Add sugar → Cooking with stirring → When mixture starts leaving the container surface add cardamom and coconut shreds → Mix thoroughly → Transfer the mass on smooth surface of tray smeared with fat → Spread in desired thickness and allow to set → Spread some coconut shreds over it → Cutting into shape of Burfi → Pack in attractive cardboard box (sweets dibba) → Use/sale

24.7.1.7 Processing of ripe papaya

Nectar

Recipe

Pulp 20%, total soluble solids 12%, acidity 0.3% and sodium metabisulphite 0.1%.

Preparation technique

Ripe fruit → Washing → Peeling → Cutting into halves → Removal of seeds → Passing through pulper → Pulp → Mixing with syrup solution (sugar + water + citric acid according to recipe) → Addition of preservative → Bottling → Crown corking → Pasteurization for 20 min in boiling water → Cooling → Storing

Squash

Recipe

Pulp 1 kg, sugar 1.5 kg, water 1 L and sodium metabisulphite 2 g.

Preparation technique

Ripe fruit → Washing → Peeling → Cutting into halves → Removal of seeds → Passing through pulper → Pulp → Mixing with strained syrup solution (sugar + water + acid heating just to dissolve the sugar and straining) → Addition of preservative by dissolving in small quantity of squash → Filling into clean sterilized bottles → Capping → Storing

Jam

Recipe

Pulp 1 kg, sugar 0.75 kg, water 100 mL and citric acid 2 g.

Preparation technique

Ripe fruit → Washing → Peeling → Cutting into halves → Removal of seeds → Passing through pulper → Pulp → Mixing with sugar → Cooking → Addition of citric acid → Cooking continue till desired consistency → Judging of end point (68% TSS) → Filling into clean and sterilized jam bottle → Capping/sealing → Labelling → Storing

Toffee

Recipe

Pulp 1 kg, sugar 600 g, glucose 100 g, skim milk powder 160 g and butter or fat 100 g.

Preparation technique

Ripe fruit → Washing → Peeling → Cutting into halves and removal of seed → Passing through pulper → Pulp → Cooking up to one-third → Mix other ingredients → Cooking up to desired consistency (till it starts leaving the side of container) → Transferring on smooth surface or tray smeared with fat → Spreading the mass (in thickness of 0.5–0.75 cm) → Allow to set → Cut the sheet into pieces of toffee size → Wrapping in butter paper → Filling in glass jar or tin → Sealing → Storage

Sauce

Recipe

Papaya pulp 1 kg, sugar 50 g, salt 12 g, onion (chopped) 40 g, garlic (chopped) 10 g, ginger (chopped) 10 g, red chillies powder 10 g, hot spices 15 g, acetic acid 4 mL and sodium benzoate 1 g.

Preparation technique

Ripe fruit → Washing → Peeling → Cutting into halves → Removal of seed → Passing through pulper → Pulp → Cooking pulp with 1/3 sugar → Tie spices in muslin bag and dipping in pulp and pressing occasionally while cooking → Cooking continue up to 1/3 of original volume of pulp → Removal of spice bag → Adding salt and remaining sugar → Cooking up to desired consistency → Addition of acetic acid and sodium benzoate → Filling hot into sauce bottle → Crown corking → Pasteurization (25–30 min) → Cooling → Storage

24.8 Litchi

Litchi is famous for its excellent quality, pleasant flavour, juicy pulp with attractive colour. Litchi fruit contains vitamins A, B and C and minerals such as calcium, phosphorus and iron.

24.8.1 Products

Litchi is processed into pulp, beverage, dehydrated litchi nut, frozen litchi, canned litchi and alcoholic beverage. The techniques for preparation of various products are as follows.

24.8.1.1 Pulp

Preparation technique

Ripe fruit → Washing → Peeling → Destoning (stone removal) → Crushing of pulp/Mincing into fine mass → Heating with little water (up to boiling)→ Addition of citric acid (1%) → Filling hot into sterilized clean bottles → Sealing → Processing in boiling water for 25 min → Air cooling → Storing in cool and dry place

Litchi pulp can be aseptically packed and stored at 2–3°C for preparation of litchi beverage. Use of 1000 ppm of KMS and storage at low temperature is ideal to check the browning of litchi pulp.

24.8.1.2 RTS beverage

Recipe

Pulp 10%, total soluble solids 12%, acidity 0.3% and SO_2 70 ppm.

Preparation technique

Ripe fruit → Washing → Peeling → Removal of stone → Addition of water in flesh in ratio of 1:0.25 → Passing through pulper → Pulp → Mixing with syrup solution (sugar + water + citric acid, heating just to dissolve the sugar) → Addition of SO_2 and mixing → Bottling → Crown corking → Pasteurization in boiling water for 20 min → Cooling → Storing

24.8.1.3 Nectar

Recipe

Pulp 20%, total soluble solid 13%, acidity 0.3% and SO_2 70 ppm.

Preparation technique

Ripe fruit → Washing → Peeling → Removal of stone → Addition of water in flesh in ratio of 1:0.25 → Passing through pulper → Straining → Pulp → Mixing with syrup solution (sugar + water + citric acid, heating just to dissolve the sugar and strained) → Addition of SO_2 and mixing → Bottling →

Crown corking → Pasteurization in boiling water for 20 min → Cooling → Storing

24.8.1.4 Squash

Recipe

Pulp 25%, total soluble solid 50%, acidity 1.2% and SO_2 350 ppm.

Preparation technique

Ripe fruit → Washing → Peeling → Removal of stone → Addition of water in flesh in ratio of 1:0.25 → Passing through pulper → Straining → Pulp→ Mixing with syrup solution (sugar + water + citric acid, heating just to dissolve the sugar and strained) → Addition of SO_2 inform of sodium metabisulphite and mixing → Bottling → Capping → Storing

24.8.1.5 Canned litchi

Preparation technique

Firm ripe fruit of suitable variety → Washing → Peeling → Removal of stone → Blanching in hot water (75°C for 30 s) → Filling into plain or SR lacquered cans → Covering with 30° brix syrup containing 0.05% citric acid → Exhausting (till centre temperature of can reaches to 82°C) → Sealing→ Processing in boiling water for 10 min → Cooling immediately in cold water (8–10°C) → Storing

24.8.1.6 Dehydrated litchi nut

Preparation technique

Ripe fruit of suitable variety (Bedana and China) → Washing → Peeling → Dipping in 2% KMS solution for 16 h → Draining → Loading on trays → Dehydration (Cross-flow dehydrator) at 55–60°C for 16 h (up to moisture content below 10%) → Packing → Storing

24.8.1.7 Frozen litchi

Preparation technique

Filling into cans/suitable containers → Covering with sugar syrup containing 0.05% ascorbic acid → Freezing at –18°C → Storing

24.8.1.8 Alcoholic beverage

The litchi can be processed into alcoholic beverage (wine) yielding 6.5% alcohol. The wine prepared from yeast strain PC and EC-III-8 is light yellow, acidic and rose flavoured with good taste has better potential for wine industry.

24.9 Aonla (Indian goose berry)

The fruit is one of the richest sources of vitamin C. It contains a chemical substance known as gallic acid, which retards the oxidation of vitamin C; hence, it has antioxidant property. Fruit is therefore, rich source of vitamin C in both fresh and processed form. Fruit has also fair source of vitamin B_1 and B_2 and rich source of minerals such as iron, calcium and phosphorus. The aonla fruit is valued high among indigenous medicines in India. It is acidic, cooling, refrigerant, diuretic and laxative. Dried fruit is useful in haemorrhage, diarrhoea, chronic dysentery, diabetes, jaundice, dyspepsia, cough, piles and disease associated with blood and dermatitis (skin disease).

24.9.1 Product

Aonla is a sour and astringent fruit, hence, not popular as table fruit. It has great potentiality for processing into number of food, medicinal and cosmetic products.

24.9.1.1 Food products

Fruits can be processed into number of food products such as preserve, candy, toffee, jam, herbal jam, jelly, fruit bar, sweets, sauce, pickles, chutney and beverages such as pulp, juice, RTS, squash, herbal syrup, tea, etc. The techniques for preparation of these products are as follows.

Preserve

Recipe
Fruits 1 kg and sugar 1–1.25 kg.

Preparation technique
Mature fruits → Washing → Pricking → Dipping in alum solution (2%) for 24 h → Washing → Blanching (in boiling water) for 5 min → Steeping in 40% syrup solution for 24 h → Steeping in 50% syrup solution for 24 h → Steeping in 60% syrup solution for 24 h → Steeping in 70% syrup solution for 3–4 days → Preserve → Packing in glass jar/plastic jar (pulpet) → Storage

Osmotic dehydrated segments

Preparation technique
Aonla fruits → Washing → Pressure cooking for 10 min → Cooling → Separation of segments and removal of stone → Dipping in 70% TSS Syrup for 24 h → Raising TSS twice to 70% after every 24 h → Draining → Dehydration for 3 h → Storage

Candy

Recipe

Aonla fruit 1 kg and sugar 1.25 kg.

Preparation technique

Mature fruits → Washing → Pricking → Dipping in alum solution (2%) for 24 h → Washing → Blanching (in boiling water) for 5 min → Steeping in 40% syrup solution for 24 h → Steeping in 50% syrup solution for 24 h → Steeping in 60% syrup solution for 24 h → Steeping in 70% syrup solution for 3–4 days → Preserve → Draining quickly from sugar syrup → Hot water rinsing for 2 second → Drying up to 15–20% moisture → Candy → Packing in glass jar/plastic jar or polyethylene bag → Storage/marketing

Toffee

Recipe

Aonla pulp 1 kg, sugar 750 g, glucose 100 g, skim milk powder 150 g and Butter 50 g.

Preparation technique

Pulp → Heating → Concentrating up to one-third volume → Mixing with sugar glucose, butter and milk powder → Cooking up to compact solid mass → Removing from fire → Adding colour and essence → Mixing → Spreading mass uniformly (0.5–0.75 cm thickness) on a table with stainless steel top/tray smeared with butter → Allow to cool and set 2–4 h → Cutting into cubes → Wrapping in butter paper → Storage

Jam

Recipe

Pulp 1 kg, sugar 0.75 kg, citric acid 1.5 g and water 150 mL.

Preparation technique

Aonla fruits → Heating in boiling water (10 min) → Separation of segments and removal of stone → Addition of water in ratio of 1:0.75 → Passing through pulping machine → Pulp → Mixing with sugar → Cooking up to desired consistency → Addition of citric acid → Judging of end point (TSS 68%) → Filling into clean sterilized bottles → Capping/sealing → Storing

Herbal jam

Recipe

Aonla pulp 1 kg, sugar 0.75 kg, citric acid 2 g, asparagus juice 200 mL and Nagauri Ashaw gandh powder 50 g.

Preparation technique

Pulp → Mixing with Asparagus juice and Ashaw gandh powder → Addition of sugar → Cooking → Addition of citric acid → Juging of end point → Filling into sterilized bottle → Capping → Storing

Jelly

Recipe

Strained juice 1 L, sugar 0.75 kg and citric acid 1.5 g.

Preparation technique

Aonla fruit (mature) → Washing → Cutting into pieces/slices → Removal of stone → Boiling with water (one and half times the weight of fruit for 20–30 min) → Boiling → Addition of citric acid → Straining of extract → Pectin test for addition of sugar (alcohol test or jell meter test) → Addition of sugar → Cooking → Judging of end point (temperature test 105°C or TSS 65% or sheet or drop test) → Removal of scum/foan → Filling hot in clean and sterilized bottles → Capping → Storing

Fruit bar

Recipe

Aonla pulp 1 kg, sugar 150 g, citric acid 1 g and KMS 1 g.

Preparation technique

Aonla fruit → Washing → Heating in boiling water for 10 min → Separation of segments → Removal of stone → Addition of water (in ratio of 1:1) → Passing through pulping machine → Pulp → Mixing with sugar, citric acid and KMS → Spreading on tray → Drying in cross-flow drier at 60°C (until can be taken out in the form of sheet) → Cutting of sheet into small bar → Wrapping in cellophane paper → Packing in polythene pouches → Storing

Sweets

Recipe

Aonla shred 1 kg, sugar 1 kg, water 0.5 L and melon seed 100 g.

Preparation technique

Aonla fruit → Washing → Grating into shred → Little drying/squeezing → Adding in sugar syrup (sugar + water boiling and straining) → Cooking up to desired consistency → Addition of melon seed → Making in shape of laddu and burfi → Little drying in shade → Packing in attractive cardboard box (sweet dibba) → Use/sale/storing (up to 1 month)

Sauce

Recipe

Pulp 1 kg, sugar 75 g, salt 10 g, onion 50 g, garlic 5 g, ginger 10 g, red chillies powder 5 g, hot spices 10 g, acetic acid 2 mL and sodium benzoate 0.25 g.

Preparation technique

Aonla fruits → Washing → Heating in boiling water for 10 min → Separation of segments and removal of stone → Addition of water in ratio of 1:1 → Passing through pulper → Straining → Pulp → Mixing with one-third sugar (25 g) → Cooking → Adding extracts of onion, garlic, ginger, chillies and hot spices while cooking → Adding acetic acid and remaining sugar → Testing of end point for desired consistency → Addition of salt → Addition of sodium benzoate (by dissolving in water) → Bottling → Crown corking → Processing in boiling water for about 20 min → Cooling→ Storing

Pickle

Recipe

Aonla 1 kg, salt 150 g, Nigella seed 10 g, red chilli powder 10 g, fenugreek 30 g, turmeric powder 10 g, cumin powder 50 g and oil 350 mL.

Preparation technique

Aonla → Washing → Blanching till it become soft → Separation of segment and seed removal → Frying spices in oil → Mixing with segments → Frying for 5 min → Mixing salt → Filling into jar → Keeping in sun for a week → Storing

Chutney

Recipe

Aonla fruit 1.25 kg, sugar 1 kg, salt 50 g, ginger 15 g, hot spices 25 g, red chillies 10 g and glacial acetic acid 10 mL.

Preparation technique

Mature fruits → Washing → Steam for 15 min in pressure cooking → Pass through pulper → Fine pulp → Mix with all ingredients except acetic acid → Cook the mixture to a desired consistency → Add glacial acetic acid → Filling into glass bottles → Capping/sealing → Cooling → Storing

RTS (beverage)

Recipe

Aonla pulp 10%, ginger juice 2%, total soluble solids 11%, acidity 0.25% and SO_2 70 ppm.

Preparation technique

Aonla pulp + Ginger juice → Mixing with syrup solution (sugar + water + citric acid, heating and straining) → Addition of preservative → Bottling → Crown corking → Pasteurization → Air cooling → Storing

Squash

Recipe

Pulp 25%, total soluble solids 50%, acidity 1% and SO_2 300 ppm.

Preparation technique

Mixing with syrup solution → Addition of preservative → Mixing → Bottling → Capping → Labelling → Storing

Supari (chewing product)
Supari prepared is light in colour, soft in texture having good amount of vitamin C. It can be a very good alternative for pan mashala, which have adverse effect on human health.

Preparation technique
Aonla fruit → Blanching → Separation of segments → Cutting the segments into four pieces → Mixing with common salt (2.5%) → Keep overnight → Removal of leachet if any → drying of pieces in dehydrator at 60°C (up to 5–6% moisture) → Packing in polythene pouches → Store at room temperature

Herbal tea powder
Herbal tea stimulates appetite and strengthen digestive system, nervine tonic and improves sense organs.

Recipe
Dried aonla 1 kg, dried bahera 100 g, pipali 50 g, sonth 100 g, cinnamon powder 50 g, clove powder 5 g, tulsi powder 5 g and cardamon 10 g.

Preparation technique
All ingredients → Mixing thoroughly → Grinding into powder → Packing in polythene pouches → Sealing → Storage. Tea can be prepared by boiling 3 cup water + 1 teaspoon full tea powder and filtered. No milk is used. Sugar may or may not be added.

Cider
Aonla cider is refreashing health drink, which contains 10% total soluble solids and 4% alcohol with some polyphenols (0.4%) and ascorbic acid.

Preparation technique
Aonla juice (ameliorated) → fermented with yeast (*S. cerevisiae* variety ellipsoideus Montrachet strain) → Siphoning of clear fermented juice → Maturation → Bottling → Storage/marketing (up to 1 year)

24.9.1.2 Medicinal products

Medicinal products of aonla used for treating chronic dysentery haemorrhage, diabetes, bronchitis, fever, diarrhoea, dyspepsia, cough, scurvy, jaundice, anaemia, piles dermatitis disease, associated with blood and preventing aging. Fruits are used in various Aurvedic preparations such as Chavanprash, Triphla, Triphla churn, Amalki churn, Amalki grith, Amalki rasayan, Amalki awaleh, Dhatri lauh, diabetes powder, Mahatikt grith, Bavasir nasak, Mahausidhi and Amrit kalash. The technique for preparation of some of the products is as follows.

Chavanprash

Recipe

Bael root, Araribark of Sonapan, Gambhar root bark, Pathal root bark, Bari and chhoti kateri root, Gokharu, Shal purnomul, Pushti parni, Balamul, Kankarsingi, Pushkarmul, Vasamul, Mashparni, Jiwanti, Punarwa, Guruch, Pipali, Haritki, Draksha, Small Cardemom, Kaknasa, Agarkasht, White Sandal, Nagarmotha, Kachur, Bikshari kand, Neel kamal, Ridhi, Bridhi jiwak, Rishmak Menda, mahamenda, kakoli, kshir kakoli – 50 g each.

Water 13 L, fresh aonla 6 kg, Banslochan 200 g, Pipali (big) 200 g, cinnamon 100 g, cardamom (small) 50 g, cassia 50g, Nag kesar 50 g, ghee (cow) 300 g, honey 300 g and sugar 6 kg.

Preparation technique

Decoction ingredient → Cuts the ingredients into small pieces. Put the pieces into aluminium/steel bhagauna → Add water and cook it up to ¼ mass → Strained with the help of muslin cloth → Boilthe fresh aonla till it becomes soft and remove stone → Prepare the pulp of segments → Put fat (ghee) into steel bhagauna and little heating → Add aonla pulp and fry till pulp becomes brown/reddish and releases ghee → Take out from fire → Add sugar in strained decoction and cooking → When the syrup become concentrated (2 tar), add fried pulp of aonla and mix it thoroughly → Take out from fire and cool it → Add banslochan, Nagkesar, Pipali, cinnamon, cardamom, cassia, by making fine powder → Add honey in the last after cooling the product → Packing the chavanprash in suitable container → Storing

Amalki churn

This is useful in acidity, blood, aging, etc. The technique for preparation of Amalki churn is as follows.

Preparation technique

Aonla fruits → Drying → Breaking → Removal of seed → Grinding into fine powder → Packing in small glass bottle/plastic bottles (pulpit) → Storing

Aonla churan

Recipe

Aonla powder 100 g, citric acid 3 g, common salt 8 g, black salt 15 g, asafoetida 1 g, fennel powder 1 g, ajwain 0.5 g, black paper 2 g, cumin seeds powder (roasted) 1 g, ginger 1.5 g and sugar 15 g.

Preparation technique

Ingredients → Grinds the ingredients finally → Straining through 80–100 mesh sieve → Mixing thoroughly → Packing the churns in air tight container/pouches → Sealing → Storing

Triphala powder

Recipe

Dried aonla 1 kg, dried Bahera 1 kg and dried harad 1 kg.

Preparation technique

Ingredients (aonla, bahera, harad) → Removing of stone/seed of each ingredients → Grinding separately to make powder → Mixing of each powder in equal quantity → Packing in glass bottles/pouches → Sealing → Storing

Diabetes powder

Recipe

Dried aonla 1 kg, Guruch 1 kg and turmeric 1 kg.

Preparation technique

Dried aonla, guruch and turmeric → Grinding into fine powder → Straining/sieving → Packing in glass bottles or polythene pouches → Sealing → Storing

Dhatri Lauh Churn (powder)

Recipe

Aonla powder 1 kg, Lauh bhasm 500 g, Mulethi powder 250 g and Aonla juice 250 mL.

Preparation technique

Aonla powder + Lauh bhasm + Mulethi powder → Mixing above ingredients thoroughly with the hand → Mix little aonla juice properly → Repeating the process 6–7 times → Packing in glass bottles → Sealing → Storing

24.10 Pomegranate

The fruit has sweet-acidic taste and rich in vitamin B_2 (riboflavin) and minerals such as calcium and iron. Fruit juice is very digestive and cooling. It is useful in fever, gastric problem and patient suffering from leprosy.

24.10.1 Products

Pomegranate fruits can be processed into juice, squash, syrup, wine, anardana and powder.

24.10.1.1 Juice

Preparation technique

Ripe fruit → Washing → Cutting into halves → Seed separation → Juice extraction with basket press or spiral type screw press → Heating in flash pasteurizer (79–82°C) → Cooling → Settling for 24 h → Racking up and filtering/decanting → Juice → Heating at 80°C → Bottling hot juice → Crown crocking → Pasteurization at 80°C for 30 min → Cooling → Storage/marketing. Juice can also be preserved by addition of 600 mg, sodium benzoate/L of juice.

24.10.2 Squash

Recipe
Juice 25%, sugar 45%, acid 1%, benzoic acid 600 ppm. Ingredients calculated for 1 L of juice are 2 kg sugar, 1 L water, 10 g citric acid and 4 g sodium benzoate.

Preparation technique
Fully ripe fruit → Washing → Cutting into halves → Removal of grains → Extraction of juice → Straining → Addition of syrup solution (sugar + water + citric acid, heating just to dissolve the sugar and straining) → Mixing → Addition of sodium benzoate by dissolving in little squash → Mixing→ Bottling → Capping/sealing → Storing/marketing.

24.10.1.3 Syrup

Recipe
Juice 25%, sugar 68%, acid 1.3%, ingredients calculated for 1 L of juice are sugar 2.75 kg, water 0.5 L and citric acid 10 g.

Preparation technique
Fully ripe fruit → Washing → Cutting into halves → Removal of grains → Extraction of juice → Straining → Addition of syrup solution (sugar + water + citric acid, heating just to dissolve the sugar and straining) → Mixing → Addition of sodium benzoate by dissolving in little syrup → Mixing → Bottling → Capping/sealing → Storing/marketing.

24.10.1.4 Wine

Preparation technique
Ripe fruit of pomegranate → Washing → Sorting (diseased and cracked fruits were discarded) → Separation of aril → Juice extraction → Adjusting to 22–23° brix (using sucrose) → Addition of diammonium hydrogen phosphate (0.05 g/100 mL) → Adjusting of acidity of juice 0.7% or 3.5 pH → Pasteurization at 82–85°C for 30 min → Cooling → Inoculation with culture of *S. cerevisiae* CFTRI-101 (at 2% level for 48 h) → Incubation at 26 ± 2°C up to 15 days → Pasteurization of fermented juice/wine at 82–85°C for 30 min → Clarification (using 0.1% bentonite and centrifuge) → Wine → Bottling → Storage

24.10.1.5 Anardana (dried arid)

Preparation technique

Sour type pomegranate → Cutting into halves → Separation of grains → Drying through solar or sun drying for 15 h or by hot air drier (6 h) to a moisture level of 16–18%. It is used in curries, chutney and other culinary preparation.

24.10.1.6 Powder

Preparation technique

Fruits → Washing → Cutting into halves → Separating grains → Steam blanching the grains (8 h) → Sulphuring with burning of 10 g/kg of grain/anardana → Drying in cabinet drier at 58–60°C for 20 h → Grinding the grains with mixy → Sieving with 30 mesh sieve → Packing in 260 g ALP pouches → Storage at 60% relative humidity. The powder can be used in churn form or with milk.

24.11 Jackfruit

It is the largest among the edible fruit and gives more yield than any other fruit tree. The immature or tender fruit is very popular as vegetable and appears in the market in spring when common vegetables are scarce and very expensive. Ripe fruits are good source of sugar, minerals and pectin with fair amount of vitamin A. Fruit has several medicinal values. The unripe fruit is acrid, astringent and carmative. The ripe fruit is laxative, cooling, fattening and useful in treating biliousness.

24.11.1 Products

Fruit can be processed into number of products such as pickle, canned jackfruit, jelly and beverages.

24.11.1.1 Pickles

Pickle in oil

Recipe

Raw/mature fruit pieces 1 kg, mustard oil 250 mL, salt 110 g, red chillies powder 15 g, turmeric powder 10 g, coriander powder 15 g, mustard powder 15 g, fennel powder 15 g, cumin powder 10 g and glacial acetic acid 20 mL.

Preparation technique

Raw/mature fruit → Washing → Peeling → Cutting into pieces (3 cm thick) → Blanching (5 min) in 10% salt + 0.5% turmeric solution →

Draining → Shade drying → Mixing with ingredients and half quantity of fried oil → Filling into clean jar → Addition of remaining oil → Capping → Storing

Sweet pickle

Recipe

Raw/mature fruit pieces 1 kg, jaggery/sugar 250 g, salt 100 g, red chillies powder 15 g, aniseed 10 g, black pepper 10 g, cardamom 10 g, onion (chopped) 60 g, clove (head less) six in numbers, vinegar 125 mL and mustard oil 250 mL.

Preparation technique

Raw/mature fruit → Washing → Peeling → Cutting into desirable pieces (3 cm thick) → Blanching in 10% salt solution → Draining off → Shade drying → Mixing with fried ingredients (except jaggery/sugar and vinegar) → Frying for 5 min → Cooling → Filling into jar → Addition of jaggery/sugar + vinegar by making paste → Capping → Storing

Pickle in vinegar

Recipe

Raw/mature fruit pieces 1 kg, vinegar 1 L, sugar 0.75 kg, water 0.75 L, hot spices 5 g, coriander powder 1 g, salt 100 g, mustard powder 1 g and ginger (grinded) 2 g.

Preparation technique

Raw/mature fruit → Washing → Peeling → Cutting into suitable pieces (3 cm thick) → Blanching in salt solution (50 g/L of water) for 5 min → Washing with plain water → Shade drying → Prepare solution of vinegar + water + sugar + cook slowly → Tie all spices in muslin bag and put in so that extract of spices mixed with vinegar solution → Cooling (takeout spice bag) → Mixing with jackfruit pieces in ratio of 1:1 → Filling of pickles into container (clean jar) → Capping → Storage in cool and dry place

24.11.1.2 Bulbs canning

Preparation technique

Firm ripe fruits → Washing → Cutting lengthwise → Removing gummy core → Separating bulbs from rind → Trimming the top and bottom of the bulbs → Removing seeds → Filling of prepared bulbs (500–550 g) into plain cans A2$^{1}/2$ → Covering with hot syrup containing citric acid 10 g/kg of syrup living 0.6 cm head space → Exhausting (till the temperature at the centre of can reaches 82°C) → Sealing of cans → Processing in boiling water for 30 min → Cooling cans in cold water → Storing cool and dry place

24.11.1.3 Jelly

Jelly can be prepared from waste material outer rind, inner soft portion and trimmings of the bulbs. These are rich in pectin.

Recipe
Extract 1 L, sugar 1 kg and citric acid 7 g.

Preparation technique
Rind (outer portion) + inner soft portion + bulb trimmings → (Removing central core and outer prickly layer of the rind) → Addition of water (in equal weight) → Boiling (30 min) → Addition of citric acid while boiling → Filtering through sieve/muslin cloth → Collecting extract → Extracting once again by boiling the residue again with half the quantity of water for 15 min → Mixing the both extracts → Keeping for settling → Decanting clear extract → Testing of pectin (alcohol or jell meter test) → Addition of sugar and citric acid → Cooking the mixture till desired consistency → Judging of end point (temperature of boiling mass reaches 105°C) → Filling the product into clean and sterilized bottles → Capping/sealing → Storing in cool and dry place

24.11.1.4 RTS beverages

Recipe
Pulp 10%, total soluble solids 12% and acidity 0.3%.

Preparation technique
Ripe fruit → Washing → Peeling → Cutting lengthwise → Removing gummy core and separating the bulb from rind → Removing seeds → Extraction of pulp (flakes and water in ratio of 1:0.25) → Mixing with syrup solution (sugar + water + citric acid heating just to dissolve sugar and straining) → Addition of 0.1% sodium metabisulphite → Mixing → Bottling → Crown corking → Pasteurization 100°C for 15 min → Cooling → Storing/marketing.

24.11.1.5 Squash

Recipe
Pulp 25%, total soluble solid 50% and acidity 1%.

Preparation technique
Ripe fruit → Washing → Peeling → Cutting lengthwise → Removing gummy core and separating the bulb from rind → Removing seeds → Extraction of pulp (flakes and water in ratio of 1:0.25) → Mixing with syrup solution (sugar + water + citric acid heating just to dissolve the sugar and straining) → Addition of sodium metabisulphite 350 ppm or 0.7 g/L of finished products → Bottling → Capping/sealing → Storing/marketing

Jackfruit pulp can also be used for making jam, chutney, sauce and leather. The partially boiled mature unripe flesh can be sun dried and can be used by reboiling during off-season.

Seeds of jackfruit can be converted into flour, which has potential for food formulation because of its good functional properties such as solubility, foamability, absorption and emulsification capacity.

24.12 Ber

The fruit is rich in vitamins C, A and B complex. It is also rich in calcium and iron. It is blood purifier, appetizer and helps in indigestion, cough and asthma.

24.12.1 Product

Ber can be processed to prepare juice, carbonated beverage, preserve, candy, slices and dried ber.

24.12.1.1 Juice

Preparation technique

Juicy variety → Washing → De-stoning/stone removal → Extraction of juice in juicer → Allow to stand the juice at 4°C for 2 h → Removal of scum with the help of stainless spoon → Passing through muslin cloth (four layers) → Filtering through ordinary filter or after removing the scum centrifuge at 500 rpm for 5 min → Juice (40% recovery). A good quality RTS and carbonated beverage can be prepared from ber juice.

24.12.1.2 Dried slices

Preparation technique

A delicious product like dried fig can be prepared from ber fruits. The technique for preparation is as follows:

Fruits → Washing → Cutting into chips with the help of slicer → Blanching of chips in boiling water containing 2% calcium chloride for 3 min → Sulphuring (2 g/kg), fumigation for 1 h → Steeping in syrup (containing 50% sugar and 1% citric acid) for 3 days → Removal of chips from syrup and drying in sun for 3 days → Pressing the product under kitchen press → Packing → Storage/use.

24.12.1.3 Ber preserve

Recipe

Mature fruit 1 kg and sugar 1 kg.

Preparation technique
Firm ripe fruit → Washing → Pricking → Steeping in 2% salt solution containing 0.2% KMS for 2 days → Blanching in water till it becomes soft → Steeping in syrup of 40% TSS for 24 h → Steeping in syrup of 50% TSS for 24 h → Steeping in syrup of 60% TSS for 24 h → Steeping in syrup of 70% TSS for 1 week → Draining quickly → Packing → Covering with fresh syrup of 68% TSS → Capping→ Storing/use

24.12.1.4 Candy

Recipe
Ber fruit 1 kg and sugar 1.25 kg.

Preparation technique
Ripe but firm fruits → Washing → Removing of floaters → Pricking → Blanching (5 min) → Steeping in syrup of 50% and 60% to total soluble solids for 24 h → Steeping 4–5 days in syrup of 70% TSS → Draining → Hot water rinsing → Shade drying → Packing in polythene bag → Storing/marketing

24.12.1.5 Dried ber

Preparation technique
Selection of variety → Ripe fruit → Washing→ Blanching in boiling water for 30 min → Sulphuring for 3 h → Drying at 50–60°C (up to 15–20% moisture) → Product yield 20–25% → Packing → Storage/marketing

24.13 Bael

The fruit is a hard-shelled berry famous for its medicinal properties due to marmelosin content. The fruit is rich in riboflavin (vitamin B_1), carbohydrates and has fair amount of vitamins A and C and minerals. The mature fruits are astringent, and digestive and stomachic are usually prescribed for dysentery and diarrhoea. The ripe fruit is tonic, restorative, laxative and good for heart and brain.

24.13.1 Product

Raw or mature green fruits are processed for candy and preserve. Ripe fruits can be processed in quality beverage, jam, toffee, powder and other products.

24.13.1.1 Preserve

Recipe
Bael cubes 1 kg, sugar 1.25 kg and citric acid 2 kg.

Preparation technique

Mature green fruits → Washing → Cutting in the form of ring → Removal of shell, seed and mucilage after boiling in water → Pricking → Cutting into pieces/cubes → Boiling in water till it becomes soft → Draining → Steeping in 50% syrup → (half sugar + 1 L water + citric acid) for 24 h → Steeping in 60% syrup solution (24 h) → Steeping in 72% sugar syrup solution for (3–4 days) → Packing in jar → Storing

24.13.1.2 Candy

Recipe

Shelled fruit 1 kg and sugar 1.25 kg.

Preparation technique

Mature green fruit → Washing → Removal of shell → Cutting into slices or pieces (2.5 cm thick) → Pricking both sides → Soaking in water for 24 h → Blanching (5–10 min) in water containing edible colour → Steeping in syrup of 50% and 60% TSS for 24 h → Steeping in syrup of 70–72% TSS for 3–4 days → Draining → Hot water rinsing (1–2 s) → Shade drying → Packing in polythene bag → Storing

24.13.1.3 Pulp extraction and storage

Preparation technique

Ripe fruit → Washing → Breaking → Removal of shell and seeds → Addition of water to the pulp in ratio of 1:1 → Mixing → Heating at 80–85°C for a minute → Passing through pulping machine → Pulp → Adjusting total soluble solids (20–25%) and acidity (0.5%) → Addition of SO_2 (400–500 ppm) → Mixing → Packing in bottles → Sealing → Storing

24.13.1.4 RTS (beverage)

Recipe

Pulp 10%, total soluble solids 11%, acidity 0.25% and SO_2 70 ppm.

Preparation technique

Ripe fruit → Washing → Breaking → Removal of shell and seeds → Addition of water to the pulp (in ratio of 1:1) → Mixing → Heating (at 80°C for a min) → Passing through pulper → Pulp → Mixing with strained sugar syrup solution → Addition of preservative→ Homogenization → Bottling → Crown corking → Pasteurization (in boiling water for 20 min) → Air cooling → Storing

24.13.1.5 Squash

Recipe

Juice 25%, sugar 45%, acidity 1% and sodium metabisulphite 350 ppm.

Preparation technique

Ripe fruit → Washing→ Breaking → Removal of shell and seeds → Addition of water to the pulp (in ratio of 1:1) → Mixing → Heating (at 80°C for a minute) → Passing through pulper → Pulp → Mixing with strained sugar syrup solution (sugar + water + citric acid, heating just to dissolve the sugar and straining) → Addition of preservative and mixing → Bottling→ Capping → Storing

24.13.1.6 Cider

Recipe

Juice, sugar, preservative and yeast.

Preparation technique

Ripe fruit → Washing → Breaking → Removal of shell and seeds → Pulp extraction → Addition of KMS 0.2 g/kg of mass → Addition of sugar to raise total soluble solids to 22% → Addition of pure wine yeast → Addition of 0.02–0.05% ammonium hydrogen phosphate (food for yeast) → Fermentation (till 0 or 1% TSS) → Filtering clear liquid ageing/maturation (in oak wood barrel) → Heating of mature cider to 66°C → Cooling → Filtering → Bottling → Crown corking → Pasteurizing at 60°C for 30 min → Cooling → Storing

24.13.1.7 Mixed jam

Recipe

Bael pulp 500 g, mango pulp 500 g, sugar 750 g and citric acid 2 g.

Preparation technique

Bael + mango pulp → Mixing → Addition of sugar → Cooking → Addition of citric acid → Cooking continue till desired consistency → Judging of end point (TSS 68%) → Filling into clean sterilized bottles → Capping/sealing→ Storing

24.13.1.8 Toffee

Recipe

Pulp 1 kg, sugar 400 g, glucose 50 g, skim milk powder 100 g and butter 80 g.

Preparation technique

Pulp → Cooking up to 1/3 → Mixing of sugar, glucose, milk powder and ½ amount of butter → Cooking up to end point → Addition of remaining half of butter → Cooking up to desired consistency (83% TSS) → Addition of sulphur dioxide (1000–1500 ppm) → Spread on aluminium tray (in 0.5 cm thickness) → Cooling → Cutting into pieces of suitable size → Drying at 60°C for 4 h (9–10% moisture) → Wrapping in butter or moisture proof paper → Packing in polythene pouches → Storing

24.13.1.9 Powder

Preparation technique
Ripe fruit → Washing → Breaking and removal of shell → Pulping through pulper → Pulp → Mixing with KMS (1500 ppm) → Spreading on tray in thin layer → Drying up to 10% moisture → Cutting/breaking thin layer into pieces → Drying up to 3–4% moisture → Grinding into powder form → Packing in moisture proof container → Storing

24.14 Jamun

Fruit is purplish red and has good nutritive and medicinal value. It is rich source of iron, pectin with fair amount of ascorbic acid. Fruit is used as an effective medicine against diabetes, heart and liver trouble. The seed powder of jamun reduces the sugar in the urine and helps in dysentery.

24.14.1 Product

Fruits can be utilized for processing of an excellent quality of juice, vinegar, cider, wine, jelly, RTS beverage and squash.

24.14.1.1 Juice

Preparation technique
Ripe fruits → Washing → Grating → Heating up to 70°C → Passing the heated mass through a basket press → Juice → Heating to 85°C → Cooling (30–35°C) → Addition of sodium benzoate (500 ppm) or pasteurization → Storage

24.14.1.2 Vinegar

Preparation technique
Ripe fruit → Washing → Addition of little water → Heating → Crushing while heating → Juice extraction through muslin cloth by pressing → Adjusting sugar about 12% either by adding the sugar or diluting the juice with water → Heating (pasteurized) up to boiling point → Filling into glass carboy/earthen pot/wooden barrel up to three-fourth of their capacity → Allow to cool → Add pure wine yeast (From Winery/Chemist's shop) at the rate of 1.5 g/L → Mixing → Plugging the mouth of carboy or barrel loosely with cotton wool or muslin cloth to escape the carbon dioxide gas → Allow the fermentation at 22–27°C for 3–4 weeks to complete (indicates 0–1% total

soluble solids) → Store the fermented juice/wine for 1–2 weeks for sedimentation → Straining through muslin cloth/siphoning the clear liquid into clean carboy up to three-fourth in capacity → Adjusting of alcohol content of fermented liquid to 7–8% by dilution with water (because acetic acid bacteria do not grow at a higher concentration of alcohol) → Add unpasteurized vinegar or mother vinegar in ratio of 1:10 and mixed well → Plug the carboy loosely to allow sufficient aeration (film of vinegar bacterial formed on surface of fermenting liquid should not be disturbed) → Maintain the temperature of liquid at 21–27°C for 10 weeks to complete the fermentation (vinegar is produced by oxidizing alcohol by acetic acid bacteria) → Siphon vinegar and filter through a thick cloth leaving at the bottom of container a turbid liquid (can be used as mother vinegar for fresh fermentation) → Ageing or store for 3–6 months (because fresh vinegar is turbid liquid has a raw biting taste) in carboy or barrel to develop good flavour and aroma → Siphon the vinegar again and filter for clarification → Fill the vinegar into clean sterilized bottle → Crown corking → Pasteurization in hot water at 70–75°C for 15 min → Air cooling → Storing

24.14.1.3 Cider

Preparation technique

Ripe fruits → Washing → Crushing → Juice extraction → Addition of KMS (0.2 g/kg material) → Addition of sugar to raise total soluble solids 22% → Addition of pure wine yeast → Addition of 0.02–0.05% ammonium hydrogen phosphate as food for yeast → Allow fermentation → Filter clear liquid → Ageing (Maturation) → Heating of mature cider to 66°C → Cooling→ Filtering→ Bottling→ Crown corking → Pasteurization at 60°C for 30 min → Cooling → Storing

24.14.1.4 Wine

Preparation technique

Ripe fruits → Washing in water → Crushing with hand without damaging seeds → Addition of boiling water in ratio 1:1 to kill yeast and bacteria → Cooling of hot must and mashing → Sugar is added (200 g/kg of fruit) to raise total soluble solids 23% → Addition of yeast nutrient in form of diammonium phosphate (0.2%) and sulphur dioxide (150 ppm) in form of KMS (23 g) → 24 h old starter is inoculated to the must at 2% level and allowed to ferment at room temperature (starter is prepared by making a malt solution by adding 20% sugar, 0.03% tartaric acid, 2% malt extract, 2% yeast extract, 0.2% citric acid, 0.2% diammonium phosphate in distill water and medium is brought to boiling, cooled and inoculated with 7 days old culture of *S. cerevisiae* var. *ellipsoideus* and maintained on MGYP medium)

→ After fermentation add 0.25% pectin enzyme → Kept for fermentation (4 days) → Pressing through muscling cloth and removal of seeds and Pomace → Keep it for settling → Racking of wine into clean glass bottles of 1 L capacity and filled up to the brim → Maintaining of SO_2 in bottles at 150 ppm → Sealing bottles air tight → Storing at room temperature (20–35°C) for maturation

24.14.1.5 Jelly

Recipe

Pulp 1 kg, sugar 0.75 kg and citric acid 2.0 g.

Preparation technique

Firm ripe fruit → Washing → Addition of water (1/2 times the weight of fruits) → Boiling (20–30 min or till softening) → Addition of citric acid while boiling → Straining of extract → Testing of pectin (alcohol or jell meter test) → Addition of sugar as per pectin test → Boiling up to desired consistency → Judging of end point (sheet/drop/temperature test 105°C) → Removing scum → Filling hot into clean sterilized bottle → Capping/sealing → Storing

24.14.1.6 RTS beverage

Recipe

Juice 15%, total soluble solids 12%, acidity 0.3% and benzoic acid 120 ppm.

Preparation technique

Ripe fruit → Washing → Addition of water (1:0.5) → Heating up to softening → Crushing → Seed removal → Passing through pulper → Straining the juice → Testing for sugar and acidity → Mixing with syrup solution (sugar + water + citric acid, heating just to dissolve the sugar and straining) → Addition of sodium benzoate as preservative → Mixing → Bottling → Crown corking → Pasteurization in boiling water for about 20 min → Air cooling → Storing

24.14.1.7 Squash

Recipe

Juice 1 L, sugar 1.25 kg, water 0.5 L, sodium benzoate 2.75 g and citric acid 15 g.

Preparation technique

Ripe fruit → Washing → Addition of water (1:0.5) → Heating up to softening → Crushing → Seed removal → Passing through pulper → Straining the juice → Mixing with syrup solution (sugar + water + citric acid, heating just to dissolve the sugar and straining) → Addition of sodium benzoate as preservative → Mixing → Bottling → Capping → Storing

24.15 Phalsa

The fruit is drupe with deep reddish brown colour and sub-acid taste. It has fair source of vitamins A and C and minerals particularly phosphorus and iron. The fruits have cooling effect and stomachic. It helps in curing inflammation, heart and blood disorders, fever and constipation. Its cultivation is favoured around big cities where fruits find a ready and quick sale because of its poor keeping quality.

24.15.1 Products

Fruits have attractive colour and pleasing flavour; hence, they are most suitable for processing into quality beverages such as RTS, squash and syrup.

24.15.1.1 RTS (beverage)

Recipe
Juice 10%, total soluble solids 12%, acidity 0.3% and benzoic acid 120 ppm.

Preparation technique
Ripe fruits → Washing → Addition of water in ratio of 1:0.5 → Heating up to softness → Crushing → Passing through pulper for juice extraction → Straining of juice → Mixing with syrup solution (sugar + water + citric acid as calculated, heating just to dissolve the sugar and straining) → Addition of preservative (sodium benzoate)→ Mixing → Bottling → Crown corking → Pasteurization → Air cooling → Storing.

24.15.1.2 Squash

Recipe
Juice 25%, total soluble solids 50%, acidity 1.2% and benzoic acid 600 ppm.

Preparation technique
Ripe fruits → Washing → Addition of water in ratio of 1:0.5 → Heating up to softness → Crushing→ Passing through pulper for juice extraction → Straining of juice → Mixing with syrup solution (sugar + water + citric acid as calculated, heating just to dissolve the sugar and straining) → Addition of preservative (sodium benzoate) → Mixing → Bottling → Capping/sealing → Storing

24.15.1.3 Syrup

Recipe
Juice 25%, sugar 68% and acid 1.3%.

Preparation technique
Ripe fruits → Washing → Crushing → Heating with addition of little water → Juice extraction or passing through pulper → Straining → Juice

→ Calculation of sugar, water and citric acid for syrup solution (sugar + water + citric acid heating just to dissolve the sugar and straining) → Mixing with juice → Filling into clean sterilized bottle → Capping → Storage

24.16 Karonda

The fruit is berry and its taste is sour and astringent. It is one of the richest sources of iron and contents fair amount of vitamin C. Fruit has antiscorbutic properties and is very useful for cure of anaemia. It is mostly grown as protective hedge and in home garden.

24.16.1 Products

Karonda fruits are astringent in taste, hence, not popular as table fruit. It is processed into quality products. Raw or mature fruits are most suitable for making an excellent quality preserve, candy, jelly, pickle and chutney. Ripe fruits can be processed into squash and syrup. Fruits may also be dried for preparing the condiments.

24.16.1.1 Preserve

Recipe
Mature fruit 1 kg and sugar 1 kg.

Preparation technique
Fruits → Washing → Slitting for seed removal → Steeping in 2% salt solution containing 600 ppm (KMS) for 24 h to bleach → Washing → Pricking → Blanching in water containing 0.05% erythrosine and 0.25% citric acid to fix colour → Steeping fruit in syrup of 50% total soluble solids for 24 h → Steeping in 60% TSS for 24 h → Steeping in 70% TSS for 24 h → Packing in glass jar/plastic jar (pulpet) → Capping → Storing

24.16.1.2 Candy

Recipe
Fruit 1 kg and sugar 1 kg.

Preparation technique
Fruits → Washing → Slitting for seed removal → Steeping in 2% salt solution containing 600 ppm (KMS) for 24 h to bleach → Washing → Pricking → Blanching in water containing 0.05% erythrosine and 0.25% citric acid to fix colour → Steeping fruit in syrup of 50% total soluble solids for 24 h → Steeping in 60% TSS for 24 h → Steeping in 70% TSS

for 5 days → Draining → Dipping in boiling water (1–2 s) to remove adhering sugar → Shade drying → Packing (polythene bag/glass jar) → Storing

24.16.1.3 Jelly

Recipe

Karonda fruit 1 kg, sugar 1 kg and citric acid 2 g.

Preparation technique

Mature/firm ripe fruits → Washing → Cutting in form of thin rings → Add equal amount of water → Boiling (20–30 min) → Addition of citric acid → Straining of extract → Pectin test → Addition of sugar → Cooking up to 105°C → Remove scum → Fill hot into clean and sterilized bottle → Capping → Storing

24.16.1.4 Pickle

Recipe

Karonda 1 kg, salt 200 g, red chillies powder 25 g, mustard powder 50 g, turmeric powder 10 g, fenugreek, cumin, aniseed 1 g and mustard oil 400 mL.

Preparation technique

Karonda fruits → Washing → Cutting into halves → Removal of seed → Mixing with salt → Filling into jar → Keeping in the sun for 4 days → Frying spices in oil → Mixing with fruit pieces → Storing

24.16.1.5 Chutney

Recipe

Fruit 1 kg, sugar 500 g, chilli 10 g, ginger chopped 10 g, salt 50 g, garlic chopped 10 g, hot spices 20 g and acetic acid 20 mL.

Preparation technique

Fruits → Washing → Slicing/grating → Cooking (with little water) → Addition of all ingredients except sugar and vinegar → Cooking to desired consistency → Addition of sugar → Continue cooking to desired thickness of semi-liquid form → Mixing of acetic acid → Packing into sterilizes clean and dry wide mouthed bottles → Capping/sealing → Allow to cool → Storage at ambient temperature

24.16.1.6 Squash

Recipe

Karonda juice 1 L, sugar 2 kg, water 1 L, citric acid 10 g, sodium benzoate 1 g/L of finished product and rose essence 1 mL.

Preparation technique
Select fully ripe fruits of coloured variety (Maroon) → Washing → Addition of half quantity of water (on weight of fruit basis) → Heating up to softness Extraction of juice with the help of mixy or muslin cloth → Straining → Addition of sugar syrup (sugar + water + citric acid, heating just to dissolve the sugar and straining) → Mixing → Adding essence and preservative → Mixing thoroughly → Filling into clean sterilized bottles → Capping/sealing → Storing

24.16.1.7 Syrup

Recipe
Juice 1 L, sugar 3 kg, water 0.5 L, citric acid 20 g and rose essence 1 mL.

Preparation technique
Syrup can be prepared by following the technique of squash.

24.17 Mulberry

Among the various species *Morus nigra* is grown for fruits. The fruits of this species are black/red which gives the juice of most attractive red colour.

24.17.1 Products

Fruits can be used for making jam with its soft seed and excellent quality of beverage such as squash and syrup.

24.17.1.1 Jam

Recipe
Pulp 1 kg, sugar 0.75 kg, citric acid 2 g and water 100 mL.

Preparation technique
Ripe fruits → Washing → Cutting → Addition of water → Heating → Addition of sugar → Cooking up to desired consistency → Addition of citric acid → Judging of end point (temperature 105°C) → Filling hot into clean and sterilized bottles → Cooling → Capping → Storing

24.17.1.2 Squash

Recipe
Juice 1 L, sugar 2 kg, water 1 L, citric acid 5 g and preservative (sodium benzoate) 4 g.

Preparation technique
Ripe fruits → Washing → Cutting → Addition of little water → Heating and Crushing → Juice extraction → Straining → Mixing with sugar syrup

solution (sugar + water + citric acid, heating just to dissolve the sugar and straining) → Mixing preservative by dissolving in little squash → Filling into bottles → Capping/sealing → Storing

24.18 Apple

The fruit is rich in minerals such as iron and calcium, fibres and carbohydrates. Apple helps in reducing dental caries, blood dysentery control and obesity.

24.18.1 Products

Apple fruit is processed into juice, cider, jam, jelly, chutney, preserve and fruit butter.

24.18.1.1 Juice

Preparation technique
Ripe fruit → Washing → Cutting/grating → Juice extraction by crushing with basket press → Straining → Clarification (enzymatic or with gelatin) → Filtration heating at 85°C → Filling hot into cans/bottling → Sealing → Processing at 100°C for 15 min → Cooling → Storage

24.18.1.2 Cider

Preparation technique
Apple fruits → Washing → Crushing → Extraction of juice → Addition of sugar to the juice to raise 22% total soluble solids → Addition of SO_2 (100 ppm or KMS 0.2 g/L) → Addition of wine yeast → Fermentation (temperature 18–21°C) → Addition of 0.02–0.04% ammonium hydrogen phosphate to hasten the fermentation (completed when the brix of the juice is 0–1%) → Racking → Filtration → Ageing/maturation (in oak wood barrel) → Heating to 66°C → Filtration → Bottling → Pasteurization (30 min at 60°C) → Cooling → Storage

24.18.1.3 Jam

Recipe
Apple pulp 1 kg, sugar 0.75 kg, citric acid 2.5 g and water 150 mL.

Preparation technique
Firm ripe fruit → Washing → Peeling → Grating → Removal of seed and core → Addition of sugar and water → Cooking up to desired consistency → Addition of citric acid → Judging of end point by temperature (105°C) or

total soluble solids (68%) → Filling hot into clean and sterilized bottles → Cooling → Capping/sealing → Storing in cool and dry place

24.18.1.4 Jelly

Recipe
Juice 1 L, sugar 1 kg and citric acid 2 g.

Preparation technique
Firm but not over ripe fruit of sour variety → Washing → Cutting into thin slices → Boiling with water (one and half times the weight of fruit for 20–30 min) → Addition of citric acid while boiling → Straining of extract → Pectin test for addition of sugar (alcohol test or jell meter test) → Addition of sugar → Cooking → Judging of end point by temperature (105°C) or TSS (65%) or sheet or drop test → Removal of scum foam → Add remaining citric acid → Filling hot clean and sterilized bottles → Wiping dry → Capping → Storing

24.18.1.5 Chutney

Recipe
Apple (sour) prepared 1 kg, onion (chopped) 150 g, garlic (chopped) 10 g, ginger (grated) 75 g, salt 40 g, red chilli powder 10 g, hot spices 5 g, sugar 500 g and acetic acid 30 mL.

Preparation technique
Mature apple fruits → Washing → Peeling → Removal of core and seed → Slicing/grating → Cooking (with little water) → Addition of all ingredients except sugar and vinegar → Cooking to desired consistency → Addition of sugar → Continue cooking to desired thickness of semi liquid form → Mixing of acetic acid → Packing into sterilized clean and dry wide mouthed bottles → Capping/sealing → Cooling → Storing

24.18.1.6 Preserve

Recipe
Mature fruit 1 kg and sugar 1 kg.

Preparation technique
Fully matured medium sized fruit → Washing → Peeling → Pricking with fork (preserve can also be prepared with halves by removing the core) → Steeping in 2% salt solution containing 0.1% citric acid and 0.05% KMS for 24 h (to prevent browning) → Washing → Dipping in 2% alum solution for 24 h → Washing → Blanching in water (5–8 min) → Steeping fruit in syrup of 40% TSS for 24 h → Steeping in syrup of 60% TSS for 24 h → Draining → Packing in jar → Covering fruit with freshly prepared syrup of 68% TSS → Capping/sealing → Storing.

24.18.1.7 Fruit butter

Recipe

Pulp 1 kg, sugar 500 g, spices powder (cinnamon, clove, ginger) 1 g each and essence of vanilla or lemon if required 2 mL.

Preparation technique

Fully ripe fruit → Washing → Cutting into pieces → Boiling with little water till soft → Passing through pulper → Pulp → Mixing with sugar → Cooking till desired consistency like jam → Addition of finally grinded/powdered spices, a little before the end point → Mixing thoroughly → Packing in clean sterilized dry wide mouthed bottle → Capping/sealing → Storing in a cool and dry place.

24.19 Pear

The fruit is rich in carbohydrates and minerals such as calcium and iron. It is also fairly rich in vitamins A, B and C.

24.19.1 Products

Pear fruits are processed into jam, preserve, fruit butter, canned pear, chutney, pickles, drying and wine. The techniques used for preparation of these products are as follows.

24.19.1.1 Jam

Recipe

Pulp 1 kg, sugar 750 g, citric acid 2 g and water 250 mL.

Preparation technique

Ripe fruit → Washing → Peeling → Grating/cutting → Removal of central core → Addition of water → Cooking → Addition of sugar and citric acid → Cooking continue till desired consistency → Judging of end point → Filling into clean and sterilized bottles → Capping/sealing → Storing in a dry place.

24.19.1.2 Preserve

Recipe

Fruit 1 kg and sugar 1 kg.

Preparation technique

Mature fruits → Washing → Peeling → Cutting into halves or quarters → Removal of core → Pricking → Steeping in 2% salt solution for 24 h to prevent browning and disintegration of fruit tissues → Washing and deeping in 2% alum solution for 24 h → Washing again → Blanching in water containing small quantity of sodium metabisulphite → Steeping fruit in syrup of 40% TSS for 24 h → Removal of fruit → Increasing consistency of syrup to 60% TSS by boiling → Steeping of fruit for 24 h → Repeating the process and raising syrup strength by 5% TSS to 70% TSS on alternate days → Steeping in 70% TSS for a week → Preserve → Draining → Filling in container/glass jar → Covering fruit with freshly prepared sugar syrup of 68% TSS → Sealing air tight → Storage

24.19.1.3 Fruit butter

Recipe

Pulp 1 kg, sugar 750 g, spices powder (cinnamon, clove, nutmeg) 1 g each and essence of vanilla 2 mL.

Preparation technique

Ripe fruits → Washing → Cutting into thin pieces → Boiling with equal quantity of water → Sieving for removal of seed and skin → Fine pulp → Mixing pulp with sugar → Cooking to consistency of jam → Addition of finely ground spices and mixing → Removing from fire → Filling hot into clean and sterilized bottles → Sealing → Storage

24.19.1.4 Canned pear

Preparation technique

Mature pear fruit → Washing → Peeling → Cutting length wise into four pieces → Removing core → Immersing the pieces in salt solution (2%) to prevent browning → Removing of pieces from salt solution → Washing → Filling the pieces (about 310 g) into can (butter size can) → Addition of 225 g of hot sugar syrup of 40% TSS containing 0.3% citric acid → Exhausting the cans (temperature 78–80°C) for 10 min → Sealing→ Pasteurizing in boiling water for 20 min → Removing cans and cooling → Storing in a cool and dry place.

24.19.1.5 Chutney

Recipe

Prepared fruit 1 kg, sugar 750 g, salt 60 g, turmeric 30 g, red chillies 15 g, cumin 15 g, mace powder 2 g, cinnamon (powder) 5 g, black pepper (powder) 10 g and vinegar 200 mL.

Preparation technique

Mature fruits → Washing → Peeling → Removal of core and seed → Grating/slicing → Cooking (with little water) → Addition of all ingredients → Cooking to jam consistency → Packing in clean sterilized wide mouthed bottles → Capping/sealing → Storing

24.19.1.6 Pickles

Recipe
Pear 1 kg, cinnamon, cardamom large, black pepper, cumin powder each 10 g, sugar 250 g, clove headless five in numbers and vinegar 250 mL.

Preparation technique
Firm ripe fruits → Washing → Peeling → Removal of core and seeds → Cutting length wise into four pieces → Keeping immediately in salt water to prevent discoloration → Cooking sugar, vinegar and spices for 5 min → Mixing with pear pieces → Heating till pear pieces become tender but still firm → Cooling → Filling in jars → Storage at ambient temperature in a cool and dry place

24.19.1.7 Drying

Preparation technique
Mature fruits → Washing → Peeling → Cutting into halves → Remove core → Keeping in 2% salt solution → Sulphuring 30 min or immerse for 20–30 min in 1–2% KMS solution → Draining → Drying at 60–65°C or sun drying → Packing → Storage

24.19.1.8 Wine (perry)

Wine prepared from pears is known as perry. The technique used for preparation is similar to that of apple cider.

24.20 Apricot

Fruit is highly nutritive with pleasant flavour. It is rich in β-carotene which is one of the important antioxidant nutrients. It is also rich in vitamin C, niacin, carbohydrates, protein, potassium, phosphorus and fibre. Dried apricot is high in calcium and iron content. The fruit is good for vision, skin growth, reproductive and immune system. Apricots are laxative and considered good for the patient suffering from constipation. Kernel is either sweet or bitter both have valuable by products.

24.20.1 Product

Products that can be processed from apricot are jam, jelly, beverage, osmotic dehydration, dehydrated product, fruit bar, chutney, etc. The techniques for preparation of these products are as follows.

24.20.1.1 Jam

Recipe
Pulp 1 kg, sugar 750 g, water 125 mL and citric acid 5 g.

Preparation technique
Fruits → Washing → Cutting into small pieces → Addition of water → Heating till softening of fruit pieces → Addition of sugar and citric acid → Cooking till desired consistency → Testing of end point → Filling into clean and sterilized bottle → Capping/sealing → Storing in dry and cool place

24.20.1.2 Jelly

Recipe
Juice extract 1 L, sugar 0.75 kg and citric acid 3 g.

Preparation technique
Semi-ripe fruits → Washing → Cutting and removing of stone → Addition of water just to cover the pieces → Heating/boiling till softening → Addition of citric acid while boiling → Juice extraction → Testing of pectin for addition of sugar → Addition of required sugar → Cooking → Judging of end point (temperature 105°C or TSS 65%) → Removing of scum → Filling hot into sterilized bottles → Wiping dry → Capping → Storing

24.20.1.3 Nectar

Recipe
Pulp 20%, total soluble solids 12%, acidity 0.3% and SO_2 70 ppm.

Preparation technique
Ripe fruits → Washing → Cutting and removal of stone → Passing through pulper → Pulp → Straining → Determination of TSS and acids → Addition of require amount of sugar and acid inform of syrup solution (sugar + water + citric acid, heating just to dissolve the sugar and straining) → Addition of preservative by dissolving in little quantity of nectar → Mixing/homogenization → Bottling → Crown corking → Pasteurization → Air cooling → Storing

24.20.1.4 Squash

Recipe
Pulp 25%, TSS 50%, acidity 1.3% and SO_2 350 ppm (sodium metabisulphite).

Preparation technique
Ripe fruits → Washing → Cutting and removal of stone → Passing through pulper → Pulp → Straining→ Determination of TSS and acids → Addition of require amount of sugar and acid in form of syrup solution (sugar + water + citric acid, heating just to dissolve the sugar and straining) → Mixing → Addition of preservative by dissolving in little quantity of squash and mixing → Bottling → Capping/sealing → Storing.

24.20.1.5 Osmotic dehydration

Preparation technique

Firm ripe fruits → Washing → Removing stone by giving a slight cut along the suture so that fruit retains their shape → Collecting such fruits in large buckets → Addition of strained sugar syrup of 70% TSS having 0.25% citric acid, 0.06% calcium phosphate and sodium metabisulphite 1500 ppm → Covering with lid → Keeping for 24 h → Draining → Dipping in cold water for 30 s (to remove excess of sugar syrup from fruit surface) → Spreading fruits uniformly putting cavity up over nylon net hanged 5°C m above ground → Sun drying up to 16% moisture (takes about 4–5 days) → Packing in polythene or air tight container → Storing.

24.20.1.6 Sun dried

Preparation technique

Ripe fruits → Washing → Cutting into halves → Removal of pits → Placing of halves in trays → Sulphuring → Drying 20–24% moisture → Packing into polythene bags → Storing

24.20.1.7 Dehydrated apricot

Preparation technique

Selection of suitable variety (yellow white variety) → Ripe fruits → Washing → Cutting into halves → De-stoning → Sulphuring for 20 min → Drying at 57–68°C for 10–12 h up to 15–20% moisture and product yield 15–20% → Packing → Storing

24.20.1.8 Apricot chutney

Recipe

Prepared fruits (slices) 1 kg, sugar 750 g, salt 40 g, onion (chopped) 30 g, garlic (chopped) 10 g, ginger (grated/chopped) 25 g, red chilli powder 10 g, black pepper 10 g, cinnamon powder 10 g, large cardamom 10 g, aniseed 5 g, cumin powder 10 g, clove (headless) six in number and vinegar 150 mL.

Preparation technique

Firm ripe fruits → Washing → Slicing → Removal of stone → Mixing with sugar → Cooking slowly → Tie the spices including onion, garlic, ginger in muslin bag and dip in the mixture while cooking → Continue cooking and stirring till desired consistency → Removal of muslin bag and squeezing the spice extract into mixture → Addition of vinegar and mixing → Addition of salt and mixing → Packing into clean and sterilized wide mouthed bottles → Capping/sealing → Storage at ambient temperature.

The other food products such as frozen halves, intermediate moisture food, fruit bar and fruit sauce have been developed and standardized for commercial production.

24.20.2 By-products

Apricot seed gives two types of kernels sweet and bitter. The varieties of sweet kernels are dried with stones for consumption as dry fruits. The bitter kernels are unfit for human consumption and utilized mostly for oil extraction. The oil content in apricot kernels varies from 36–62%. The oil of sweet kernel is used for cooking purpose and oil of bitter kernel used as hair oil and for illumination. Apricot oil is extensively used in joint pains and for body massage.

24.21 Plum

Fruit is rich in Vitamins A and B with fair amount of iron. Its juice is very cooling and helpful in reducing the temperature in fever.

24.21.1 Product

Fruits are processed into quality beverage such as RTS, squash and syrup, jelly, chutney, sauce and canning. The techniques for preparation of these products are as follows.

24.21.1.1 RTS beverage

Recipe

Juice 10% , total soluble 12% , acidity 0.3% and benzoic acid (sodium benzoate) 120 ppm.

Preparation technique

Ripe fruit (coloured varieties) → Washing → Addition of water in ratio of 1:0.5 → Heating 80°C → Crushing → Removal of stone → Passing through pulper → Straining → Juice→ Mixing with strained sugar syrup solution → Addition of preservative → Mixing/homogenization → Bottling → Crown corking → Pasteurization at 80–90°C for 25 min → Air cooling → Storing in a cool and dry place

24.21.1.2 Squash

Recipe

Juice 25%, sugar 50%, acid 1.2% and sodium benzoate 600 ppm.

Preparation technique
Ripe fruits → Washing → Cutting → Removing stone → Passing through pulper to extract the juice → Straining → Mixing with sugar syrup solution (sugar + water + citric acid, heating just to dissolve the sugar and straining) → Addition of preservative by dissolving in little squash and mixing → Filling into clean sterilized bottles → Capping/sealing → Storing

24.21.1.3 Syrup

Recipe
Juice 25%, sugar 68% and acid 1.3%.

Preparation technique
Ripe fruits → Washing → Cutting → Removing stone → Passing through pulper to extract the juice → Straining → Mixing with sugar syrup solution (sugar + water + citric acid, heating just to dissolve the sugar and straining) → Filling into clean sterilized bottles → Capping/sealing → Storing

24.21.1.4 Jelly

Recipe
Juice extract 1 L, sugar 750 g and citric acid 2.5 g.

Preparation technique
Firm ripe fruits → Washing → Cutting and removal of stone → Addition of water just to cover the fruit pieces → Heating → Addition of citric acid → Extraction of juice → Testing of pectin → Addition of required sugar → Cooking → Judging of end point (temperature 105 °C) → Removing scum → Filling of jelly into clean and sterilized bottle → Capping/sealing → Storing.

24.21.1.5 Plum chutney

Recipe
Pulp 1 kg, sugar 500 g, salt 10 g, onion chopped 25 g, garlic chopped 10 g, ginger chopped 20 g, red chilli powder, black pepper powder, cinnamon powder, cumin powder, cardamom, any seed powder 10 g each and acetic acid 15 mL.

Preparation technique
Plum fruit → Washing → heating with little water for softening → Pulp extraction and removal of seed and skin) → Addition of all ingredients except sugar and acetic acid → Cooking → Addition of sugar → Cooking to semi-liquid form/desired consistency → Mixing of acetic acid → Packing into sterilized clean and dry wide mouthed bottles → Capping/sealing→ Storing

24.21.1.6 Sauce

Recipe

Pulp 1 kg, sugar 100 g, salt 20 g, onion chopped 50 g, ginger chopped 25 g, Garlic chopped 10 g, red chilli powder 10 g, clove five numbers headless, black pepper, cardamom large, cinnamon 10 g powdered each, vinegar 40 mL and sodium benzoate 0.7 g/kg sauce.

Preparation technique

Ripe fruits → Washing → Cutting → Removal of seed→ Cooking pulp with onion and ginger till softening → Rubbing pulp and straining → Cooking with one-third quantity of sugar → Putting spice bag in pulp and pressing occasionally → Cooking to one-third of original volume of pulp → Removal of spice bag → Adding remaining sugar and salt → Cooking one-third to its original volume → Addition of vinegar/acetic acid and preservative → Filling hot into bottles → Crown corking → Pasteurization (85–90°C for 30 min) → Cooling → Storage at ambient temperature.

24.21.1.7 Canning

Preparation technique

Fruits → Washing → Pricking → Filling into lacquered AR can (A2½) → Filling syrup of strength 40° brix → Exhausting can at 82–100°C for 6–10 min or until temperature in centre of can reaches about 79°C → Sealing of can → Processing in boiling water 20 min → Cooling→ Storing in a cool and dry place.

24.22 Strawberry

The fruit is rich in vitamin C and minerals such as iron, potassium and sulphur.

24.22.1 Products

Various value added products can be prepared from strawberry. Berries can be used for canning, candy, jam, jellies, sauce, syrup and frozen product. The techniques for preparation of these products are as follows.

24.22.1.1 Canning

Preparation technique

Selection of suitable variety → Firm ripe fruit → Grading → Washing → Removal of stem → Filling into AR-lacquered cans → Syruping (Hot syrup of 50% total soluble solids strength) → Exhausting → Sealing → Processing in boiling water (100°C) for 10 min for A2 cans and 15 min for A2½ cans → Cooling → Labelling → Storage.

24.22.1.2 Candy

Recipe

Fruit 1 kg, sugar 1 kg and water 1 L.

Preparation technique

Firm ripe fruits → Washing → De-capping → Preparation of sugar syrup with equal quantity of sugar and water in boiling pan and cooking syrup to a temperature of 104°C → Cooling to 94°C → Transferring strawberry into it → Place wire-mesh tray over it and set aside for 24 h → Cooking the syrup up to 70% TSS → Steeping the strawberry for 2–3 days → Hot water rinsing to remove adhering sugar → Shade drying → Packing in waterproof container or polythene bag → Storage/marketing.

24.22.1.3 Jam

Recipe

Pulp 1 kg, sugar 750 g, citric acid 2 g and water 250 mL.

Preparation technique

Ripe fruits → Washing → Crushing → Addition of water → Heating up to softening → Addition of sugar → Cooking and addition of citric acid → Judging of end point → Filling into clean and sterilized bottle → Capping/sealing→ Storing in a cool and dry place.

24.22.1.4 Jelly

Recipe

Juice extract 1 kg, sugar 0.75 kg and citric acid 2 g.

Preparation technique

Firm ripe fruits → Washing to remove dirt/dust → Decapping berries → Extraction of juice by crushing fruits and boiling with water for 5–10 min → Addition of citric acid while boiling → Straining of extract → Pectin test (alcohol or jelmeter test) for required amount of sugar → Addition of required quantity of sugar → Cooking → Judging of end point (temperature 105°C or 65% TSS or sheet test) → Removal of scum foam→ Filling hot into clean and sterilized bottles → Wiping of bottles with cloth → Capping → Storage.

24.22.1.5 Syrup

Recipe

Juice/pulp 1 kg, sugar 2.75 kg, water 0.5 L, citric acid 15 g.

Preparation technique

Fully ripe fruit → Washing → Crushing → Juice extraction → Straining → Addition of sugar syrup solution (sugar + water + citric acid, heating just to dissolve the sugar and straining) → Mixing → Filling into syrup bottle → Capping → Storing in a cool and dry place

24.22.1.6 Sauce

Recipe

Pulp 1 kg, sugar 210 g, chilli powder 10 g, salt 16 g, glacial acetic acid 5 mL and sodium benzoate 0.25g/kg of finished products.

Preparation technique

Ripe fruits → Washing in running tap water → Removing calyx → Passing through pulping machine → Pulp → Mixing with sugar, chilli powder and salt → Cooking in medium flame → Adding vinegar (when the content reaches to 30° brix) → Cooking continue till the final TSS of 37° brix → Cooling at room temperature → Addition of sodium benzoate → Packing in glass bottles/polypropylene pouches → Capping of bottles or sealing of pouches → Storage.

24.22.1.7 Frozen strawberries

Preparation technique

Firm ripe fruits → Washing → Packing in polythene bag with covering of 50% sugar syrup → Sealing → Arranging in cartons → Freezing at –40°C → Storage at –20°C. Strawberry is also used for preparation of juice and wine and for flavouring the ice-cream.

The recent development in fruit processing are IQF process for freezing which require less time to freeze, development of retortable pouches in place of tin can which improved product quality, aseptic processing for superior quality of products, osmotic process which removes 30–50% water without heating and development of new products such as aonla based herbal products, oil less pickle, dehydrated ripe mango slices, fruit bar, cereal flakes, baby foods and blends. There are tremendous possibilities in export market. Fruit-based exportable processed products are pulp, slices, concentrate, powder, pickles, jam, confectionary products such as candied fruit, glazed fruit, toffee and aonla-based medicinal products.

24.23 Capegoose berry

Capegoose berry is rich in Vitamins C and P. Fruit contains good amount of iron. The acidic pulp has pleasant flavour.

24.23.1 Products

Fruit can be processed into quality jam, jelly and chutney.

24.23.1.1 Jam

Recipes

Fruit 1 kg, sugar 750 g, water 100 mL and citric acid 1.5 g.

Preparation technique

Ripe fruit → Removal of covering → Crushing and heating with water → Addition of sugar and citric acid → Cooking up to desired consistency → Judging of end point → Filling into clean and sterilized jam bottles → Capping/sealing → Storing

24.23.1.2 Jelly

Recipe

Juice extract 1 L, sugar 1 kg and citric acid 1 g.

Preparation technique

Firm ripe fruit → Removal of covering → Washing → Addition of water (about 0.5 L) → Heating up to softening → Addition of citric acid → Straining the extract → Testing of pectin → Addition of sugar → Cooking into desired consistency → Judging of end point (temperature 105°C) → Removing scum → Filling into clean and sterilized bottles → Capping/sealing → Storing.

24.23.1.3 Chutney

Recipe

Gooseberry 1 kg, onion 50 g, garlic 5 g, sugar 500 g, salt 10 g, hot spices 5 g, acetic acid 30 mL.

Preparation technique

Gooseberry → Removal of covering → Washing of berry → Cut into halves → Add sugar and mix with ingredient (except acetic acid) it → Cooking till desired consistency → Add acetic acid → Remove from fire → Fill into clean and sterilized bottles → Capping/sealing→ Storing.

25

Vegetable products and processing technique

Vegetables are an indispensable part of human diet. These are the natural source of protective food supplying all the nutrients, specially vitamins, minerals and crude fibre. Vegetable production not only contributes to food and nutritional security but also to income generation. A variety of vegetables are produced in the country. Plant parts normally used as vegetable include roots, tubers, bulbs, fruits, flower, seeds, stems and shoots. Vegetables being perishable in nature processing is very vital to reduce the post-harvest losses. Common vegetables and tier products are given in following sections.

25.1 Potato

Potato is one of the most important world's food crops. The potato produces more carbohydrates, minerals, fibre and vitamins per unit area and time than other major food crops. Potato has the highest potential to mitigate problems of hunger and malnutrition.

The varieties which have been found suitable for processing are Kufri Chipsona-1 (21–24% dry matter), Kufri Chipsona-2 (21–25% dry matter), Kufri Chipsona-3 (19–20% dry matter), Kufri Surya (19–20% dry matter), Kufri Himsona (22–24% dry matter) and Kufri Frysona (21–23% dry matter).

25.1.1 Products

Potato can be processed into a number of products like dehydrated chips, fried potato chips, dehydrated sticks or cubes, canned potato, flour, granules, diced potato, starch, wine etc.

25.1.1.1 Dehydrated chips

Preparation technique

Fully mature potato → Washing → Peeling (abrasion peelers) → Trimming (removal of eyes) → Cutting into 1-cm thick slices → Blanching in hot water [containing salt and potassium metabisulphite (KMS)] or steam for 4 min → Rinsing and dewatering dehydration at 60°C (hot air dryers) → Packing → Storing

25.1.1.2 Fried potato chips (wafers)

Preparation technique

Fully mature potato → Washing → Peeling (by abrasion peelers) → Trimming (defective portion) → Slicing → Drying (drum dryers) → Frying→ Salting and spicing → Packing → Storing

25.1.1.3 Frozen potato chips (French fries)

Preparation technique

(Kufri, Surya and Kufri Frysona) → Removal of defective and small tuber → Washing → Peeling → Removing of defective portion → (Green portion and discoloured area) → Cutting into strips (with strip cutter) → Removing excess moisture → Frying (into fryers) → Defatting by passing the product over a vibrating screen → Cooling → Inspection (dark, overfried or defective pieces should be removed) → Packing → Freezing (belt freezer) → Storing

25.1.1.4 Dehydrated sticks or cubes

Preparation technique

Fully mature potato → Washing (soak tanks or rotary washers) → Peeling → Cutting into sticks or cubes → Dewatering → Drying for 3–4 h (moisture level to around 10%), further drying (bin dryer) to bring down moisture up to 5% → Cooling → Packing → Storing

25.1.1.5 Canned potato

Preparation technique

Fully mature potato → Sorting → Peeling → Cutting → Blanching for 3 min → Cooling → Filling into cans → Brining (2% brine) → Exhausting till the temperature in centre of can reaches 79°C → Sealing → Processing → Cooling → Storing (used in food preparation)

25.1.1.6 Granules

Preparation technique

Fully mature potato → Washing → Preparation of dough → Addition of pre-prepared granules in proper ratio → Drying in fluidized bed Dryer → Granules → Packing → Storage

25.1.1.7 Potato flour

Preparation technique

Fully mature potato → Washing → Peeling (abrasion peelers) → Dicing → Soaking overnight in solution of salt and sodium metabisulphite → Soaked pieces are granulated in a mincer and pressed → Drying → Grinding of dry granules in a plate mill → Flour → Packing →Storing

25.1.1.8 Potato starch

Preparation technique

Potato (even off grade) → Washing thoroughly → Preparation of dough by grinding with the help of machine → Mixing with water to dilute the thickness → Mixing with KMS (500 ppm) → Allow to flow on sloppy table → Starch settled down on table and water passed away → Collection of starch → Drying → Packing → Storage (used in food preparation, cosmetics, paper and textiles)

25.1.1.9 Potato wine

Preparation technique

Potato starch → Conversion in glucose by hydrolysis → Addition of yeast for fermentation under controlled condition → Alcoholic matter → Distillation → Alcohol (concentration can be increased as per standards)

25.1.1.10 Diced potato

Preparation technique

Mature potato ⟶ Washing → Peeling → Cutting into rectangular shape → Blanding → Dip in 500 ppm of sulphur dioxide solution containing 0.1% citric acid for 15–20 min → Keeping into trays → Drying in dehydrator → Packing in polythene bag → Storage/marketing (used in soup mixture and with other vegetables)

25.2 Sweet potato

Sweet potato is one of the most important food crops, which produces more calories than rice, wheat and maize. Sweet potato is principal source of starch which is used in production of industrial starch, syrup and alcohol. Besides rich in protein, minerals (potassium and calcium), pectin and vitamins, sweet potato contains selective nutritional components such as dietary fibres, carotene and flavanoids which play an important role in human nutrition.

25.2.1 Products

Sweet potato is mainly consumed as fresh boiled roots. Sweet potato can be processed into dried chips, flour, frozen sweet potato and canning. Sweet potato can also be processed into puree (baby food), sugar syrup, pectin, pigments, ethanol and citric acid. The other food items which can be prepared from sweet potato are porridge, crisps, relish, chapattis, doughnuts, buns, crackies, cake, etc. The roots starch and vines rich in protein and fibre are used as animal feed.

25.2.1.1 Dried chips

Preparation technique

Select only health roots → Cleaning, peeling and trimming → Washing → Remove surface water by keeping in sun (10 min) → Slicing/chipping (uniform pieces) → Soaking (in clean water for 90 min) → Drying (either sun dried for 4–6 h or dehydrated up to 10% moisture) → Packing (polypropylene sacks) → Storage/marketing

25.2.1.2 Flour

Preparation technique

Dried chips as prepared above → Grinding/milling → Flour → Packing in polythene bags or tins → Storage in a cool and dry well ventilated place (wooden pallets/platforms can be used to stack the packed sweet potato products to prevent moisture)

25.2.1.3 Frozen sweet potato

Preparation technique

Fully mature sweet potato → Washing → Steaming → Removal of peel → Slicing in suitable shape → Dipping in 0.4% citric acid + 10% lemon juice for 4–5 s → Removal of slices → Filling in plastic bag → Freezing → Storage

25.2.1.4 Canning

Preparation technique

Fully mature sweet potato → Washing → Steaming (20–30 min) → Peeling → Cutting into desired thickness (13 mm) → Filling into cans (2½) → Addition of 2% salt solution or syrup solution (30–40° brix) → Exhausting → Sealing → Processing (145 min) → Cooling → Storage

25.3 Elephant foot yam

Elephant foot yam is very popular due to its high yield potential. Elephant foot yam also known as *suran/jimmikant* is rich in starch and carotene. It contains alkaloids, tannins and steroids which have pharmaceutical values. It is very helpful in curing of piles, dysentery, asthma, swelling of lungs, vomiting and abdominal pain. It is blood purifier and paste of tuber applied externally relief pain in arthritis.

25.3.1 Product

25.3.1.1 Pickle

Recipe

Yam 1 kg, mustard (*rye*) powder 20 g, onion 50 g, cumin seed powder 6 g, hot spices 6 g, ginger 50 g, turmeric powder 3 g, salt 60 g, red chillies powder 10 g and mustard oil 200 mL.

Preparation technique

Elephant foot yam → Washing → Peeling → Cutting into small pieces → Boiling of pieces in hot water till softening → Draining and drying → Frying the pieces in mustard oil till browning → Draining from oil → Grinding onion and ginger and frying in mustard oil → Addition of all spices and little frying → Addition of fried yam and mixed thoroughly → Addition of remaining heated oil → Addition of acetic → Filling into jar → Capping → Keeping in sun for few days → Storage

25.4 Tomato

Tomato is popular vegetable known for its high nutritive value. It is rich source of minerals (calcium, magnesium, phosphorus, iron and potassium), vitamins (A and C) and organic acids.

25.4.1 Products

Tomato is processed for number of products such as ketchup, chilli sauce, chutney, pickles, crush, canned tomato, juice, cocktail, soup, paste and puree.

25.4.1.1 Ketchup

Recipe

Tomato pulp 1 kg, onion chopped 60 g, ginger chopped 10 g, garlic chopped 5 g, sugar 75 g, salt 10 g, red chilli powder 5 g, cinnamon, cardamom, aniseed, cumin, black pepper powder 10 g each, clove headless 5 number, glacial acetic acid 5 mL and sodium benzoate 0.25 g/kg of finished product.

Preparation technique

Fully ripped red tomatoes → Washing → Trimming if any green portion → Cutting into pieces → Washing → Trimming if any green portion → Cutting into pieces → Washing → Trimming if any green portion → Cutting into pieces → Washing → Trimming if any green portion → Cutting into pieces → Heating (80°C) for 5 min → Crushing → Extraction of pulp → Straining → Cooking strained pulp with one-third of sugar → Putting spiced bag (onion, garlic, ginger chopped + red chilli powder and hot spices) in pulp and pressing occasionally → Cooking to one-third of original volume of pulp → Removal of spice bag after squeezing in pulp → Addition of remaining sugar and salt → Cooking to desired consistency → Judging of end point for total soluble solid (TSS = 28%) → Addition of acetic acid and sodium benzoate → Filling hot (88°C) into bottles → Crown corking → Pasteurization for 30 min at 85°C → Cooling → Storing in a cool and dry place

25.4.1.2 Tomato chilli sauce

Recipe

Tomato pulp 1 kg, onion paste 50 g, garlic paste 30 g, sugar 100 g, salt 10 g, hot spices 10 g, red chilli powder 5 g, sodium benzoate 0.25 g/kg of finished product and acetic acid 5 mL.

Preparation technique

Fully ripped red tomato → Washing → Dipping the fruit in boiling water for a minute → Cooling by immersing in cold water → Removal of skin → Crushing → Cooking pulp with one-third quantity of sugar till desired consistency → Putting spices bag and pressing occasionally → Cooking up to one-third of original volume of pulp → Removing spice bag after squeezing in pulp → Addition of remaining sugar and salt → Cooking → Judging of end point (TSS = 25–27%) → Adding acetic acid and sodium benzoate → Filling hot into bottles → Crown corking → Pasteurization at 90°C for 30 min → Cooling → Storing at ambient temperature in a cool and dry place

25.4.1.3 Chutney

Recipe

Tomato 1 kg, sugar 500 g, salt 25 g, onion 100 g, ginger10 g, garlic 5 g (grinded), red chilli 10 g, hot spices 20 g (cinnamon, black pepper, cardamom, aniseed, cumin powder), vinegar 100 mL and sodium benzoate 0.5 g/kg of finished product.

Preparation technique

Fully ripped red tomato → Washing → Blanching → Keeping in cold water to crack the skin → Peeling → Crushing → Addition of ingredients (except salt and vinegar) → Cooking to desired consistency → Addition of salt and vinegar → Heating for 5 min → Addition of sodium benzoate → Feeling hot into clean and sterilized bottles → Capping → Levelling → Storage in a cool and dry place/marketing

25.4.1.4 Tomato pickle

Recipe

Ripe tomato 1 kg, ginger chopped 50 g, garlic chopped 10 g, salt 75 g, red chillies, mustard (rye) powder and cinnamon 10 g each, vinegar 250 mL and mustard oil 300 mL.

Preparation technique

Firm ripe tomato → Washing → Blanching (5 min) → Cooling in water → Peeling → Cutting into 4 pieces → Frying of all ingredient in little oil (except vinegar) → Mixing with pieces → Heating for 2 min → Cooling → Addition of vinegar and remaining oil → Filling into jar → Capping → Storing

25.4.1.5 Tomato crush

This is different from pure and paste in having skin and seeds.

Preparation technique

Fully ripped red tomato → Washing → Removal of green portion, if any → Cutting into pieces → Boiling and crushing the pieces or blending in blender (for uniform pulp inclusive of skin and seeds) → Boiling till the mass reduced to one-third/thick paste → Addition of acetic acid (5 mL/kg of paste) → Boiling for 5–8 min → Addition of 0.4 g KMS and 0.2 sodium benzoate after dissolving in small quantity of water separately (for 1 kg of finished product) → Mixing thoroughly → Filling hot in wide mouth glass bottles/jars → Sealing → Storing in cool and dry place

25.4.1.6 Canned tomato

Preparation technique

Fresh firm ripe and uniform-sized tomatoes → Washing → Dipping the fruit in boiling water for a minute → Cooling in cold water → Removal of core (from stem side), skin and black tip (at the blossom end of the fruit) → Packing into can (A2$^1/_2$) up to the top → Addition of salt and sugar (5 g each) → Filling with boiling water → Exhausting (until the temperature reaches at the centre of cans 82°C) → Sealing → Processing for 40 min in boiling water → Cooling the cans using cold water stream → Storing in a cool and dry place

25.4.1.7 Tomato juice

Recipe

Juice 1 L, sugar 50 g, salt 10 g, citric acid 2 g and sodium benzoate 1 g.

Preparation technique

Fully ripped red tomato (juicy variety) → Washing → Removing stem and green portion if any → Cutting into 4–6 pieces → Crushing/chopping →

Heating at 70–90°C for 5 min → Extraction of juice through machine or by sieving → Mixing with salt, sugar and citric acid → Homogenization → Heating at 88°C for a minute → Filling hot into sterilized bottle or cans → Sterilization in boiling water for 30 min → Cooling → Storing in cool dry place

25.4.1.8 Tomato cocktail

Recipe

Juice 1 L, clove 0.3 g, cumin seed, black pepper, cardamom, cinnamon 1 g each (power), red chilli 0.05 g powder, vinegar (10% acetic acid) 60 mL, salt 9 g and lime/lemon juice 10 mL.

Preparation technique

Tomato juice (strained) → Cooking for 20 min by putting the spices into bags and covering vessel → Addition of stained lime juice, salt and vinegar → Heating at 88°C → Filling into clean and sterilized bottle → Crown corking → Sterilization for 30 min (100°C) → Cooling → Storing in a cool and dry place

25.4.1.9 Tomato soup

Recipe

Tomato juice/pulp 1 kg, salt 10 g, sugar 15 g, flour/starch 5 g, onion chopped 15 g, garlic chopped 5 g, cinnamon, headless cloves, dry ginger, cardamom, black pepper, cumin (all spices in powder form) 0.5 g each, sodium bicarbonate 1 g and cream/butter 10 g.

Preparation technique

Fresh, firm and red tomatoes → Washing → Cutting into pieces → Heating for 10 min till the skin separate out from the pulp → Straining the pulp and removing the seeds and skin → Addition of sodium bicarbonate paste (sodium bicarbonate +little water and making of paste) → Mixing properly → Boiling and stirring → Packing of all the spices in muslin bag and putting the bag in juice while boiling → Preparation of paste of butter and flour/starch → Adding in concentrated juice → Cooking to desired consistency and stirring → Adding sugar and salt → Boiling for 2–3 min → Removal of spice bag → Filling into plain cans (A-1 tall cans) → Sealing → Processing for 45 min at 115°C (or 0.7 kg/cm^2 in pressure cooker) → Cooling the cans → Storing at ambient temperature in cool and dry place

25.4.1.10 Tomato paste

Preparation technique

Fully ripped red tomato → Washing → Cutting into pieces → Crushing → Heating at 90°C for 5 min → Extraction of juice/pulp → Cooking to desired consistency → Judging of end point (TSS = 25%) → Filling hot into cans/bottles → Sealing → Sterilizing in boiling water for 20 min → Cooling → Storing in cool and dry place

25.4.1.11 Tomato puree

Preparation technique
Fully ripped red tomato → Washing → Cutting into pieces → Crushing → Heating (90°C) for 5 min → Extraction of juice and/pulp → Cooking to desired consistency → Judging of end point (TSS = 9–12%) → Filling hot into cans/bottles → Sealing → Sterilizing in boiling water for 20 min → Cooling → Storing in cool and dry place

25.5 Brinjal

Brinjal is the most popular widely cultivated vegetable crop. It is good source of vitamin B (thiamine and riboflavin) and minerals (calcium, iron and phosphorus). Brinjal fruits have medicinal property and useful against liver trouble and high blood cholesterol due to linoleic and linolenic fatty acids.

25.5.1 Products

Brinjal fruits are mostly consumed in various culinary preparations such as fried, boiled, roasted, etc. Fruits can be pickled and dehydrated.

25.5.1.1 Pickle

Recipe
Ingredients used for pickle are brinjal 1 kg, red chilli powder 20 g, turmeric powder 20 g, cumin powder 15 g, mustard powder 15 g, coriander powder 20 g, salt 100 g and mustard oil 200 mL.

Preparation technique
Brinjal fruits (small-sized long fruited varieties) → Washing → Draining → Removal of stalk with calyx → Cutting into suitable sized pieces → Boiling in 2% salt solution for 5 min → Draining of water → Shade drying → Mixing pieces with spices → Filling in jar → Addition of oil after heating and cooling → Keeping in sun for a week → Capping → Storage

25.5.1.2 Dried brinjal

Preparation technique
Select mature and tender brinjal → Washing → Removal of stalk → Slicing (6 mm thickness) → Dipping the pieces in 0.5% KMS solution for 90 min (to

prevent browning) → Removal from solution → Draining → Drying at 50°C for 9 h → Packing → Storage

25.6 Chilli

Chilli also known as hot pepper is an important spice and vegetable. Chilli is grown in many parts of the country and their consumption is also very high. The fresh green chilli is rich in vitamins A and C, and fibre. It is also rich in vitamin P, niacin and minerals such as potassium, phosphorus, magnesium, sulphur and iron. The septa and placental tissue contain the pungent principle known as capsaicin. Green chillies eaten with food stuffs increase the flow of saliva by stimulating the taste and act as an appetizer. Chilli also produces stress resistance. Chillies are very useful as a cure for appetite, digestion and mitigate flatulence. It is also useful in cure of colic, diarrhoea, dropsy, gouts and toothaches. It has tonic and carminative action when it is taken with food.

25.6.1 Products

Chillies can be processed into powder, dry green chillies, pickle, sauce, etc.

25.6.1.1 Drying/dehydrated red chillies

Preparation technique

Chillies (dark red parts) → Ashing → Drying at 50–60°C/sundrying → Packing → Storing

25.6.1.2 Chilli powder

Preparation technique

Red coloured chillies → Washing → Removal of stalk → Drying → Grinding → Sieving → Packing in polythene bags → Sealing → Storing

25.6.1.3 Red chillies pickle

Recipe

Red chillies 1 kg, dry mango powder (*amchur*) 250 g, salt 150 g, coriander powder 50 g, nigella seeds 15 g, aniseed powder 20 g, fenugreek powder 20 g, hot spices 50 g, mustard (ground) 100 g and mustard oil 500 mL.

Preparation technique

Red chillies → Washing → Draining and drying (1 h) → Removal of stem → Making incision → Removal of seeds → Mixing all spices and seeds → Frying in oil → Cooling → Filling into chillies → Packing in jar → Addition of oil (after heating and cooling) → Capping → Keeping for 2 weeks → Storing/using

25.6.1.4 Green chillies pickle

Recipe

Green chillies 1 kg, garlic 100 g, mustard (rye) powder 50 g, turmeric powder 50 g, lime juice 500 mL, fenugreek 25 g and mustard oil 500 mL.

Preparation technique

Green chillies → Washing → Drying → Removal of stem → Making incision (longitudinal) → Mixing all spices in little lime juice → Mixing with chillies → Filling into jar → Addition of lime juice and oil → Keeping in sun for few days → Storage in cool and dry place

25.6.1.5 Dry green chillies

Preparation technique

Green chillies → Washing → Pricking → Blanching in boiling water for a minutes → Draining → Immersing in 2% sodium hydroxide solution for 10 min → Draining → Drying up 5% moisture → Packing → Sealing → Storing

25.6.1.6 Chilli sauce

Recipe

Green chillies 1 kg, carrot 250 g, potato 250 g, sugar 50 g, salt 50 g, hot spices 50 g and glacial acetic acid 5 mL.

Preparation technique

Green chillies (remove stem), carrot (scrapping and washing), potato (peeling) → Boil chilli carrot and potato in little water or cooking in pressure cooker → Mix together → Sieving/straining → Mixing of strained hot spices with the mixture of chillies, carrot and potato → Cooking till desired consistency → Addition of salt → Addition of acetic acid → Heating for 5 min → Filling into clean sterilized bottles → Capping/crown corking → Storing

25.7 Cabbage

Cabbage is rich source of vitamins A, B and C. It has good amount of minerals such as phosphorus, calcium, potassium, iron and sulphur. It is also very rich in fibre. The flavour in cabbage head is due to the presence of sinigrin (glycosides). Cabbage is helpful in curing digestion, diarrhoea and celiac troubles.

25.7.1 Products

Cabbage can be processed into canned products, canning, frozen product, drying, wafers and pickle.

25.7.1.1 Canned cabbage

Preparation technique

Suitable varieties of cabbage → Washing → Cutting into section → Blanching in steam for 2 min → Cooling → Filling into A2½ SR lacquered can → Brining with 2% salt solution → Exhausting → Sealing → Processing at 116°C for 35 min → Cooling in plain water → Labelling → Storage

25.7.1.2 Cabbage sauerkraut

Preparation technique

Mature cabbage head → Removing core → Removing outer leaves → Washing → Cutting into fine shreds → Keeping shreds in jar/container → Addition of salt (2.5%) → Covering the mouth of containers with plastic cover and allowing fermentation at 16–20°C for a week → Removing of scum → Draining of juice → Pasteurization of shreds at 75–80°C for 10 min → Filling hot into sterilized wide mouthed bottles → Addition of drained out juice which has been pasteurized at 90°C → Capping/sealing → Storing

25.7.1.3 Fermented cabbage with carrot

Recipe

Cabbage 1 kg, carrot 1 kg, salt 50–60 g and mustard powder 20–30 g.

Preparation technique

Mature cabbage heads and orange coloured carrots → Washing → Removal of outer leaves of cabbage and scrapping of carrot hairs → Washing → Cutting of cabbage and carrots into fine shreds → Mixing of both shreds in ratio of 1:1 → Filling into clean jars → Addition of salt (2.5%) and mustard powder (1.5%) → Shaking whole mass daily (up to 10–14 days) and allow to ferment → Capping of jar → Storing fermented vegetable jar/containers in shade and dry place

25.7.1.4 Cabbage wafers

Recipe

Cabbage 1 kg, urad dal 0.25 kg, cumin seeds 20 g, ginger 50 g, green chillies 25 g and salt 20 g.

Preparation technique

Soaking of urad dal at night → Draining → Grinding to a thick paste → Addition of salt → Keep a side → Washing of whole cabbage and shredding → Grinding of ginger and chillies and make paste → Addition of shredded cabbage, cumin seeds and ginger, chilli paste to dal paste → Spread damp cloth in the sun → Making of paste into small balls and dropping on cloth → Drying for 2–3 days → Sprinkle some water on back of the cloth and separating wafers → Drying again → Packing in tins → Sealing airtight → Storage/marketing

25.8 Cauliflower

Cauliflower is grown for its white tender curd which is rich in carbohydrate, vitamins A and C and minerals such as phosphorus, potassium, sodium, calcium and iron.

25.8.1 Products

Cauliflower is processed into pickle, mixed pickle with turnip and carrot, dried cauliflower, canned cauliflower and frozen cauliflower. The techniques for preparation of these products are as follows.

25.8.1.1 Pickle

Recipe

Cauliflower 1 kg, ginger pieces 50 g, onion pieces 50 g, salt 75 g, red chillies powder 40 g, cumin seed 5 g, cloves 5 g, cinnamon 5 g and mustard oil 150 mL.

Preparation technique

Cauliflower curd → Washing → Cutting into pieces → Blanching (5 min) → Draining → Drying (half an hour, keep a side) → Grinding of all spices and frying → Frying onion, ginger and spices in mustard oil till browning → Addition of cauliflower pieces → Addition of salt → Mixing thoroughly and take out from fire → Filling into jar → Keeping the jar in sun for few days → Addition of acetic acid (60–100 mL) → Shaking → Capping → Storing/marketing

25.8.1.2 Mixed pickle with turnip and carrot

Recipe

Cauliflower pieces 300 g, carrot pieces 350 g, turnip pieces 350 g (total 1 kg), sugar 200 g, onion 150 g, garlic10 g, red chillies power 30 g, salt 50 g, mustard (rye) powder 40 g, mustard oil 250 mL and acetic acid 10 mL.

Preparation technique

Cauliflower, carrot and turnip → Washing → Cutting into pieces → Blanching for 5 min in boiling water → Draining on cloth and drying for half an hour → Frying onion, ginger and garlic in small quantity of mustard oil → Addition of all ingredients (except spices and salt) → Mixing → Addition of sugar in form of solution → Addition of spices and salt → Mixing → Addition of acetic acid → Shaking → Filling into jars → Capping → Storage

25.8.1.3 Dried cauliflower

Preparation technique

Cauliflower → Removal of stalk and covering leaves → Break flower into pieces of suitable size → Blanching for 4–5 min and immersing in 1% KMS solution for an hour → Draining → Drying at 55–60°C sundrying → Packing → Storage

25.8.1.4 Canned cauliflower

Preparation technique

Suitable variety of cauliflower → Removal of stem and leaves → Washing → Breaking into pieces → Soaking in cold brine → Blanching for 3 min → Exhausting at 90°C for 10 min → Sealing → Processing at 116°C for 20 min → Cooling in plain water → Labelling → Storage

25.8.1.5 Frozen cauliflower

Preparation technique

Mature head of cauliflower → Washing → Cutting into bits → Blanching (2 min) → Cooling → Soaking in 0.05% KMS solution for 4 min → Draining → Packing in polythene bag → Sealing → Arranging in cartons → Freezing at 1–5°C → Storage at –18°C

25.9 Okra

Okra is rich in minerals and fibre. It contain high amount of iodine which is useful in prevention of goitre. The dry seed of okra is rich in edible oil and protein. Okra helps in renal colic, leucorrhoea and general weakness. The raw fruit of okra consumed on an empty stomach every morning nourish the body, cure peptic ulcer and in increasing the semen content.

25.9.1 Products

Okra can be dried product and caned. The techniques for drying and canning are as follows.

25.9.1.1 Dried okra

Preparation technique

Tender green fruits of okra → Washing → Removal of both ends → Cutting into slices (6 mm thick) → Blanching in boiling water (5 min) → Sulphiting in 0.25% KMS solution for 30 min (0.5 L solution for a kg of slices) → Drying at 60°C (up to 5% moisture)/sundried → Packing → Storage/marketing

25.9.1.2 Canned okra

Preparation technique

Tender green fruits of okra → Removal of cap → Blanching in 1% salt solution for 2–3 min → Filling into A2$^{1}/_{2}$ can → Exhausting → Sealing → Processing at 116°C for 35 min → Cooling → Labelling → Storing/marketing

25.10 Pea

Pea is mainly grown for its green pods and mature dry seeds. Pea is a rich source of protein, amino acid, sugar, vitamins A, B and C and minerals such as calcium, iron and phosphorus.

25.10.1 Products

Peas can be dried, canned, frozen and used for pickle preparation. The techniques for preparation of these products are as follows.

25.10.1.1 Drying

Preparation technique

Peas → Washing → Removal of shell → Collection of grains → Blanching/steaming (3–4 min) → Immersing in KMS solution (0.5%) → Draining → Drying (60–65°C) or sundrying → Packing → Storage

25.10.1.2 Canning of peas

Preparation technique

Suitable varieties of peas → Shelling → Washing → Blanching (4 min) → Grading for maturity (Blanched peas immersed in plain water. Small immature grain floated should be discarded) → Filling into A$^{1}/_{2}$ lacquered can (550 g/can) → Brining 400 g/can [1% salt (35 g) and 2% sugar (75 g) + 3.5 L water] → Exhausting at 90°C for 10 min or till the centre of the can records temperature 75–82°C → Sealing → Processing at 116°C for 45 min → Cooling in plain water → Labelling → Storing

25.10.1.3 Frozen peas

Preparation technique

Suitable variety of peas → Washing → Shelling → Washing → Blanching (4 min) → Cooling → Grading for maturity density gradient (immersing grain in 10% brine solution, floaters are immature peas and sinkers are mature grains) → Further grading of mature peas (Floaters in 9% solution are A grade in 13% solution B grade and in 15% solution C grade) → Packing in polythene bag → Sealing → Arranging in cartons → Freezing at –1°C to –5°C → Storage at –18°C

25.10.1.4 Pickles

Recipe

Green peas grains 1 kg, sugar 200 g, salt 75 g, onion 100 g, ginger 30 g, red chillies powder 10 g, mustard seed powder 10 g, fenugreek powder 10 g, mustard oil 250 mL and vinegar 250 mL.

Preparation technique
Peas grains/seed → Blanching in boiling water for 2 min → Draining → Spreading on cloth so that water dries up/dewatering → Grinding onion, garlic and ginger to fine paste and keep a side → Heating of oil and adding onion, garlic and ginger paste → Frying → Adding mustard and fenugreek powder and frying till brown → Adding vinegar and peas → Heating for 5 min → Adding remaining ingredients → Heating for 10 min → Cooling → Filling into bottles/jar → Capping → Storing

25.11 Onion

It is known as the queen of the kitchen. The pungency in onion is due to allyl propyl disulphide (volatile oil). Onion has fair amount of vitamin B and folic acid. It is very rich in potassium, calcium, phosphorus and iron. This is also a rich source of amino acid and anthocyanins. Onion has high medicinal values. It is very useful for people suffering from high cholesterol, lethargy, feebleness and lack of vitality. Dropsy, kidney, coronary heart disease, lever cirrhosis, diabetes, tuberculosis, asthma and heart strokes are the major diseases and disorders which are cured by regular use of onion.

25.11.1 Products

Onion can be dehydrated, powdered and used for making pickle. The techniques for preparation of these products are as follows.

25.11.1.1 Dehydrated onion (flakes/rings)

Preparation technique
Select sound, clean, undamaged bulbs having 5 cm diameter or above → Washing in agitated water to remove dirt/dust → Removal of tops and tail → Removal of outer dry scales → Cut into 4- to 5-mm thick shreds → Dipping in 5% salt solution → Draining → Drying at 60°C or sundrying → Packing → Storing

25.11.1.2 Onion powder

Preparation technique
Selection of white and pungent variety → Grading (preferably small sized or less than 5 cm diameter → Washing → Removal of outer leaves → Peeling → Cutting into 0.25-cm thick slices → Immersing in 5% common salt solution for 10 min → Draining → Drying at 60–65°C for 12 h → Powdering (moisture content 4%) → Packing → Storing

25.11.1.3 *Onion pickle*

Recipe

Onion (small preferably white variety) 1 kg, vinegar 1 L, salt 250 g, red chilli powder 10 g, cardamom and cumin (powder) each 10 g and cloves 5 in number.

Preparation technique

Onion → Peeling → Blanching (5 min) → Filling into jar → Addition of salt → Keeping for 2–4 h → Draining water → Addition of vinegar and spices → Mixing → Capping → Storing

25.12 Garlic

This is very important herb and valuable spice crop. It is mainly used for flavouring and seasoning vegetable and meat dishes. Garlic is rich in carbohydrates, protein, calcium, phosphorus, potassium and magnesium. The green form of garlic is very high in ascorbic acid content. Garlic helps in absorption and digestion of food. It has anthelmintic, antiseptic, carminative and natural antibiotic properties.

25.12.1 Products

Garlic is dehydrated, powdered and used for making pickle. The techniques for preparation of these products are as follows.

25.12.1.1 *Dehydrated garlic*

Preparation technique

Garlic → Peeling the clove → Cutting into 5–6 mm thick shreds → Dipping in salt solution (5%) for 10 min → Drying at 60°C or sundrying → Packing → Storing

25.12.1.2 *Garlic powder*

Preparation technique

Garlic bulbs → Scrubbing manually with mild pressure → Removal of papery skin and separation of cloves → Washing of cloves → Slicing or pressed between rolls to form flakes → Drying of flakes (tunnel dryers or continuous belt dryer) up to 6% moisture → Powdering → Packing in polythene bags (air tight to prevent moisture absorption) → Storing

25.12.1.3 *Garlic pickle*

Recipe

Garlic clove 1 kg, lime juice 1 L, fenugreek powder 40 g, red chilli powder 20 g, salt 400 g and mustard oil 400 mL.

Preparation technique
Garlic clove → Shelling of garlic clove → Cutting of lime and extraction of juice → Filling of the lime juice into jar → Addition of salt → Addition of garlic after frying in oil → Addition of chillies and fenugreek powder → Mixing thoroughly → Capping → Storing

25.13 Carrot

Carrot is very rich in vitamin A and has fair amount of vitamin B_1 and B_2, it is also good source of calcium, magnesium and iron. It is very useful in jaundice and preventing stone formation in kidney. Its carotene is sometimes used for colouring butter and other foods.

25.13.1 Products

Carrot can be processed into number of products such as carrot powder spice carrot juice, dried carrot, carrot shred, carrot preserve/candy, burfi, canned carrot, carrot jam, carrot pickle, etc. The techniques for preparation of these products are as follows.

25.13.1.1 Carrot powder

Preparation technique
Carrot → Washing → Pilling → Boiling (90 min) → Crushing → Addition of ascorbic acid (0.4 g/kg) → Puree with 8% RE → Drying in drums under vacuum at 85°C → Packing (water vapour proof boxes or drum) → Storage (below 25°C preferably 15°C) or at lower temperature 0–10°C

25.13.1.2 Spice carrot juice

Recipe
Grated carrot 1 kg, common salt 32 g, mustard powder 3 g, good quality vinegar 62 g and red chillies powder 1.5 g.

Preparation technique
Selection of deep orange variety → Washing → Removal of hairy parts → Chopping of two ends → Scrapping to remove the inedible parts → Grading → Mixing of ingredients thoroughly → Packing the mass earthenware pitchers up to the brim → Covering with lid → Storing in a cool and dry place for about a month → Pressing the juice → Straining → Allow the strained juice to stand in closed and deep container for few days → Decanting the clear juice and staining → Addition of sodium benzoate (300 mg/L of beverages) → Mixing thoroughly → Filling into clean stylized bottles → Crown corking → Storage (dilute the beverage 2–3 times with water before use)

25.13.1.3 Dried carrot

Preparation technique
Carrot → Washing → Removal of stalk and tips → Cut into 10-mm thick slices → Blanching (2–4 min in 2% common salt solution) → Drying at 60–65°C or sundrying → Packing → Storing

25.13.1.4 Shred

Recipe
Carrot 1 kg, sugar 1 kg and water 0.5 L.

Preparation technique
Carrot (orange coloured) → Washing → Removing → Top and bottom portion → Removing hairs through scrapping → Making of shreds → Blanching in boiling water for 4 min → Draining → Keeping in sugar syrup solution (sugar + water, heating and straining) → Little heating → Keeping overnight → Removing of shreds from syrup after 24 h → Draining → Drying in tray → Packing in polythene bag → Storing. The shreds can be used for making *halwa* during off-season.

25.13.1.5 Preserve

Preparation technique
Select suitable variety (orange-yellow) of tender carrot having soft pith → Removal of green leafy portion → Scrapping thin peel → Washing → Pricking → Cutting into suitable pieces → Washing again → Blanching for 2–3 min→ Draining → Steeping in strained sugar syrup of 40% TSS for 24 h → Removal of pieces → Boiling of syrup to 60% of TSS → Steeping pieces for 24 h → Removal of pieces → Boiling of syrup to 70% TSS → Steering in syrup for few days (4–5) → Draining → Filling into jar/container → Covering preserve with 68% freshly prepared and strained sugar syrup → Capping/sealing → Storage

25.13.1.6 Candy

Prepare preserve as mentioned above → Drained carrot pieces from syrup → Dipping in boiling water (1–2 s) → Removal from water and shade drying → Packing → Storage/marketing

25.13.1.7 Carrot burfi

Recipe
Carrot 1 kg, sugar 450 g, milk 0.5 L, fat (*ghee*) 200 g, dry fruits (cashew nut, raisins) 50 g and cardamom 1 g.

Preparation technique
Orange-yellow variety of carrot → Scrapping → Washing → Grading → Cooking with milk till dryness of milk → Frying in fat (*ghee*) → Addition of sugar,

dry fruits and cardamom → Spreading in trays after smearing fat → Allow to set → Cutting into shape of burfi → Packing in cardboard box → Sale/use

25.13.1.8 Canned carrot

Preparation technique

Selection of orange yellow variety → Scrapping → Washing → Cutting longitudinal or slices (1–2 cm thick) → Blanching for 5 min → Filling into plain 2½ can → Brining (2% salt solution) → Exhausting at 90°C for 10 min → Sealing → Processing at 116°C for 25 min → Cooling in plain water → Labelling → Storing

25.13.1.9 Jam

Recipe

Pulp 1 kg, sugar 500 g, citric acid 2 g and water 150 mL.

Preparation technique

Carrot → Washing → Removal of hairs by scrapping → Removal of green top portion → Grading → Addition of sugar and water → Heating → Addition of citric acid → Cooking till desired consistency → Judging of end point → Filling into clean and sterilized bottles → Capping/sealing → Storing

25.13.1.10 Pickle

Recipe

Carrot 1 kg, salt 60 g, red chillies powder 25 g, rye (whole) 25 g, ginger 25 g, onion (grated) 25 g, rye (crushed) 25 g, turmeric 10 g, cumin 5 g, clove 5 g, sugar/gur 250 g, mustard oil 150 mL and vinegar 250 mL.

Preparation technique

Carrot → Washing → Scrapping → Cutting medium-sized pieces → Blanching in boiling water for 6–8 min → Grinding of all hot spices and mixing together → Frying of ginger and onion in little mustard oil → Mixing of spices and carrot on slow fire → Making of thick syrup with sugar or gur and little water → Addition of vinegar in thick syrup → Addition of mixed syrup and vinegar with spiced carrot → Packing into clean jar → Addition of remaining mustard oil → Keeping in sun for 4–5 days → Capping → Storing

25.13.1.11 Fermented carrot with cabbage

Recipe

Carrot and cabbage in ratio of 1:1 (1 kg each) salt 50–60 g and mustard powder/rye 20–30 g.

Preparation technique

Select good carrot roots and cabbage heads → Peel carrots, wash and make shreds and remove outer leaves of cabbage and cut them finally into shreds in ratio of 1:1 → Mix the shreds of vegetables and putting jars/containers → Add salt and mustard powder → Shaking whole mass daily up to 2 weeks → Fermented product → Storage in a cool and dry place

25.13.1.12 Frozen carrot

Preparation technique

Orange yellow variety → Washing → Scrapping of skin → Cutting (2 cm pieces) → Blanching (2 min) → Packing in polythene bag → Sealing → Arranging in cartons → Freezing at –1°C to –5°C → Storage at –18°C

25.14 Radish

Radish is rich in minerals such as calcium, phosphorus, potassium and vitamin C. Radish tops are the good source of protein. Leafy tops are also rich in vitamins A, B and C. Its use in diet increase appetite and prevents constipation. It is very useful in liver and gall bladder troubles and patients suffering from jaundice. The root of radish is useful in urinary problem, piles, enlargement of spleen and gastric troubles.

25.14.1 Product

Radish is processed in to pickle. The technique for preparation is as follows.

25.14.1.1 Pickle

Recipe

Sliced, radish 1 kg, salt 100 g, sugar 50 g, turmeric powder 10 g, cumin powder 10 g, coriander powder 10 g, red pepper powder 10 g, mustard seed powder 50 g and vegetable oil 50 mL.

Preparation technique

Radish → Removal of tops and tips → Washing → Cutting into thin slices → Add all the mixed spices (powdered spices) → Add salt and sugar → Mixed properly → Fry in little oil → Packed in glass jar → Storing

25.15 Watermelon

This is a common man's fruit used as desert fruit. Fruit juice is very delicious, refreshing and has cooling effect. This is very rich in minerals particularly in potassium, phosphorus, iron and magnesium. Watermelon cures enlargement of spleen, ulcers, asthma, bronchitis, jaundice, anaemia, dyspepsia and constipation. It is purgative, antipyretic and carminative in action.

25.15.1 Products

Watermelon is processed into rind pickle, jam and squash. The techniques for preparation of these products are as follows.

25.15.1.1 Rind pickle

Recipe

Melon rind pieces 1 kg, sugar 200–250 g, vinegar 250 mL, salt 10 g, cinnamon 2–5 cm long and cloves 10 in number.

Preparation technique

Melonrind (strip) → Remove the pink portion → Cut melon rind in square of 5 cm pieces → Keep in aluminium pan → Add salt → Cover with water → Boiling until rind becomes tender → Draining → Chilli the rind pieces in cold water for about a hour → Keep pieces overnight → Add vinegar syrup (by boiling vinegar and sugar together) → Add cloves and cinnamon tide in bag → Simmer until rind becomes soft → Remove spice bag → Pack hot pickle in sterilized jars → Cover with boiling syrup → Sealing → Storing

25.15.1.2 Jam

Recipe

Fruit juice 74%, sugar 55%, fresh ginger 0.8%, pectin 0.4% and citric acid 0.7%.

Preparation technique

Watermelon fruit → Washing → Removing skin/rind → Cutting the flesh into small pieces → Removing seeds → Mashing pieces into pulp → Straining through muslin cloth → Dry mixing of pectin with little grinded sugar → Mixing of juice, sugar, citric acid and fresh ginger in a stainless steel sauce pan → Boiling of mixture and stirring → Addition of pectin dry mix near the end of boiling process → Judging of end point through TSS (68%) or temperature (106–108°C) → Filling of jam into sterilized jars → Capping → Cooling in water around 55°C (the water should be kept below the lid of jar) → Wipping of bottles after removing from water → Storing in a cool and dry place

25.15.1.3 Squash

Recipe

Juice 1 L, sugar 900 g, citric acid 2 g and sodium benzoate 2 g.

Preparation technique
Select ripe watermelon → Washing → Cutting → Removal of pulp/flesh → Extraction of juice → Mixing with sugar and citric acid → Heating at 80–85°C → Removal from fire → Addition of preservative and mixing → Filling into bottles → Capping → Storage at cool and dry place

25.16 Bottle gourd

Bottle gourd is rich in vitamin B_1, niacin, carbohydrate and minerals such as potassium, calcium and iron. It is also rich in many amino acids which are vital in our diet. Bottle gourd has high therapeutic values. It has curative properties such as cooling, diuretic and sedative. It is a cardiac tonic, useful in removing cough, biliousness and indigestion.

25.16.1 Products

Bottle guard is processed into powder and candy. The techniques used for preparation of these products are as follows.

25.16.1.1 Powder

Preparation technique
Fresh, tender greenish bottle gourd → Washing → Preparation of shreds → Blanching (80–85°C) for 3 min → Cooled → Sulphiting (steeping shreds in 1% KMS solution for 15 min) → Drying of shreds up to 5% moisture. Drying ratio (15:1) (in cross flow cabinet dryer at 55°C for 3 h) → Grinding (in mill) → Sieved → Packing in polythene bags of 300 gauge → Stored at room temperature (2 months)

25.16.1.2 Candy

Preparation technique
Bottle gourd → Washing → Peeling → Removal of seeds and fluffy portion → Cutting into small pieces (1.5 × 0.5 cm size) → Blanching in hot water (80–85°C for 3 min) → Cooled → Syruping (increase concentration slowly) → Removal of pieces from syrup → Washing mildly → Drying in cabinet dryer at 45–50°C up to 15–16% moisture content → Packing in polythene bags of 300 gauge → Storing

25.17 Bitter gourd

Bitter gourd contains vitamin C and fair amount of vitamin A. It is good source of phosphorus, calcium and potassium. It is full of medicinal properties. It has anti-carcinogenic and anti-leukaemia properties. It improves digestion, removes germs from stomach, and helps in diabetes, piles and jaundice.

25.17.1 Products

Bitter guard can be dehydrated and used for making pickle. The techniques used for preparation of these products are as follows.

25.17.1.1 Dehydrated product

Preparation technique

Bitter gourd → Washing → Removal of stalk and tips → Cut into 6-mm thick slices → Blanching in boiling water (8 min) → Drying at 60°C or sundrying → Packing → Storage

25.17.1.2 Pickle

Recipe

Bitter gourd 1 kg, red chilli powder 20 g, turmeric powder 20 g, cumin powder 20 g, mustard (rye) powder 15 g, coriander powder 20 g, salt 100 g and mustard oil 120 mL.

Preparation technique

Bitter gourd → Washing → Draining → Making longitudinal incision → Filling salt in it → Keeping in sun for half an hour → Washing with clean water → Draining and squeezing → Boiling in salted water for 5 min → Draining and drying → Filling some spices in bitter gourd and some spreading on it → Filling into jar → Addition of heated and cooled oil → Capping → Storage

25.18 Pointed gourd

This is dioecious crop. This is very nutritious and rich in protein, dietary fibres and minerals such as potassium, phosphorus, calcium and iron. It is also fairly rich in vitamins A and C.

25.18.1 Product

Pointed guard can be used for making sweet. The technique for preparation of sweet is as follows.

25.18.1.1 Sweet

Recipe

Pointed gourd 1 kg, khoya 900 g, sugar 500 g, whole milk powder 100 g, green pistachios 20 g, almond 20 g and cardamom powder 2 g.

Preparation technique
Green mature pointed gourd → Washing → Peeling → Slitting lengthwise → Removes seeds carefully → Dropping in boiling water and cooking for 2 min → Draining the water or carefully squeeze out water → Roasting of khoya till it becomes light pink and cool it → Mix milk powder crushed almond, pista, cardamom and saffron strands → Stuff this mixture into each pointed gourd → Prepare sugar syrup of one thread consistency → Add stuffed pointed gourd in syrup → Cooking for 2 min → Take out pointed gourd carefully and keep on mesh or plate (to drain excess syrup) → Packing of pointed gourd sweet in cardboard boxes for sale/use

25.19 Ash gourd

Fruit is rich source of vitamin C, dietary fibre and minerals such as potassium, calcium, magnesium and sodium. Fruit juice is very useful in treating various ailments such as peptic ulcer, insanity epilepsy and blood sugar.

25.19.1 Products

An excellent quality of preserve, candy and bari can be prepared from mature fruits of ash gourd. The technique used for preparation is as follows.

25.19.1.1 Preserve

Preparation technique
Select fully mature with firm pulp of ash gourd → Washing → Cut length wise large pieces → Remove seeds and fluffy portion → Pricking → Cutting into pieces of suitable size → Soaking in lime water (60 g lime/L for 24 h to harden texture) → Washing to remove lime → Soaking in alum solution (2%) for 24 h → Washing again → Draining → Blanching in water containing little KMS to bleach → Steeping in strained sugar syrup of 40% TSS for a day → Removal of ash gourd pieces → Boiling of syrup to 60% TSS → Steeping of ash gourd for a day → Removal of pieces → Boiling of syrup to 70% TSS → Steeping of pieces in 70% TSS for a week → Draining → Preserve → Filling into jar → Covering preserve with freshly prepared sugar syrup of 68% TSS → Sealing → Storage

25.19.1.2 Candy

Preparation technique
In case of candy, raising of sugar syrup strength to 75% of TSS → Steeping of ash gourd pieces in syrup for a week → Draining of ash gourd pieces from syrup → Dipping in boiling water for a second to remove adhering syrup → Shade drying → Packing → Storage

Recent development in vegetable processing are individual quick freezing for small size vegetables like pea, carrot, cauliflower and other vegetables, osmotic dehydration of vegetables, minimal processing of salad vegetables, leafy vegetables, tubers and other vegetables (available in super market) are the recent development. Ready to eat vegetable curries, frozen vegetables such as green peas, okra, carrot, etc., vegetable-based soup powder and mixed vegetable pickles with improved recipe are some of the new products. Frozen vegetables such as green peas, okra, carrot, cauliflower, potato and tomato-based product, vegetable-based soup, garlic and onion powder have better potential for export.

25.20 Mushroom products and processing technique

Mushroom is most important microbes used as a source of human food. Mushroom is a rich source of protein, vitamins, minerals and also a good source of energy. This is an ideal food for diabetes because of low content of fat and carbohydrates. Button mushroom (*Agaricus bisporus*) is the most important among the cultivated species. It has superior texture and cooking quality and is easily digestible. Other commonly cultivated species of mushroom are oyster mushroom, paddy straw mushroom, milky mushroom, black year mushroom and giant mushroom.

25.20.1 Products

This is highly perishable. Mushroom can be processed into number of quality products such as canned mushroom, ketchup/sauce, pickles, dehydrated, steeping, preservation, soup powder, weaning foods and frozen mushroom.

25.20.1.1 Canned mushroom

Preparation technique

Selection of button mushroom → Sorting → Washing → Trimming → Washing → Blanching for 4 min → Pre-soaking for 30 min in 2% salt containing 0.1% citric acid 100 mg percent ascorbic acid → Draining → Filling in SR A2½ cans → Covering with hot brine solution (2% brine containing 0.1% citric acid) → Exhausting at 85°C for 5 min → Sealing immediately → Sterilization at 116°C for 35 min → Cooling in plain water → Labelling → Storage at ambient temperature

25.20.2 Mushroom sauce

Recipe

Mushroom 1 kg, red chillies powder 5 g, cinnamon powder 5 g, mixed spices 10 g, salt 25 g and vinegar 500 mL.

Preparation technique

Mushroom → Sorting → Washing → Cooking with vinegar for a short time → Allow to stand for 6 days → Making in to fine pulp → Addition of spices and salt → Cooking up to desired consistency → Filling hot into bottles → Crown corking → Pasteurization (85°C) for 30 min → Cooling → Storing

25.20.1.3 Mushroom pickle

Recipe

Mushroom 1 kg, salt 100 g, red chilli powder, aniseed powder, cumin powder, fenugreek powder 5 g each, turmeric powder 10 g, coriander powder 10 g, black pepper powder 2 g, cinnamon powder 1 g, garlic paste 25 g, vinegar 100 mL and mustard oil 350 mL.

Preparation technique

Mushroom → Sorting → Washing → Trimming → Frying with spices in little oil till dryness → Cooling → Addition of salt and vinegar → Filling into glass jar → Addition of oil to cover pieces → Capping → Sealing → Storing

25.20.1.4 Dehydrated mushroom

Preparation technique

Mushrooms → Sorting → Washing → Trimming → Slicing into halves → Blanching (water containing 2% salt and 0.1% citric acid) for 3 min → Pre-soaking (solution containing 1000 ppm SO_2 and 0.1% citric acid) for 30 min → Draining → Spreading in trays → Drying at 50–65°C for 5 h/up to 5–10% moisture → Sweating → Packing in polythene bag → Storing at ambient temperature

25.20.1.5 Steeping preservation

Recipe

Salt 2%, sugar 2%, citric acid 0.5%, ascorbic acid 1% and KMS 0.1%. Ratio of mushroom to solution of above chemical is 1:2.

Preparation technique

Button mushroom → Sorting → Washing → Blanching in boiling water for 3 min → Draining → Filling into containers → Covering with above mentioned chemical solution (preparing solution by mixing the mentioned ingredients in mushroom to solution ratio of 1:2) → Capping → Storing (up to 6 months) at room temperature

26

Spice products and processing technique

Spices are used for flavouring, seasoning and imparting, aroma in foods. India is known as the home of spices, producing a wide variety of spices such as black pepper, cardamom, ginger, garlic, chilli, turmeric, onion and a variety of tree and seed spices. Spices and herbs have tremendous importance in everyday life, as ingredients in food, alcoholic beverage, medicine, perfumery, cosmetic and colouring. Spices are credited with preservative, antioxidant, appetizing and digestive properties. Common spices and their products are discussed in the following sections.

26.1 Black pepper

The dried mature but unripe berry is obtained from climbing vine. It is one of the most important spices of India called king of spices. It is widely used and contributes flavour and taste. Black pepper has antifugal, antimicrobial and antioxidant properties. It is an essential ingredient of most curry powder and spices extracts. It has effective cure for dyspepsia, malaria, delirium tremors, haemorrhoids, etc. It is used as preservative for meat packers, canning, pickling, baking, confectionary and preparation of beverage.

26.1.1 Products

Pepper is processed into number of products such as black pepper, white pepper, dry green pepper, dehydrated green pepper, black green pepper, cured green pepper, frozen green pepper, freeze-dried green pepper, decorticated black pepper, powder pepper, pepper oil, pepper oleoresin and piperine. The techniques for preparation of important products are as follows.

26.1.1.1 Black pepper

Preparation technique

Fresh green pepper berries → Cleaning → Blanching (in perforated vessel or gunny bag and deep in boiling water for 1 min) → Draining → Drying in sunlight (3–4 days) → Packaging → Storing

26.1.1.2 White pepper

Preparation technique

Suitable varieties → Harvested at full ripe berries → Despiking → Selection of black berries of uniform size → Soaking in water (tank) → Changing water after 24 h up to 7 days → Removal of outer skin → Drying in sunlight → Packaging → Storing

26.1.1.3 Dry green pepper

The steps involved in the preparation of dry green pepper are as follows:

Fresh tender green pepper → Blanching → Draining → Drying → Packaging → Storage

26.1.1.4 Dehydrated green pepper

The steps involved in dehydrated green pepper are as follows:

Harvesting pepper 10–15 days before maturity → Boiling in water for 10 min or steaming → Draining → Drying (oven/microwave) till wrinkled appearance → Packaging → Storing

26.1.1.5 Green pepper in brine (bulk packaging)

Preparation technique

Whole spikes (immature spike about 4–5 months old) → Washing of spikes and berries in running water → Steeping in fresh water containing chlorine (80–100 ppm) to avoid mould during storage → Filling in PVC jerry cans of 20–35 L capacity → Covering with 16% brine containing 0.25% citric acid and 100 ppm SO_2 → Packaging → Storing

26.1.1.6 Canned green pepper

Preparation technique

Freshly harvested green pepper → Despiking → Washing of berries → Filling into cans → Covering with brine containing 2% common salt and 0.6% citric acid → Exhausting of cans → Cans sealing → Heat processing → Cooling in water → Storage

26.1.1.7 Bottled green pepper

The steps involved in preparation of green pepper are as follows:

Fresh pepper spikes → Cleaning → Bottling → Covering with 10% brine containing 2% acetic acid → Capping → Storing

26.1.1.8 Cured green pepper (dry packed)

Preparation technique

Freshly harvested spikes (slightly under mature green berries) → Despiking of tender green berries → Cleaning in water → Draining → Steeping in saturated brine solution containing chemical → Draining of berries → Packing in suitable flexible package → Storing

This product is better than dehydrated green pepper and cheaper than canned and bottled green pepper.

26.1.1.9 Frozen green pepper

Preparation technique

Green pepper berries → Cleaning → Blanching → Cooling → Covering in 2% brine containing 0.25% citric acid and ascorbic acid (to serve as antioxidant) → Frozen → Packing in suitable flexible pouches → Storage/marketing

26.1.1.10 Freeze-dried green pepper

Preparation technique

Green pepper berries → Cleaning → Washing → Blanching → Cooling (water cooled) → Deep frozen to –40°C → Vacuum-shelf drying under an ultra low pressure (5 μ) → Packaging → Storing

26.1.1.11 Decorticated black pepper

The steps involved in preparation of decorticated are as follows:

Black pepper → Mechanical decortications of outer skin → White pepper packing → Storing

26.1.1.12 Powdered pepper (black/green pepper)

The steps involved in preparation of powdered pepper are as follows: dehydrated green pepper/dehydrated black pepper → Powdering to uniform mesh → Packing → Storing

26.1.1.13 Pepper oil

It is used in perfumery and in flavouring of sausages, canned meat, soups, sauces, some beverages and liquors. It finds uses in medicine. The technique of preparation is as follows:

Black pepper → Crushing to coarse powder → Steam distillation → Essential oil colourless or pale green (2.5–3.5%)

26.1.1.14 Pepper oleoresin

Oleoresin is used for flavouring sauces, sausages, chutney, etc., in commercial scale. The technique for the preparation of oleoresin is as follows:

Black pepper → Ground pepper → Extraction with organic solvents (acetone or ethanol or dichloroethane) → Oleoresin (10–13%)

26.1.1.15 Piperine

The quality component of black pepper is piperine contribute pungency and volatile oil responsible for the aroma and flavour. It is really soluble in alcohol and on hydrolysis splits into piperidine and piperic acid. Crude piperine occurs from 4% to 10% and true piperine 5–6%. Piperine has been used to impart a pungent taste to brandy.

26.2 Cardamom

Cardamom is used for flavouring various preparations of food, bakery, confectionery and beverages such as tea, coffee and chocolates. It is used as an aromatic stimulant, carminative and antioxidant. Cardamom is an essential ingredient of digestive stimulants.

26.2.1 Products

Cardamom is processed for bleached cardamom, cardamom seed and powder, essential oil and oleoresin.

26.2.1.1 Bleached cardamom

Both fresh and dried capsules can be used for bleaching. The technique use for blanching is as follows.

Fresh capsule bleaching

Preparation technique

Fresh capsule → Soaking in 20% potassium metabisulphite solution containing 1% hydrogen peroxide for a hour → Draining → Drying (golden yellow colour) → Packing → Storage

Dried capsule bleaching

Preparation technique

Dried capsule → Steeping in bleaching agents (bleaching powder/sulphur dioxide/potassium metabisulphite/hydrogen peroxide) → Draining → Drying → Packing bleached cardamom has better keeping quality but it has low volatile oil content

26.2.1.2 Seed and powder

Cardamom seeds are chewed to prevent bad smell in mouth, indigestion, nausea and excessive watering in mouth (phrosis). Powdered seed of cardamom boiled with tea water gives a very pleasant aroma to tea. This can be used as medicine for scanty urination, diarrhoea, dysentery, palpitation of heart and depression. The technique used for preparation is as follows:

Capsules → Decorcating seeds → Seeds → Grinding → Powder → Packing (laminated) → Storage/sale

26.2.1.5 Cardamom oil (essential oil)

It is produced in small quantity. Technique for production is by steam distillation of crushed fruits or powdered seeds of cardamom. Oil content is about 8–11%. The essential oil is used in flavouring of processed food and in certain liquid products such as cordials and liquors. It is also used in perfumery.

26.2.1.6 Oleoresin

The technique used for its production is by solvent extraction. Oleoresin is mainly used to meat products such as sausages. It is used as a soluble spice. It is also used in flavouring of processed food.

26.3 Turmeric

Turmeric has several uses. It is used as condiment in vegetables, meat, fish and pickle preparation. It is stomachic, tonic and blood purifier. Curcumin, the yellow colouring pigment, is gaining popularity with ban on artificial colour in food industry. In pharmaceuticals, it is valued as carminative or anti-cancerous, anti-inflammatory and for antiseptic properties. Turmeric is useful in treating gall stones, diabetes and skin infection. Turmeric is also used in cosmetic.

26.3.1 Products

Turmeric is processed for powder, volatile oil and oleoresins. Turmeric oleoresin contains 30–35% curcumin which is the main colouring agent.

26.3.1.1 Turmeric powder

Turmeric is valued for its aroma and colour. The powder is mostly consumed domestically for culinary purpose. It is used in manufacture of curry powder, spice mixture, pickle, soup, etc. The technique for preparation is as follows:

Dried, polished and coloured rhizome cut into pieces/taken to disintegrator → Pulverising → Grinding/powdering by milling or with hand operated chakki → Sieving (300 microsieve) → Packing in sacks/polyethylene packs/foil/tin containers → Sealing of bags/tin container → Storage/marketing

26.3.1.2 Oleoresin

Oleoresin is highly viscous orange, brown product containing 30–35% curcumin, 15–20% volatile oil and has characteristics turmeric aroma. Turmeric oleoresin finds application in meat and fish products, pickles, dairy products and confectionary. Curcumin pigment has application in colouring of foods. The technique used for extraction is as follows:

Turmeric powder → Extraction with help of solvent (acetone/alcohol/ethylene dichloride) → Distillation of extract → Recovery of solvent → Blending → Packing → Storing/marketing

26.3.1.3 Essential oil

The oil content varies with maturity, method of curing and condition of distillation. The oil is an orange-yellow liquid. The dried rhizome yields 5–6% of oil and fresh ones give about 0.25%. The technique used for obtaining essential oil is by steam distillation of crushed rhizomes.

26.4 Ginger

Ginger is an important spice crop of the world. It is one of the oldest spices known for its distinct flavour or aroma and pungency. It is valuable cash crop and contributes much towards the export earnings. Ginger is rich in carbohydrates, fibre, carotene, vitamin B_1 and B_2. It is also good source of minerals such as calcium and iron. ginger has wide range of uses such as culinary, confectionery, flavourants in alcoholic and non-alcoholic beverages and pharmaceutical preparations. Ginger is very useful in gastritis, dyspepsia, flatulence and in cold and cough as an expectorant. Ginger is stimulant, carminative and stomachic and hence, extremely valuable in colic and vomiting.

26.4.1 Products

Green and dry ginger both are processed into number of products. Green ginger is processed into preserve, candy, chocolates, beverage (alcoholic and non-alcoholic), chutney, pickles, salted ginger and ginger in brine. Dry ginger is processed into dehydrated ginger, bleached ginger, powder, oil and oleoresin.

26.4.1.1 Products of green/fresh ginger

1. Dehydrated ginger

Preparation technique

Fresh ginger rhizome → Washing → Removal of outer skin by lye treatment [deeping in boiling solution of sodium hydroxide (20%) for 5 min and placing rhizomes in 4% citric acid for 2 h and washed] or by mechanical peeling (abrasive peeling for 60 s) → Drying in a flow drier at temperature of 60°C

→ Removal of extraneous matter → Packing → Storage in a cool and dry place/marketing

2. Bleached ginger

Preparation technique
Peeled rhizomes → Cleaning → Immersing in lime solution repeatedly → Drying in sun until ginger received uniform coating of lime (calcium hydroxide) and bright colour (drying takes about 10 days) → Rubbing of product thoroughly with gunny cloth to remove remnants of skin and to provide smooth finish → Bleached/lime ginger → Packing → Storage/marketing

3. Preserve

Recipe
1 kg fresh ginger, 1 kg sugar, 1 L water and 4 g citric acid.

Preparation technique
Select large-sized tender rhizomes of low fibre content → Washing → Removal of skin/peeling and washing → Pricking of rhizomes → Cutting into cubes/suitable pieces → Blanching in boiling water till to become soft (about an hour) → Draining and drying for removal of moisture → Steeping in strained sugar syrup of 40% TSS (sugar + water + citric acid little heating and straining) for a day → Removal of pieces → Boiling of syrup to 60% TSS → Steeping pieces for a day → Removal of pieces → Boiling of syrup to 70% TSS → Steeping of pieces for 2 days → Draining → Feeling into containers → Covering with freshly prepared 68% sugar syrup →Sealing → Storing/marketing

4. Candy

Preparation technique
Ginger preserve prepared as mentioned above → Draining of ginger preserve cubes/pieces from syrup → Rinsing pieces promptly with water → Shade drying → Packing in polyethylene bag → Storage/marketing

5. Chocolate

Recipe
Ginger juice/pulp 1 L, sugar 1.75 kg, coco powder 700 g, milk 1.6 L and ghee/fat 135 g.

Preparation technique
Ginger → Washing → Cleaning/peeling → Cutting into small pieces/shredding → Extraction of juice with little water and heating or through pulping machine → Mixing with mixture of milk and sugar (boiled and concentrated form) → Mixing with ghee and coco powder → Cooking till desire consistency → Spreading little ghee in tray and spreading of cooked mixture over it → Allow to cool and set → Cutting into suitable pieces → Wrapping in butter papers →

Packing in glass jar or polyethylene pouches → Capping the jar or sealing the bag → Storing/marketing

6. Non-alcoholic beverages

Ginger soft drink

Recipe
Ginger juice 2%, total soluble solid 11% and acid 0.3%.

Preparation technique
Fresh ginger → Washing → Peeling → Cutting into pieces → Addition of water in ratio of 1:1 → Passing through pulper/mixer → Keeping half an hour pulp/juice for sedimentation → Siphon or take clear juice → Mixing with strained sugar syrup solution (sugar + water + citric acid little heating and straining) → Addition of preservative (sodium metabisulphite) → Mixing thoroughly → Bottling → Crown corking → Pasteurization (85°C for 15 min) → Air cooling → Storage/marketing

Syrup

Recipe
Ginger juice 1 L, sugar 5 kg, citric acid 100 g and water 2 L.

Preparation technique
Fresh ginger → Washing → Peeling → Cutting into pieces/shredding → Addition of water in ratio of 1:1 → Passing through pulper → Storing juice for half an hour for sedimentation → Siphoning clear juice → Mixing with syrup solution (sugar + water + citric acid heating just to dissolve sugar and straining) → Bottling → Capping → Storage in cool and dry place/ marketing

7. Alcoholic beverages

Beer
This is alcoholic beverage prepare from ginger extracts, hopes and spices. The technique for preparation is as follows:

Ginger → Washing → Extraction → Fermentation with yeast and citric acid → Mixing with hopes (6 parts of ginger extracts + 3 parts of hopes + spices) → Boiling for 22–25 min → Filtration of syrup → Mixing with sugar → Cooling to −10°C

8. Chutney

Recipe
Ginger 1 kg, tamarind 500 g, sugar 1 kg, salt 150 g, red chilli powder 20 g, garlic 200 g, fenugreek powder 40 g, mustard powder 40 g and mustard oil 500 mL.

Preparation technique
Fresh ginger → Washing → Peeling → Grinding → Grinding of tamarind + 100 g grounded garlic → Mixing of grinded ginger + grinded tamarind and garlic → Little heating → Addition of salt → Fry remaining garlic with fenugreek and mustard powder in oil → Mixing with ginger mixture → Filling into glass jar → Capping → Storage in cool and dry place/marketing

9. Pickle

Recipe
Fresh ginger 1 kg, cumin seed, chillies and ajma 40 g each, black salt and citric acid 40 g each.

Preparation technique
Ginger → Washing → Peeling → Grating → Mixing with all ingredients → Filling into glass jar → Keeping in sun shine for 2 weeks → Stirring → Capping → Storage in cool and dry place/marketing

10. Salted ginger/ginger in brine

Preparation technique
Fresh immature ginger of low fibre content → Washing and cleaning → Soaking in 30% salt solution containing 1% citric acid → Removal of ginger from salt solution after 2 weeks → Cleaning → Preserving in cool condition → Storing in 1–2% brine containing citric acid

26.4.1.2 Products of dried ginger

Powder
The steps involved in preparation of ginger powder are as follows:

Dry ginger → Pulverizing to mesh size of 50–60 → Packing (laminated bag) → Storage in a cool and dry place/marketing

Oleoresin
Oleoresin is manufacture in India and is used in food industry. There is great demand for this product from outside.

Preparation technique
Dried ginger powder → Extraction with suitable solvents (alcohol or acetones) → Concentration of acetone extract under vacuum → Complete removal of solvent used even traces of solvent → Oleoresin (commercially known as gingerin) → Blending → Packing.

The yield and quality of oleoresin depends upon the variety, solvents used and method of extraction of oleoresin (Gingerin). Oleoresin contains mainly gingerol, with shogaol and zingerone.

Ginger oil
Ginger oil is prepared by distilling dry ginger powder. Ginger has about 2% oil, and major ingredients are sesquiterpene and zingiberene.

26.5 Garlic

This is very important herb and valuable spice crop. It is mainly used for flavouring and seasoning vegetable and meat dishes. Garlic is rich in carbohydrates, protein, calcium, phosphorus, potassium and magnesium. The green form of garlic is very high in ascorbic acid content. Garlic helps in absorption and digestion of food. It has anthelmintic, antiseptic, carminative and natural antibiotic properties.

26.5.1 Products

26.5.1.1 Dehydrated garlic

Preparation technique
Garlic → Peeling the clove → Cutting into 5- to 6-mm thick shreds → Dipping in salt solution (5%) for 10 min → Drying at 60°C or sun drying → Packing → Storing

26.5.1.2 Garlic powder

Preparation technique
Garlic bulbs → Scrubbing manually with mild pressure → Removal of papery skin and separation of cloves → Washing of cloves → Slicing or pressed between rolls to form flakes → Drying of flakes (tunnel driers or continuous belt drier) up to 6% moisture → Powdering → Packing in polythene bags (air tight to prevent moisture absorption) → Storing

26.5.1.3 Garlic pickle

Recipe
Garlic clove 1 kg, lime juice 1 L, fenugreek powder 40 g, red chilli powder 20 g, salt 400 g, mustard oil 400 mL.

Preparation technique
Garlic clove → Shelling of garlic clove → Cutting of lime and extraction of juice → Filling of the lime juice into jar → Addition of salt → Addition of garlic after frying in oil → Addition of chillies and fenugreek powder → Mixing thoroughly → Capping → Storing

26.6 Chilli

Chilli also known as hot pepper is an important spice and vegetable. The fresh green chilli is rich in vitamin A and C, and fibre. It is also rich in vitamin P, niacin and minerals such as potassium, phosphorus, magnesium, sulphur and iron. The septa and placental tissue contain the pungent principle known as capsaicin. Green chillies eaten with food stuffs increase the flow of saliva by stimulating the taste and act as an appetizer. Chilli also produces stress resistance. Chillies are very useful as a cure for appetite, digestion and mitigate flatulence. It is also useful in cure of colic, diarrhoea, dropsy, gouts and toothaches. It has tonic and carminative action when it is taken with food.

26.6.1 Products

Chillies can be processed into powder, dry green chillies, green chilli pickle, chilli powder, drying/dehydrated red chilli, red chilli pickles and sauce.

26.6.1.1 Drying/dehydrated red chillies

The steps involved in preparation of dried chillies are as follows:

Chillies (dark red parts) → Ashing → Drying at 50–60°C/sun drying → Packing → Storing

26.6.1.2 Chilli powder

The steps involved in preparation of chilli powder are as follows:

Red coloured chillies → Washing → Removal of stalk → Drying → Grinding → Sieving → Packing in polythene bags → Sealing → Storing

26.6.1.3 Red chillies pickle

Recipe

Red chillies 1 kg, dry mango powder (*amchur*) 250 g, salt 150 g, coriander powder 50 g, nigella seeds 15 g, aniseed powder 20 g, fenugreek powder 20 g, hot spices 50 g, mustard (ground) 100 g and mustard oil 500 mL.

Preparation technique

Red chillies → Washing → Draining and drying (1 h) → Removal of stem → Making incision → Removal of seeds → Mixing all spices and seeds → Frying in oil → Cooling → Filling into chillies → Packing in jar → Addition of oil (after heating and cooling) → Capping → Keeping for 2 weeks → Storing/using

26.6.1.4 Green chillies pickle

Recipe

Green chillies 1 kg, garlic 100 g, mustard (rye) powder 50 g, turmeric powder 50 g, lime juice 500 mL, fenugreek 25 g, mustard oil 500 mL.

Preparation technique
Green chillies → Washing → Drying → Removal of stem → Making incision (longitudinal) → Mixing all spices in little lime juice → Mixing with chillies → Filling into jar → Addition of lime juice and oil → Keeping in sun for few days → Storage in cool and dry place

26.6.1.5 Dry green chillies

Preparation technique
Green chillies → Washing → Pricking → Blanching in boiling water for a minute → Draining → Immersing in 2% sodium hydroxide solution for 10 min → Draining → Drying up 5% moisture → Packing → Sealing → Storing

26.6.1.6 Chilli sauce

Recipe
Green chillies 1 kg, carrot 250 g, potato 250 g, sugar 50 g, salt 50 g, hot spices 50 g, glacial acetic acid 5 mL.

Preparation technique
Green chillies (remove stem), carrot (scrapping and washing), potato (peeling) → Boil chilli carrot and potato in little water or cooking in pressure cooker → Mix together → Sieving/straining → Mixing of strained hot spices with the mixture of chillies, carrot and potato → Cooking till desired consistency → Addition of salt → Addition of acetic acid → Heating for 5 min → Filling into clean sterilized bottles → Capping/crowncorking → Storing

26.7 Nutmeg

This is a unique tree spice produces two spices nutmeg and mace. Nutmeg is the ovoid kernel which is hard and brown enclosed with in a thin shell. Surrounding this shell is the aril (scarlet in colour) which gives the mace. The mace is separated from the nut without breaking. Nutmeg is a stimulant carminative, astringent, aphrodisiac and hallucinogen. Mace is used as a culinary spice and largely as a flavouring agent for food products.

26.7.1 Product

Both nutmeg and maces are processed into number of products. Nutmeg is processed into volatile oil, nutmeg butter and volatile oil from bark and flowers. The mace products are mace oil and fixed mace oil. Fresh fleshy pericarp/fruit rind is used for making jam, jelly and pickles.

26.8 Cinnamon

Leaves of cinnamon are widely used as spice for flavouring meats, sauces and sausages. Bark is also utilized as spice as flavouring agent. It is also used as medicine and perfume. The dried bark of *Cinnamomum verum* is the true cinnamon. Cinnamon bark has carminative, stimulative, astringent and antiseptic properties. It checks vomiting and relieves flatulence.

26.8.1 Products

Both bark and leaf are processed for various products. Bark is processed for powder, oil and oleoresin. Leaf is processed into leaf oil.

26.8.1.1 Bark products

Powder
Cinnamon powder can be obtained by grinding the barks of various grades.

Oils
The bark to be distilled for oil should be kept dry since dampness encourages mould growth which affects oil composition. Hydrodistillation of chips, featherings and quillings produce cinnamon bark oil. Cinnamon bark has 0.25–2.5% oil in it. Oil of superior quality can be obtained from inner portion of bark. Lower quality of oil is obtained from broken quills, chips and bark. Bark oil contains high percentage of cinnamaldehyde (65%) and low content of eugenol (5–10%).

Oleoresin
Oleoresin is extracted from powdered cinnamon bark using solvent such as acetone/ethylene dichloride. Cinnamon has about 7–10% oleoresin.

26.8.1.2 Leaf product

Leaf oil
The raw materials used for leaf oil production are leaves after trimming the cut stems and those obtained from pruning. The leaves are usually allowed to dry for a few days before distillation. Leaves contain 0.5–1.5% oil. The oil contains high percentage of eugenol (70–80%). It is used in dental preparation.

26.9 Clove

Various food products are flavoured with cloves. Food-processing industries use both whole and ground form of cloves in various preparations. Clove oil is used in perfumeries, pharmaceuticals and flavouring industries. Clove oleoresin is also used in food-processing industries. Clove is used as stimulant carminative and local antiseptic.

26.9.1 Product

Clove buds are processed for oil. The oil can be obtained by hydro or steam distillation of whole or broken buds. Distillation method and distillation time affect both the oil yield and its characteristics. Combined water and steam distillation produce better recovery of oil than steam alone. Clove buds yield 16% oil. The main constituents of oil are eugenol, eugenol acetate and caryophyllene. Oil can also be obtained from steam (4–5%), mother cloves (6.5%), leaf (1–2%) and roots (6%).

26.10 Kokum

It has originated in the tropical forest of Western Ghats of India. Kokum fruit has various uses. It is used as fish preservative and as a flavouring substitute. Kokum seed contains about 35% fat which is edible, nutritive, demulcent, astringent and emollient. It is also used in pharmaceuticals preparation and cosmetic products. Kokum rind is the richest sources of natural pigment anthocyanin (2–3%). Kokum fat is used in chocolates and confectionary preparations. It is also used in manufactured of soap and candle.

26.10.1 Products

Kokum is processed into number of products such as dried green kokum rind, kokum syrup, dried ripe kokum rind and kokum agal (brine kokum juice).

26.10.1.1 Dried green kokum rind

The steps involved in preparation of dried green kokum rind are as follows:

Green kokum fruit → Washing → Cutting into four longitudinal pieces → Drying in sun → Packing→ Storage

26.10.1.2 Dried ripe kokum rind

Preparation technique

Ripe fruit → Washing → Drying in sun or cabinet drier at 60°C → Treating with brined kokum juice → Drying (drying and treating repeated five times, drying ratio of ripe kokum fruit in a cabinet drier is 6.2..1 and sun drying 7.7 ..1) → Packing → Storage

26.10.1.3 Brined kokum juice (kokum agal)

Preparation technique
Ripe fruit rind/pulp → Mixing with 16% common salt → Keeping the mixture for 8 days → Stirring time to time → Packing in glass bottles or food-grade polythene → Storage

26.10.1.4 Kokum syrup (Amrit kokum)

Preparation technique
Fresh ripe kokum rind → Addition of sugar in ratio 1:2 (kokum and sugar) → Straining of mixture through muslin cloth → Addition of sodium benzoate (610 mg/kg of syrup) → Addition f common salt and cumin powder according to taste → Packing in food-grade polythene containers or glass bottles → Storage

26.11 All spice (pimento/pimenta)

All spice is an ever green tree. It is a tree spice. It combines the composite flavour and aroma of four spices, that is, clove, nutmeg, cinnamon and black pepper. It bears berries which are similar to black pepper. The dry unripe fruit is the spice of commerce. This is used for flavouring of meats, sauces, canned foods, confectionaries and pickles. All spices are aromatic, stimulant, digestive and carminative. Powdered fruits are used against dyspepsia, diarrhoea and flatulence. It is also used in preparation of tonics and purgatives. The dried berries give oil. The oil contains mainly eugenol. There is good market for berry oil and it is being used widely in food industry, perfumery and pharmacy.

26.11.1 Products

Dried berries of all spice are processed as whole spice, ground spice, berry oil, leaf oil and oleoresin.

26.11.1.1 Ground spice

The steps involved in the preparation of ground spice are as follows:

Dried whole all spice → Cleaning → Grinding → Sieving → Packing → Storage

26.11.1.2 Berry oil

Berry oil has yellow to yellowish red colour and possesses the characteristics colour and flavour of all spice. The principal constituent of the oil is eugenol (65–89%). There is good market for berry oil. The oil is used in food, cosmetic and pharmaceutical industries. It is used for flavouring condiments and food products such as canned foods, meat, etc. It is used in manufacture of cosmetics such as soap, shave lotion, etc. It has uniform quality and avoids microbial contamination, hence, better substitute of ground spice. The oil is used as stimulant and carminative. The technique used for obtaining oil from all spice berries is as follows:

Dried berries → Crushing (crushed berries) → Steam distillation (about 10 h) → Oil (3.3–4.5%) → Packing → Storage/marketing

Oil can also be obtained by super critical fluid extraction (SCFE).

26.11.1.3 Leaf oil

Oil can be obtained from leaf which has inferior quality in terms of odour and flavour. It is used as substitute for expensive berry oil. Oil has eugenol as main component. Leaf oil is obtained from dry leaves. The steps involved in obtaining leaf oil are as follows:

Leaves → Drying → Dried leaves → Steam distillation → Leaf oil (0.7–3.0%) → Packing → Storage/marketing

26.11.1.4 Oleoresin

Oleoresin is comprised of both volatile and non-volatile resins. To obtain complete flavour of all spice non-volatile components (oleoresin) should be extracted using organic solvents. Oleoresin prepared from ground spice by extraction with suitable solvents. The solvents should be totally removed from the final product by distillation under vacuum or by SCFE technology. Oleoresin is used as a source of flavouring in wide variety of food products.

26.12 Coriander

Coriander is an annual herb. It is native of Mediterranean centre. It is mainly cultivated for its fruit and tender green leaves. The fruit have a fragrant order and pleasant aromatic taste. The dried ground fruits are extensively used in preparation of curry powder, pickling spices, sausages and seasoning. The young plants and their leaves are also used in soup, sausages, chutney and as dressings. The seeds are used in medicine as diuretic, carminative, refrigerant and aphrodisiac.

26.12.1 Products

Coriander is processed in ground spice, essential oil, oleoresins and curry powder.

26.12.1.1 Ground spices

These are incorporated in food dishes more uniformly as compared to whole spice. The whole spices are milled to a certain degree of fineness and packed for marketing. This is mainly used by the food processors.

26.12.1.2 *Curry powder*

It is prepared by grinding the mixture of several spices such as coriander, fenugreek, cumin, black pepper, chillies, fennel, etc. There is great demand for curry powder by consumers.

26.12.1.3 *Essential oil*

Essential oil is the aromatic, volatile components present in coriander. It provides the characteristic aroma of coriander. It is extracted through steam distillation. The technique used for extraction of essential oil is as follows:

Clean, dried coriander → Comminuted → Charging into stainless steel vessel equipped steam inlet, vapour outlet, condenser and separator assembly → Introducing live steam below the charge which rises through the plant → Volatile oil is condensed and separated from water → Oil drying → Packing in full tight containers → Storage in a cool and dry place/marketing

26.12.1.4 *Oleoresin*

Oleoresin gives complete flavour and non-volatile resinous fraction present in coriander. The resinous fraction comprises of fixative, natural antioxidant and pigment. This is the true essence of spice. The technique for preparation of oleoresin is as follows:

Clean, dried coriander → Commuted → Subject to distillation → Volatile essential oil (gives aroma of the spice) → Deoiling → Drying → Grinding (Finer) → Extraction with suitable food-grade solvents (hexane/ethylene dichloride) → Non-volatile taste principles (aroma and taste) → Blending of aroma and taste fraction → Oleoresin

26.13 Cumin

Cumin is an annual herb cultivated for flavouring vegetables, pickles, soup and for pleasant aroma. Cumin seeds are largely used as condiments and in all mixed spices and curry powders. Seeds are extensively used in medicines as stimulant, carminative, stomachic, dyspepsia and astringent. Essential oil (volatile oil) is used in perfumery and for flavouring beverage (liquors, cordials, etc.). Seeds are rich in protein, fat, carbohydrates and minerals.

26.13.1 Products

Cumin seed is processed for grounded spice, curry powder, essential oil and oleoresin.

26.13.1.1 Ground spice

Ground spices are produced by grinding or milling of clean and dried cumin seed. Curry powder is prepared by grinding the cumin seed with various spices.

26.13.1.2 Essential oil

Cumin seed yields 2–3% essential oil. Essential oil is extracted through solvents such as acetate, ethyl alcohol or by distillation such as steam and hydrodistillation. The flavour of the oil is warm bitter and curry like.

26.13.1.3 Oleoresin

Oleoresin of cumin is a free flowing liquid, yellowish brown in colour and contains 10–30 mL volatile oil/100 g. Roasted seeds are also used for oleoresin extraction. Oleoresin is extracted from deoiled spice which is dried and grounded by suitable food-grade solvents such as hexane, ethyle dichloride, etc. Oil and oleoresin of cumin seed are used in seasoning for snacks, soups, stews, cheese, pickles and meat products.

26.14 Fennel

Seeds are aromatic with a pleasant taste and widely used for flavouring and garnishing material in culinary preparation. It is also used for chewing. They are used against diseases affecting chest, spleen, kidney and cure of colic pain. Seeds are rich in protein (9.5%), minerals (13.4%) and also rich in vitamins such as A, thiamine, riboflavin niacin and C. The seeds contain essential oil which is used as flavouring agent in manufacture of pickles, cakes, perfumes, soap, liquors and cough drop.

26.14.1 Product

Fennel is processed for curry powder and volatile oil. Curry powder is prepared by mixing and grinding with other spices. Volatile oil is obtained by steam distillation or with solvent extraction. Fennel seeds contain 0.7–1.9% volatile oil. The chief constituents of oil is anethole (50–70%), and fennel seeds also contain 9–13% fixed oil. The volatile oil is used for manufacturing cordials and fennel water which is given to infants as medicine. I t is also used for scenting soap and flavouring material for cakes.

26.15 Fenugreek

Fenugreek is an annual herb. It is cultivated as leaf vegetable, condiment and as medicinal plant. The fresh tender leaves and stem are consumed as culinary vegetable and seeds are mainly used as spice for flavouring dishes. It has high medicinal value as carminative, tonic, emollient, diuretic, antidiabetic, demulcent and astringent. It prevents constipation, stimulates spleen and liver, and reduces blood level of glucose, total cholesterol and triglycerides. Fenugreek seeds are rich in protein, minerals fibres and vitamins. Seed contains steroid diosgenin (0.4–1.3%) which is used as an oral contraceptive.

26.15.1 Products

Fenugreek is processed into seed powder, curry powder, volatile oil and oleoresin or fixed oil.

26.15.1.1 Seed powder

Fenugreek is grown to release the flavour. The dried seed is milled or ground into powder to uniform mesh and packed curry powder.

26.15.1.2 Curry powder

Fenugreek is one of the principal odorous constituents of curry powder in India. It is prepared by grinding the mixture of several spices such as fenugreek, coriander, fennel, cumin, turmeric, chillies, garlic and black pepper. There are different types of mixes known as garam masala, meat masala, channa masala, etc. This is used for specific food preparations. Market for this is growing fast.

26.15.1.3 Volatile oil

Volatile oil content of the seed is very low (0.02%). This can be obtained with steam distillation or by solvent extraction.

26.15.1.4 Oleoresin

Seed contains 7% fixed oil. Oleoresin represents the overall flavour profile of the spice. The oleoresin is therefore designated as the true essence of the spice and can replace spice powders in food products without impairing any flavour characteristics.

Oleoresin is generally extracted or produced by solvent extraction. Solvent extraction yields oleoresin of fenugreek with strong maple like aroma and bitter taste. The bitterness is due to the presence of trigonelline and choline alkaloids. Steroid saponins isolated from the seeds are useful to reduce plasma cholesterol levels. Oleoresin obtained from fenugreek seed is used in preparation of imitation maple flavour, run flavours and as a flavouring agent in pharmacy. It is also used in seasoning for processed food such as meat, curry mixes, etc. Saponins and fibre of fenugreek are ingredients in health foods.

26.16 Anise

Anise is an annual herb. The crop is grown for its seed. Seeds are used for flavouring food, confectionaries, beverages and liquor industries. Seeds are rich in volatile oil which is used in perfumery, soaps and other toilet articles. Oil is also used in medicine as an aromatic carminative to relieve flatulence and as an ingredient of cough syrup. It is also used in preparation of gripe water. Oil has also an insecticidal and fungicidal property.

26.16.1 Product

26.16.1.1 Essential oil

Seeds are processed into essential oil. Essential oil is used in perfumery, soaps, other toilet articles, dental preparation and mouth washes. It is also used in medicine. The techniques used for preparation are as follows:

Mature/ripe seed → Cleaning → Crushing → Steam distillation → Oil (aniseed oil 2–3%) → Packaging → Storage

26.17 Ajwain

Ajwain is an annual plant. It has aromatic smell and pungent taste. It is widely used as a spice in curries. It has medicinal value as a stimulant, antispasmodic and carminative. It is also used as a households remedy for indigestion. Large quantities of ajwain are used in India.

26.17.1 Product

Ajwain is processed for two types of oil: (i) essential/volatile and (ii) non-volatile oil.

26.17.1.1 Essential oil

Oil of ajwain can be obtained by steam distillation which has importance in medicine on account of the presence of thymol. Ajwain essential oil is principal source of thymol. The techniques used for its extraction of oil are given below:

Clean and dried seeds → Crushing → Steam distillation → Oil (2.5–4.0%)

26.17.1.2 Thymol

Thymol can be separated from oil in the form of crystal which is sold as ajwain ka Phul/Sat ajwain. This is used in medicine as antiseptic in surgery and used in treatment of hook worm disease. Thymol is an excellent mouth wash and it is constituent of many tooth paste. It is also used in cholera. Thymol is obtained by treating ajwain oil with aqueous alkaline solution and regenerating thymol by extraction with ether or steam distillation. The other technique used for extraction of oil is by using a subcritical liquid carbon dioxide. This technique gives better quality of oil. The ground seed is extracted with liquid carbon dioxide at 60 bars pressure and temperature of 10–15°C. The yield of oil obtained at this temperature and thymol content both are higher than steam distillation technique. The ajwain seeds are rich in fatty oil. It contains 26% fatty oil.

26.18 Celery

Celery is an aromatic herbaceous plant. It is grown for its leaves and seed. Its seeds are used as spice. Seeds are rich in essential oil and oleoresin. Celery seed is used to flavour soups, salad, vegetable juices and Sauces, meat seasoning, chewing gums, ice cream and baked foods. In medicine, seeds are used for ailments such as rheumatism, arthritis, nervousness, asthma, liver disorders and induce menstruation. It is also stimulant and tonic. The oil is used as nerve tonic and in digestive mixture. In India, it is commercially important more for its seed, which have a good aroma and find ready export market.

26.18.1 Products

26.18.1.1 Leaf/stalk-based product

Dehydrated celery
Dehydrated celery products are (i) stalk dice (10 mm), (ii) leaf and stalk flakes, (iii) stalk and leaf granules and (iv) celery powder. These dehydrated products are utilized to flavour soups, canned tuna fish, stuffings and stewed, tomatoes and garnishing on potato salad and meat sauceses.

Celery stalk products
Celery stalk products are (i) celery flakes, which are, used in dry soup mixes, canned soups, sauces and stuffings; (ii) granulated/powdered celery which are used for canned and frozen sauces and dry mixes for soups; and (iii) cross-cut and diced celery which is used in canned and frozen soups and salad mixes.

Celery juice blends
Tomato juice blend from fresh celery leaves and tomatoes can be prepared which has good market.

Freeze-dried celery
Cross-cut slices of celery stalks are prepared in freeze-dried form. This form has better shape and crispness.

Celery herb (leaf oil)
Volatile oil from celery leaves can be extracted through distillation. This celery herb oil is different from seed oil. This oil can be used in food industry.

Celery-chaff oil
This can be also extracted by distillation. This oil has coarser odour and flavour than the celery seed oil.

26.18.1.2 Seed-based products

Seed oil
The celery seed oil is obtained by steam distillation. Seed gives 2–3% pale-yellow volatile oil with a persistent odour. This is valued both as fixative and ingredient of perfumes, pharmaceuticals preparation and medicines. The aroma of celery seed oil is spicy, slightly fatty, fruity, penetrating and very persistent.

Seed oleoresin
The oleoresin of celery seed is prepared by extraction of crushed dried celery seeds with suitable volatile solvents such as food-grade hexane or ethylene dichloride. It is filtered and desolventization under vacuum. The celery seed oleoresin is a green liquid having volatile oil content 9 mL/100 g. This is easier to handle in the preparation of tinctures and extracts. This is very popular product because of easy to store, no microbial and fungal contamination, no enzymatic problem and more stable than whole are ground spices.

Celery salt
Celery salt is prepared by mixing finely ground table salt (75%) with ground celery seed/celery seed oleoresin/ground dried celery stems (25%).

26.19 Asafoetida

Asafoetida is a dried latex or gum oleoresin obtained from underground rhizome/taproot or rootstocks of several species of *Ferula*. The various species of genus *Ferula* are distributed from Mediterranean region to central Asia, Europe and North Africa. In India, Arabian physicians introduced it. Asafoetida is extensively used in India for flavouring curries, sauces and pickles. It is considered stimulant, carminative and expectorant. It is used as uterine tonic and very useful remedy for asthma, whooping cough and chronic bronchitis, indigestion and colic. It is one of the most effective remedies for treating hysteria, flatulence and nervous disorders. It has antibiotic properties and inhibits the growth of microbes.

26.19.1 Products

26.19.1.1 Powder and tablets

The raw materials required are gum arabica, starch and asafoetida. Gum arabica and starch are available in India but asafoetida has to be imported from Afghanistan or Iran. Mixer and mill tableting machine are used for preparation, which are available indigenously.

Recipe
1 kg asafoetida, 1 kg starch, 3 kg gum arabica (powdered).

Preparation technique
Starch + Gum → Mixing (in mixer) → Slurry of asafoetida (prepared by soaking of asafoetida in water) → Mixing properly → Addition of more gum and mixing continued in the mixer → Compound asafoetida → Powdering in mill to obtain powder → Powder can be used for making tablets → Packing either in powder form or tablets → Storage

26.19.1.2 Volatile oil

The oil of asafoetida is obtained by the steam distillation of gum resin. Its yield varies from 10% to 17%. The chief constituents of oil are secondary butyl propenyl and disulphide that give a disagreeable odour. It is mainly used in flavouring and pharmaceutical industries.

26.19.1.3 Hingashtaka

This is used in ayurvedic system of medicine. The product contains asafoetida as one of the important ingredients.

26.20 Saffron

Saffron consists of tri-lobed and orange coloured stigma of *Crocus sativus* is one of the most expensive spices. Saffron plants when in full blossom (October-November in moonlight night) present a wonderful fascinating sight. It is used as food flavourant and colourant. The principal colouring agent in saffron is crocin glycoside. It is also famous for its medicinal properties. It is an important ingredient of Ayurvedic and Unani systems of medicine in India. This is used in exanthematous diseases, fever, enlargement of liver and spleen. It is stimulant, warm and dry in action and helps in urinary, digestive and uterine troubles. In Homeopathy, the mother tincture prepared from saffron and its useful dilution is used in various human disorders such as eyes, nose, head, throat, stomach, sleep problems and male and female organs. Its oil is used in external application in uterine sores and mixing with ghee is effective in diabetes.

26.20.1 Product

Saffron is a very expensive spice and not much attention has been given to the manufacture of any processed products. Saffron yields essential oil (1.4%) and fixed oil (13.4%).

Crocin is the chief colouring pigment in saffron. Saffron dried between 35°C and 50°C in solar dryer or in oven dryer give highest concentration (15–17%) of this pigment.

The main flavouring component of saffron is safranal, which is found 60% in the oil.

A product known as *Zarda* is manufactured for religious purpose in flavouring and colouring of foods and perfumery. Saffron is also utilized in preparation of various medicines.

The type of unit in spice-processing sectors are garlic paste and powder, onion powder, chillies powder and pickle, turmeric powder, ginger, soft drink, paste and powder, oil, candy and beer, ground spices and dried spices. Recent development in spices processing are essential oil, oleoresins, dehydrated green pepper and its powder, ginger oil, ginger beer liquid soluble spices, emulsions, encapsulated spices and natural colouring agents from turmeric, chilli and saffron. The antioxidant property of curcumin, piperine from pepper, zingiberene from ginger, anticholesterol and antidiabetic properties of garlic, onion and fenugreek can be exploited to brighten the future of Indian spice industry.

27

Sugarcane products and processing technique

Sugarcane is the main source of sugar and holds a prominent position as a cash crop. Sugar has high potential for export. Sugarcane products are the source of instant energy.

27.1 Products

Sugarcane is processed for sugar, gur, khandsari, juice and molasses. Molasses is used for alcohol and alcoholic drink such as rum. It is also used in various gur-based nutritive products and fortified foods.

27.1.1 Sugarcane juice (beverage)

Preparation technique
Sugarcane (fresh juicy and mature) → Juice extraction with the help of cane crusher (horizontal power crusher) → Clarification (with the help of deola at juice pH 6.0) → Filtering → Addition of preservative additives and flavours in required quantity → Incubation at desired temperature for about a week → Bottling (200 mL capacity) → Crown corking → Storing/marketing

27.1.2 Alcoholic beverage (rum)

Rum is a spirit distilled from molasses.

Preparation technique
Molasses → Making a mash of molasses → Addition of natural yeast plus special strains → Fermentation of sugar in molasses → Alcohol mash → Distillation (in coffee stills) → White rum

Dark rum can also be prepared. Dark rum is coloured because of highly refined sugarcane syrup of caramel is added.

27.1.3 Jaggery (gur)

Jaggery is a pure, wholesome, unrefined whole sugar. This is a traditional sweetener and snack food of India which is nutritionally superior to refined sugar. Jaggery is the medicinal sugar. It purifies the blood, prevents rheumatic afflictions and disorder of bile. Jaggery of good quality is in demand not only in India but also in abroad. Jaggery is prepared from sugarcane juice and is very widely used in daily food preparation. The demand for jaggery is steadily growing many folds in the urban and rural areas. There are several applications of jaggery and market for jaggery is round the year. Jaggery produced in different parts of the country has different physical and chemical characteristics. Jaggery is considered as a complete food due to having nutritional and medicinal values. Jaggery contains sucrose 72–78 g, fructose 1.5–7.0 g, glucose 1.5–7.0 g, calcium 40–100 g, iron 10–13 g, vitamin A 3.8 mg, vitamin B_1 0.01 mg, vitamin B_2 0.06 mg, vitamin B_6 0.01 mg, vitamin C 7 mg, vitamin E 111 mg, protein 280 mg, water 1.5–7.0 mg, calories 312 mg/100 g of jaggery.

The specification for cane jaggery (grade I) is – sucrose 80%, reducing sugar 10%, moisture 5%, water insoluble matter 1.5%, sulphated ash 3.5%, sulphur dioxide 50 ppm, total sugar as invert sugar 90%. Jaggery is of various types such as solid jaggery, powder jaggery and liquid jaggery.

27.1.3.1 Solid jaggery

Preparation technique

Fresh sugarcane → Cleaning of cane (dry leaves, trashes, green tops, roots, mud, clods, etc.) → Extraction of juice (crushing of cane with horizontal power crusher gives 60–70% juice) → Juice settling (in juice settling tank covered with thick layered cloth and allowed to remain for 1 h) → Filtration (some impurities such as ions, colloid, dirt of soil, waste, wax, etc.) with 1 mm cloth/wire mesh sieve → Boiling (in pan) and stirring → Herbal clarification (deola/okra juice) → Removal of brownish foam come at the top till golden colour of jaggery is obtained → Boiling up to desired thickness → Moulding frame → Natural cooling and drying → Formation of moulded jaggery cubes → Packing in polyester–polyethylene packets (250 g) → Storing (bin)/marketing

27.1.3.2 Liquid jaggery

Liquid jaggery locally known as pak. It is a semi-solid syrup-like product. Liquid jaggery is highly nutritious, easily digestible and increases palatability of food. It is rich in various minerals and it can be used confectionary. It has also medicinal properties. Liquid jaggery contains water 30–35%, sucrose 40–60% invert sugar 15–25%, calcium 0.3%, iron 8.5–10 mg/100 mg, protein 0.1–0.15 mg/100 mg, vitamin B_1 14 mg/100 mg.

Preparation technique

Mature fresh sugarcane → Cleaning → Crushing as early as possible (horizontal-three roller crusher) → Juice settling → Filtration of impurities (two-stage filtration using 2 and 0.5 mm screens) → Settling of juice for removal of sediments (tank with taper bottom and two-valve system) → Clean juice → Boiling of juice → Addition of filtrants (lime 150–200 g/1000 L of juice and okra plant mucilage 2 kg/1000 L of juice) → Removal of black scum → Liquid jaggery stage (removal of golden scum and addition of edible oil 150 mL/1000 L) → Settling for 9 days and addition of citric acid 0.04% + KMS 0.01% → Filtration (with nylon two-layer filter) → Liquid jaggery → Boiling (45–50°C) → Bottling (clean and sterilized glass bottles) → Capping/sealing airtight → Storing/marketing

27.1.3.3 Powder/granular jaggery

Granular jaggery has longer shelf life up to 3 years. It has medicinal and nutritive value and fetches higher price. It has also good scope for export.

Preparation technique

Mature sugarcane → Cleaning → Crushing (crusher) → Juice → Settling in tanks (impurities) → Filtration of juice → Keeping in boiling pan 1000 L capacity → Addition of lime and oil spray → Removal of scum at 80–85°C → Liquid → Cooling pan → Cold thick slurry → Rubbing with wooden scrappers → Powder jaggery → Natural drying → Packing → Storing/marketing

27.1.3.4 Table sugar

Sugar has 99.5 g sucrose, 0.05 g total minerals 0.2–0.05 g moisture and caloric value 398/100 g of sugar. Sugar is prepared from granular jaggery. The technique for preparation of granular jaggery is mentioned above. The granular jaggery is further refined to make table sugar of various grades.

27.1.3.5 Value-added products of jaggery

Chocolate, chikki, patti with ramdana and puffed rice, gajak, rewari, til laddoo, etc., are the jaggery-based value-added products. These are very popular in rural as well as in urban areas.

Jaggery chocolate

Ingredients

Cocoa powder 19%, skim milk powder 30%, butter 20%, soya flour 30%.

Preparation technique

Freshly prepared jaggery (before setting) → Putting into pre-heated pan → Addition of ingredients → Mixing up to desired time → Preparation of chocolate mould (by applying a thin layer of melted butter on its surface) → Pouring of chocolate mix in the mould → Cooling till it sets → Removing chocolate from mould and putting on a aluminium foil → Natural drying of chocolate up to 24 h (from the time of pouring in the mould) → Wrapping of chocolate after natural drying in aluminium foil → Packing in polythene bag → Sealing → Storage/marketing.

Various gur-based nutritive product and fortified food and alcoholic drink are the new development in sugarcane processing.

28

Tea, coffee and cocoa beverage

28.1 Tea

Tea is the most important refreshing, drink in many countries. India tops the list in production and export of tea. Fresh tea leaves contain polyphenols (22.2%), caffeine (4.3%), protein (17.2%), fibre (27%), starch (0.5%) and ash (5.6%). Fresh tea leaves also contain little carotene, riboflavin, niacin, pantothenic acid and ascorbic acid. It is rich in sodium (44 mg/100 g) and potassium (2160 mg/100 g).

28.1.1 Tea processing

28.1.1.1 Black tea

Steps involved in manufacture of black tea are as follows:

Withering or drying till moisture content is 40% → Rolling with rolling machine or curled machine → Fermentation at 21–27°C for 2 h → Drying of fermented leaves at 87.7–93°C which contain 3–4% moisture → Sorting and grading into three grades on the basis of size that is orange pekoe - long thin leaves, pekoe – small tightly rolled, souchong – largest and coarsest → Blending of different tea to produce uniform product → Packing of blended tea in poly wood boxes lined with aluminium foil and parchment paper

28.1.1.2 Green tea

Steps involved in manufacturing green tea are as follows:

Steaming for preventing colour by inactivating the enzyme → Rolling → Drying → Packing

The beverage prepared from green tea has green yellow colour, bitter and astringent. It has higher caffeine and little aroma and flavour than black tea.

In preparing hot-water-soluble instant tea, the fermented tea leaves are extracted with hot water, centrifuged and dried in drum drier.

In preparing cold-water-instant tea, the aqueous extract is cooled to 5°C, the separated caffeine–polyphenol compound is removed by centrifugation and then dried.

28.1.2 Tea beverage preparation

A good cup of tea is sparkling clear and has maximum flavour with minimum polyphenol compounds which produce bitterness. The technique for preparation of tea beverage is as follows:

Water should be freshly boiled at 85°C in China glass or enamelled ware. Avoid metallic pot which gives metallic flavour → Add amount of tea generally one teaspoonful for 150 mL water at boiling in pot (one cup tea). Cover the pot with lid → Steeping period is about 3 min. This gives stimulating beverage which is not astringent

A very easy method for making tea is the tea bag method. In this method, water at boiling temperature is pored over tea bag or cheese cloths or paper bag. Tea bag is allowed in hot water till desired strength is obtained. Milk or lemon may be added to the tea extract for body and flavour and sugar for taste.

28.2 Coffee

Coffee produces green berries which turn red on ripe. Ripe berries are picked for processing which is used for coffee beverage. The most importance substance present in coffee is caffeine which is responsible for stimulating effect of the drink. Caffeine content varies from species to species. *Coffea arabica* contains 1–1.2% caffeine, *C. robusta* contains 1.5–2.5% caffeine and *C. liberica* contains 1.4–1.6% caffeine.

The caffeine content of a cup of coffee (150 mL) is about 100 mg. Several organic acid, volatile compounds and polyphenol substances are found in coffee. Coffee is rich in sodium (74 mg/100 g) and potassium (2020 mg/100 g). A cup of coffee has more nutritional value than a cup of tea due to more milk contents, resulting more protein and minerals.

28.2.1 Coffee processing

Coffee processing consists of removing the skin, pulp parchment and silvery skin in drier. It is the curing process that prepares the coffee beans for market. There are two methods of curing that is dry and wet methods. The steps involved in these methods of curing are as follows.

28.2.1.1 Dry methods

Coffee berries → Sundried → Outer skin and parchment dry up → Pounded and hulled → Polishing by rubbing the berries against each other and removing the outer silvery skin

28.2.1.2 Wet method

Coffee berries → Pulp removal by pulper → Mucilage removal by fermentation or added enzyme (ultrazyn) → Seeds are dried

28.2.1.3 Coffee powder

The process involved in manufacture of coffee powder is as follows:

Cured berries → Roasting of bean → Grinding of roasted beans to powder → Blending (pure coffee and French coffee containing chicory) → Packing (gas packing under CO_2 or vacuum packing)

28.2.1.4 Coffee beverage preparation

There are various methods of preparing coffee such as filtration, vacuum coffee maker, percolator and steeping. The merits and limitations of these methods are given in Table 28.1.

Table 28.1. Methods of coffee preparation.

Methods	Flavour	Tannins	Limitation
Filtration	Retains well	Extract less	Decoction may not be hot
Vacuum coffee maker	Retains well	Extraction is more	More bitter
Percolator	Loss of flavour	Extraction is more	More bitter
Steeping	Retains best	Extraction less	Flavour extraction may not be complete

28.2.2 Espresso coffee

Coffee is prepared by special machine which brew the beverage a cup at a time. It is prepared by a brewing finely ground coffee with a mixture of steam and hot water.

28.2.3 Soluble coffee

It is spray dried strong coffee brew or it can be made by freeze drying. The product is inferior in taste and aroma as compared to freshly prepared brew. Soluble coffee is packed in water proof and airtight container or aluminium foil.

28.2.4 Decaffeinated coffee

Caffeine is not tolerated by some people due to adverse physiological effects; hence, it is avoided by using decaffeinated coffee. Caffeine is removed from beans by chemical process.

28.3 Cocoa

Cocoa is made by grinding the seeds of pods of cacao tree. Cocoa contains a substance called theobromine which has stimulating properties like caffeine. Cocoa has higher protein content than coffee and tea (without milk). Cocoa gives pleasant flavour to milk. Cocoa contains protein (11.5%), starch (9%), cocoa butter (54%) and water (5%). Cocoa also contains theobromine, caffeine and aromatic oils. It also contains sodium (6 mg/100 g) and potassium 1522 mg/100 g.

28.3.1 Processing

Steps involved in preparation of cocoa beans and manufactures of powder are as follows:

28.3.1.1 Beans

Fermentation of beans for 3–5 days or mass temperature reaches to 45–60°C → Curing/drying to moisture content of 5–8%) → Cleaning and roasting at 210°C for 10–15 min

28.3.1.2 Powder

Breaking, winnowing and shell removal → Nib/germs separation → Germ-free nib → Milling → Cacao mass → Alkalization → Removal of excess moisture → Fat pressing → Press cake-cocoa butter → Breaking → Grinding → Sifting through fine silk screens → Fine cocoa powder

28.3.1.3 Preparation of cocoa beverage

Cocoa contains high amount of starch; hence, it will lumps if directly put into hot liquids such as hot water or milk. It should be mixed with small amount of cold liquid before combining with other ingredients. Cocoa is then heated to boiling and held at this temperature to gelatinize the starch. This gives body and flavour to the beverage and reduces the amount of sediments which settles from the beverage. The sugar required is added to give flavour to the cocoa. Its amount is little higher than in tea and coffee.

29
Milk products and processing technique

Milk is the most complete of all foods. It is an excellent source of protein, fat, carbohydrates, minerals and vitamins. It is universally regarded as ideal food for nourishing infants and young children. This is also good supplementary food in the diet of adults. Milk and milk products are now the second largest contributor to the agriculture produce of the country. Indian dairy industry has shown remarkable growth over the past few decades. Dairy development has been recognized as the modern India's most successful development programme. About 45% milk produced is consumed as liquid milk and remaining 55% is converted into wide range of dairy products.

29.1 Products

A variety of products can be prepared from milk. These are packed and branded pasteurized milk, chenna, cheese, paneer, cream, ice-cream, ghee, yoghurt, khoa, butter, milk powder, butter milk (packed), condensed milk, evaporated milk, infant milk food, milk toffee, etc. Whole milk powder, skimmed milk powder, condensed milk, infant milk food and confectionary-based products have better export potential.

29.1.1 Pasteurized milk

There are two methods of pasteurization: high temperature short time (HTST) system (80–85°C) and ultra high temperature (UHT) sterilization system (135°C for 2 s). UHT sterilization system is more popularly adopted for longer preservation of milk. The technique for pasteurization of milk is as follows:

Normal raw milk of good quality → Heating to 135°C for 2 s → Chilling (4°C) → Packing in pouches (aseptic polythene) → Marketing

29.1.2 Chenna

Chenna is a solid product obtained by the acid coagulation of milk at its boiling point followed by subsequent removal of whey. The technique for the preparation of chenna is as follows:

Cow milk → Boiling → Removal from fire → Addition of coagulant (old sour, chenna) → Gentle stirring till the clear coagulation is formed → Separation of coagulation mass through straining with muslin cloth → Hanging cloth containing of chenna for draining of whey → Cooling → Shaping of chenna → Packing → Marketing

29.1.3 Cheese

Cheese is a product made from curd obtained from milk by coagulating the casein (milk protein) with help of rennet enzymes in the presence of lactic acid produced by added microorganisms from which part of the moisture has been removed by cutting, cooking and pressing. Cheeses are of various types such as soft, semi–soft, hard, very hard, whey cheese and processed cheese. Among all cheese, cheddar cheese is the most popular. The techniques for preparation of various types of cheese are as follows.

29.1.3.1 Cheddar cheese

Milk (high grade preferably cow milk) → Filtration/clarification → Standardization (adjustment of fat and casein ratio 1:0.7) → Pasteurization → Addition of calcium chloride (0.1–0.3%) for compensation of loss of soluble calcium →Addition of starter (starter contains *Streptococcus lactis*/*S. cremoris*) → Mixing → Addition of colour (extracted from annatto seed) 30 mL/1000 L of milk → Addition of rennet (preparation obtained from young calf stomach) 15–20 mL/100 L of milk → Setting the curd → Cutting the curds into cubes → Cooking the curd gently (37–39°C) at the rate of 1°C in every 4 min → Draining of whey (curd cubes attained firmness) → Cheddaring (matting for 4–5 min and matted curd cut into small slabs) → Acidity of whey reaches to 0.5% → Milling (cheese mill-cutting the curd blocks into small pieces) → Salting (1–2% common powder salt on milled cheese for removal of water and improving quality → Pressing → Drying (kept in drying room for few days at 12–16°C to form rind → Paraffining/dipping in hot paraffin for few seconds (reducing loss of moisture, mould growth and insect pest) → Ripening/curing (storage of cheese for 2 months at 0–16°C) → Packing → Marketing

29.1.3.2 Soft cheese (sweet cheese)

Cow milk → Standardization (2.0–2.5% fat) → Heating to 71°C for 5 min → Addition of $CaCl_2$ culture, citric acid rennet → Incubation for setting of curd → Cutting of curd → Draining of whey and filling into cloth bag → Soft cheese (base material) → Addition of sugar and essence → Grinding and kneading → Packaging (100 g in butter paper) → Storing at 2–4°C

29.1.3.3 Processed cheese

Milk→ Coagulation of casein (milk protein) with the help of rennet (enzyme) in the presence of lactic acid produced by added microbial culture → Curd → Cutting into pieces → Cooking to remove part of the moisture → Pressing to form into block → Ripening (holding for sometime in cold storage) → Cheddar cheese → Converting into processed cheese by blending old and young cheddar cheese in a desired ratio → Cooking it in the cheese cattle with salt, etc. → Homogenous mass/processed cheese → Packing → Storing/ marketing

29.1.3.4 Cottage cheese

Milk → Bringing to setting temperature → Addition of starter → Coagulation → Cutting of curd (as it becomes jelly like and showing separation of clear whey) into cubes about 3–3.5 cm size with both horizontal and vertical cheddar cheese knives → Packing

29.1.4 Paneer

Paneer is an acid coagulated milk product from which moisture is removed by pressing. Paneer shall contain not more than 70% moisture and not less than 50% fat in dry matter. Buffalo milk is generally used due to its high total solid (TS) contents. The technique for preparation of paneer is as follows:

Milk → Standardization to 5.5–6.0% fat → Heating 85–90°C for 5 min → Cooling at 70°C → Addition of 1% citric acid solution (heated to 70°C) and stirring → Separation of clear greenish whey (after complete coagulation allow the curd to settle down) → Draining whey and scooping the curd with cheese cloth → Wrapping of curd in cloth and pressing about 10 min → Removing paneer → Immersing in water for cooling and moisture absorption → Transferring paneer into chilled water to bring the temperature 5–10°C → Removing chilled paneer from water and draining till removal of all water → Cutting into convenient sizes → Packing → Storing at refrigeration temperature/marketing

29.1.5 Cream

Cream is a fat-rich portion of milk. Cream should contain a minimum of 25% fat. Cream can be separated from milk by centrifugal or gravity method. The technique for centrifugal separation of cream is as follows:

Milk → Putting in bowl of cream separator → Subjected to centrifugal force (both serum and fat) → Skimmed milk is forced to periphery and fat portion moves towards centre → Both cream and skimmed milk which form vertical walls within the bowl → Separated by separate outlets

29.1.6 Butter

Butter is a fat concentrate which is obtained by churning cream, milk or curd. Butter may be table butter and white butter. Table butter shall contain not less than 80% by weight of milk fat, not more than 1.5% by weight of curd and not more than 3% by weight of common salt. White butter shall contain not less than 76% by weight of milk fat, not more than 1.5% by weight of curd. It has no salt and colour. The technique for preparation of table butter is as follows:

Reception of cream (separation of cream) → Neutralization of cream (partial reduction in acidity of sour cream) → Standardization of cream (adjustment of fat level in cream 30–35% in winter and 35–40% in summer) → Pasteurization of cream (HTST method 95–100°C for 15 s) → Cooling (5–10°C) → Ripening (fermentation of cream with the help of desirable starter culture) → Ageing (at least 4 h) → Churning and addition of colour and salt → Butter with 80% fat, 16% moisture, 2.5% salt and curd not more than 1.5% → Packing (boxes and tubs for bulk and 25, 50, 100 and 250 g pats for retailing) → Storage (–23°C to –29°C) → Marketing

29.1.7 Ghee

Ghee is a clarified butter prepared mainly from desi butter or cream obtained from milk of cow or buffalo. The technique for preparation of ghee is as follows:

Butter → Heating (80–85°C for 30 min in ghee boiler) → Separation into three layers → Bottom layer of butter milk 60–70% solid-not-fat (SNF) and 80% moisture removed → Top layer of floating denatured curd particles and middle layer of fat both are heated (110–120°C) → Ghee with mild flavour → Packing → Storage/marketing

29.1.8 Khoa

This is a partially desiccated whole milk prepared in open pans through the direct application of heat. The milk content of khoa should not be less than 20% of the finished product. In general, buffalo milk is preferred for khoa due to its high fat and TS content. The technique for preparation of khoa is as follows:

Milk → Boiling (in any iron container) → Stirring continuously while boiling → Scrapping of milk from all parts of the pan in contact → Vigorous stirring and desiccation are continued until the viscous product reaches a pasty consistency and start to dry up → Judging of end point (when it shows signs of leaving the sides of the pan and sticking together) → Removing the pan off the fire and working the content up and down→ Khoa (finished product is in the form of circular pats of uniform size or balls) → Marketing

29.1.9 Curd

Dahi is a fermented milk product obtained from pasteurized or boiled milk by souring with the help of lactic acid producing bacteria. The technique for preparation of curd is as follows:

Milk → Standardization to desired fat and SNF content (to avoid variation in composition) → Pasteurization (80–90°C for 15–30 min) → Cooling (22–25°C) → Inoculation with 1–3% of starter culture → Feeling in suitable containers of required capacity → Incubation (22–25°C for 16 h) → Acidity reaches 0.6–0.7% → Formation of curd → Cooling of curd (<12°C) → Storing in cold room (about 5°C)

29.1.10 Buttermilk

Buttermilk is a by-product of butter left after churning. Cultured buttermilk is prepared by culturing pasteurized skimmed milk with lactic acid and aroma producing microorganism. The main ingredient is skimmed milk or homogenized, low-fat milk having fat content of about 1.7%. The technique for the preparation of buttermilk is as follows:

Skimmed milk → Pasteurization → Cooling (22°C) → Inoculation with starter culture → Incubation at 21–24°C for 14–16 h (to ensure balanced growth of strains which produce acid and aroma-diacetyl flavour) → Agitation of the acid curd at 4.6–4.7 and titrable acidity of 0.8% as lactic acid gently and smooth → Viscous buttermilk → Cooling at 5°C → Packing → Marketing cold within 24 h

29.1.11 Shrikhand

This is a fermented milk product used as desert in India. The technique for preparation of shrikhand is as follows:

Milk → Boiling → Cooling → Inoculation with lactic acid bacteria or portion of previous day's curd → Curd → Draining (by hanging in musclin bag for 6–8 h) → Semi-solid mass (chakka) → Mixing with 45–50% sugar → Adding flavouring substance cardamom, saffron → Garnishing with nuts → Storing under refrigeration for a month or at room temperature 2–3 days/ marketing

29.1.12 Ice-cream

This is a frozen dairy product prepared by blending and processing of cream and other milk products with sugar and flavour. Ice-cream shall contain not less than 10% milk fat and 3.5% protein and 36% TSs. If ice-cream contains fruit/nuts, the content of milk fat may be reduced but not less than 8% by weight. The technique for preparation of ice-cream is as follows:

Ingredients (cream, milk products, sugar, colour, emulsifiers, stabilizers) → Calculation of amount of ingredients → Mixing of ingredients (addition of liquid materials such as cream, milk other liquid milk materials, solids as dry milk, gelatine, etc., start heating addition of sugar when mix is 50–55°C) → Pasteurizing the mix (70°C for 30 min) → Homogenizing the mix (through homogenizer, 2000–3500 psi) → Cooling the mix (0–5°C) → Aging the mix (held at low temperature for 4–24 h) → Freezing by batch method (about –4°C and 35–40% water of the mix is frozen) or continuous freezer (–6°C and 50–55% of the water of the mix is frozen) → Packing of ice-cream (carry home package-plastic cylindrical container with recloseable lid. Retail ice-cream may be packed in cups, sticks/bars → Hardening (in cold rooms or cabinets at –23°C to 29°C and held at this temperature until marketing) → Storage of ice-cream (excessive storage should be avoided) → Marketing

29.1.13 Condensed milk

Condensed milk is commonly used for full cream sweetened condensed milk. It is preserved by the addition of sugar. Condensed milk shall contain not less than 9% fat, 31% total milk solid and 40% cane sugar. The technique for preparation of condensed milk is as follows:

Reception of milk → Filtration/clarification (38–40°C) → Standardization (for desired fat and SNF ratio) → Fore warning (115–118°C) and no holding → Addition of sugar → Condensing (in vacuum pan) → Cooling (30°C) and Crystallization (seeded with 0.1–0.3% powdered lactose for forced crystallization) → Stirring and slow cooling to 15°C in an hour → Packing → Storage/marketing

29.1.14 Evaporated milk

Evaporated milk is commonly used for unsweetened condensed milk. It is preserved by heat sterilization. Evaporated milk shall contain not less than 8% fat and 25% milk solids. The technique for preparation of evaporated milk is as follows:

Reception of milk → Filtration/clarification at 38–40°C → Standardization (for desired fat and SNF ratio) → Fore warning (115–118°C) no holding

→ Condensing → Homogenization (applying pressure of 2000 psi in first stage and 500 psi in second stage) → Cooling (7°C) → Pilot sterilization test (for determining the amount of chemical stabilizer which has to be added) → Packaging (cans) → Sealing → Sterilization (116–118°C) for 15 min → Cooling (27–32°C) within 15 min → Shaking (to break down in curd which have formed during sterilization) → Storage (5–15°C) → Marketing

29.1.15 Milk powder/dried milk

Milk powder is obtained by the removal of water from milk by heat to produce solid containing 5% or less moisture. The types of milk used for drying are whole milk, skimmed milk or partially skimmed milk. While milk powder shall contains not more than 5% moisture and not less than 26% fat. Skimmed milk powder shall contain not more than 5% moisture and not less than 15% fat. Partially skimmed milk powder shall contain not more than 5% moisture and fat contain shall be between 16% and 24%. There are two methods of drying milk: (1) drum drying/roller drying and (2) spray drying. The technique for preparation of milk powder with drum drier is as follows:

Concentrated milk (about 18% TSs) → Pumping in reservoir between the two drums of roller (drying equipments) → Operating (Speed of drums are adjustable and to control the moisture content of milk powder. Average speed ranges between 12 and 20 rpm) → Formation of thin sheet of dry milk and scrapping from each drum (product is in contact with drum for about 3 s at 150°C) → Transporting to packaging station → Further reduction in particle size in a hammer mill → Sieving of ground particles through mess → Packing skimmed milk in 25–50 kg craft paper bag with plastic liner. In case of whole milk powder, gas pack in metal container. A mixture of nitrogen and carbon dioxide is used for gas packing

29.1.16 Infant milk food

Infant milk food has been formulated to meet the feeding requirements of infants who do not get sufficient feeding from their mother. Infant milk food refers to the material prepared by drying (spray drying or roller drying) of cow or buffalo or mixture of both. The milk can be modified by partial removal of fat and by the addition of various carbohydrates (sucrose, dextrose and dextrins, maltose and lactose), salts (phosphate and citrates, vitamins (A, B group, C and D) and minerals (calcium and iron infant milk foods is white with greenish ting to light cream in colour and is uniform in appearance). It should be free from any non-milk fat and extraneous matter which can be harmful to human health. The method used for manufacturing of infant milk is either by drum drying or by spray drying. This is manufactured and packed under hygienic condition.

29.1.17 Milk toffee

Milk toffee is a confectionery item which has mass consumption among children and youngsters. The ingredients required for milk toffee are milk, sodium hydrosulphite, liquid glucose, salts, colour and essence. The technique for preparation of milk toffee is as follows:

Preparation of sugar syrup → Addition of milk → Addition of sodium hydrosulphite → Boiling of mixture → Mixing of liquid glucose and salt → Stirring of boil material continuously to avoid formation of paste → Addition of colour and essence if required → Pouring of mixture in roller frames → Cooling → Cutting according to desired sizes/individual pieces → Packing → Storage/marketing

29.1.18 Milk-based beverages

Milk-based beverages are flovoured milk, milkshake, miltone and eggnog. Flavoured milk may contain cardamom, pista, chocolate, edible colours and essence. Milkshake is prepared by adding the pulp of fruit such as banana and mango. Miltone is a blend of equal part of milk and an emulsion of protein from groundnut. In eggnog, milk can be mixed with whole egg are only egg yolk to make a nourishing beverage with smooth creamy consistency.

The kinds of unit which have come up in milk processing in the country are packed and branded pasteurized milk, ghee, curd, khoa, butter, milk powder, chenna, cheese, paneer, ice-cream, cream packaged buttermilk and yoghurt. The new developments in milk processing are UHT processing of milk which is the most effective treatment to increase shelf life of milk at room temperature. The dairy industry has been tremendously transformed with the advancement of UHT processing. Continuous making plant for indigenous products like khoa, gulabjamun, ghee, chenna and paneer is the recent remarkable break through in processing of indigenous products. These innovations enable organized sector to manufacture and market indigenous milk product on industrial scale which can have a far reaching impact on dairy industry as well as social and economic condition of milk produce in the country. Bio-technological application in dairy processing improved dairy state culture, dairy enzyme, accelerated cheese ripening, efficient whey utilization and biological stabilization of dairy wastes. Application of membrane in processing of milk product is a recent break through but it is very expensive.

30

Meat and poultry products and processing technique

Meat provides high-quality protein of biological value. It is also a fair source of iron, phosphorus and vitamin A, riboflavin, thiamine and niacin. Meat industry constitutes beef and veal (cow family), buffalo, pig (pork), sheep and goat (chevon) meat, poultry, fish and value-added products.

30.1 Meat products

Meat of different food animals are chevon (goat), mutton (meat of mature sheep), lamb meat of young animals of ovine species less than 12 months of age and pork (meat of pig). These meat can be sold as fresh meat (cut pieces), frozen meat and can be converted into value-added products such as sausages, pickles, etc.

30.1.1 Frozen meat

The technique for preparation of frozen meat is as follows:

Quality livestock → Slaughtering → Deskinning → Cleaning→ Deboning → Grading → Freezing (–40°C) → Packing in corrugated boxes → Dispatching

30.1.2 Sausages

Sausages is a fermented food, usually made from ground meat, animal, fat, salt and spices (sometimes with other ingredients such as herbs), and typically packed in a casing. The technique for preparation of sausages is as follows:

Chopped meat (goat) → Chilling/partial freezing → Comminuting in meat grinder/cutter → Grind meat → Addition of potassium nitrite (for development of colour) → Curing with 2.4–3% of sodium chloride (curing salt brings the initial water activity to about 0.95 which inhabits the growth of undesired microflora and favours the growth of lactobacilli) → Blending with spices (pepper, garlic, mace, cardamom and mustard powder) → Filling into casing at low temperature 2°C → Casings should allow water evaporation → Fermentation (in ripening chamber at 22–26°C) → Addition of starter culture for lactic acid bacteria in sausages fermentation to reduce the fermentation time and improve quality → Exposed to smoking (anti-microbial activity) → Packing → Marketing

30.1.3 Pickles

Ingredients

Mutton 1 kg, ginger 220 g, onion 225 g, garlic 100 g, vinegar 350 mL, mustard oil 350 mL, cloves (no.) 10, cardamom (no.) 6, nutmeg 2 g, salt 5 g, chili powder 5 g, ground mace 2.5 g, mango powder (Amchur) 5 g. The technique for preparation of make pickle is as follows:

Meat pieces → Cut into 3–4 cubes → Simmering in large sauce pan without adding water till the liquid from the meat dries up → Keep on one side → Grind onion, garlic and ginger into paste → Fry the paste in oil till brown → Add meat pieces and mix well → Frying → Add 150 mL vinegar and all the remaining spices → Cooking for 5 min with stirring → Remove from fire, pour remaining vinegar and cool → Fill into jars → Capping airtight → Keep for a week (before use) → Storing/use

Meat processing in India has become a thrust sector for Indian industry. With growing urbanization and increasing quality consciousness, the market for scientifically produced meat products is expected to grow rapidly. There is also a growing demand for ready to eat and semi-processed meat products on account of changing lifestyles. This has also good scope for export to neighbouring countries particularly in the Middle East.

The production of value-added meat and meat products are steadily increasing. The meat-based processing units are frozen meat, sausages, luncheon, ham bacon, pickle, etc. The new development in meat processing are marinating, treatment with phosphate solution to increase water holding capacity, massaging and tumbling, hot boning, tenderization (electrical stimulation of carcasses) and particle size reduction techniques such as mincing and chopping. Integrated meat plants comprising of mechanized slaughter house, meat plant and rendering plant has been developed for export purposes.

30.2 Poultry products

Poultry forming ensures quick return; hence, poultry industry grows rapidly both for poultry meat and for eggs. There is good market for hygienically produced meat and poultry products. The egg is one of the most nutritious natural products. It is rich in protein, vitamins and minerals. Eggs are considered a complete protein because they contain all nine essential amino acids (valine, leucine, isoleucine, threonine, histidine, tryptophan, phenylalanine, methionine and lysine). Modern poultry processing plants in the country are producing dressed frozen chicken and cut parts.

30.2.1 Products

Poultry birds are dressed, frozen, canned and processed into sausages, pickles, etc. Eggs are processed into egg powder and albumen flakes. The techniques for preparation of dressed chicken and various products are as follows.

30.2.1.1 Dressed chicken

Poultry birds → Starving for about 12 h → Slaughtering → Bleeding properly → Scalding → Defeathering → Cleaning → Singeing → Venting → Eviscerating → Dressed chicken → Marketing directly

30.2.1.2 Frozen chicken

Poultry birds → Slaughtering → Bleeding properly → Scalding → Defeathering → Singeing → Venting → Eviscerating → Dressed chicken → Packing → Freezing

30.2.1.3 Canned chicken

Poultry birds → Slaughtering → Cleaning (defeathering and removal of lungs, kidneys, head and other unwanted parts) → Washing → Cutting into required sizes → Packing into sterilized cans with 3–5% brine/curried vegetables → Exhausting (15 min at 60–65°C) → Sealing of cans airtight → Processing (in retort at a pressure of 10–15 pounds for about 45 min) → Cooling of cans to room temperature → Labelling → Storage/marketing

30.2.1.4 Dehydrated chicken

Poultry meat → Cutting into pieces → Yeast in cooking for 30 min → Precooked poultry meat → Passing through meat chopper → Chopped meat → dried in a continuous drier (65–71°C for 3 h) up to 4–5% moisture → Dried poultry meat is compressed → Packed in cans

30.2.1.5 Pickles

Ingredients

Chicken 1 kg, mustard oil 1.5 kg, ginger ground 100 g, onion ground 400 g, garlic ground 200 g, turmeric powder 5 g, vinegar 80 mL, sugar (as per taste), salt 5 g, green chillies (no.) 15, chili powder 10 g. The technique for preparation of chicken pickle is as follows:

Dressed chicken → Cut into small pieces → Even size and remove bones completely → Cleaning/washing properly → Boiling in little water with little salt → Keep a side → Heat one-third of mustard oil → Addition of ginger, onion, garlic, chillies, sugar and salt → Addition of chicken → Frying on low heat till it become tender → Cooling → Mix with vinegar → Filling into cleaned jar → Pouring rest of the oil heated and cooled so that oil tops the pickle at least 2 cm → Capping the jar → Storing about 7–10 days → Using/ marketing

30.2.1.6 Sausages

Poultry meat → Chopped → Chilling/partial freezing → Comminuting in meat grinder/cutter → Grind meat → Addition of potassium nitrite (for development of colour) → Curing with 2.4–3% of sodium chloride (curing salt brings the initial water activity to about 0.95 which inhabits the growth of undesired microflora and flavours the growth of lactobacilli) → Blending with spices (pepper, garlic, mace, cardamom and mustard powder) → Filling into casing at low temperature 2°C → Casings should allow water evaporation → Fermentation (in ripening chamber at 2226°C) → Addition of starter culture for lactic acid bacteria in sausages fermentation to reduce the fermentation time and improve quality → Exposed to smoking (anti-microbial activity) → Packing → Marketing

30.2.1.7 Egg powder

Eggs → Breaking → Removal of shells → Filtering of mixture → Storing in storage tank where it is cooled down to 4°C (by means of chilled water jackets) → Drying (tubular heater) at 65°C for 8–10 min → Filtering → Passing to high pressure spray drier with the help of high pressure pump → Powder → Packing in poly-lined boxes → Storage/marketing

30.2.1.8 Egg albumen flakes

Eggs → Breaking manually/mechanically → Separation of white and yolk → Fermentation of egg white to bring down the glucose content → Straining → Drying → Packing of dried product → Storage/marketing

Recently some new products, such as heat and eat, ready to cook products and low-cholesterol egg powder, have been developed.

31
Fish products and processing technique

The fishery resources of India are grossly underutilized. A wide variety of fish are found in Indian inland waters, coastal areas and deep seas. More than 60% production of fish in India is from marine sources. Marine fish found in India include prawns, shrimps, tuna, cattle fish, mackerel, red snappers, ribbon fish and countless other varieties.

31.1 Products

Many delicious food and snack items are prepared from fish. Fishes are processed into canning, pickle, smoked fish, sausages, paste and sauce.

31.1.1 Canned fishes

Preparation technique
Fishes → Cleaning in water → Removal of head, fins, tail and other unwanted parts → Washing of remaining parts to remove blood, dirt, etc. → Cutting into desired sizes → Filling into sterilized tins/cans → Addition of tomato sauce → Exhausting (subjected to live steam) at a temperature of 80–90°C for 15–20 min → Sealing of cans airtight → Processing (treated in retort at a pressure of 10–15 lbs for 30–90 min (depending upon the type of fishes) → Taking of can out from retort and cooling → Storage/marketing

31.1.2 Canned prawns

Preparation technique
Prawns → Cleaning in water → Removal of head, fins, tail and other unwanted parts → Washing of remaining parts → Cutting into desired pieces → Blanching in 3–5% brine for 8–10 min → Filling into sterilized tins/cans → Addition of tomato sauce or brine → Exhausting (subjected to live steam) at a temperature of 80–90°C for 15–20 min → Sealing of cans airtight → Processing (treated in retort at a pressure of 10–15 lbs for 30–90 min (depending upon the type of fishes) → Taking of can out from retort and cooling → Storage/marketing

31.1.3 Pickle

31.1.3.1 Pomfret/salmon

Ingredients

Fish (pomfret/salmon) 1 kg, grated jaggery 250 g, gingelly oil 700 mL, salt as per taste 200 g, turmeric powder 5 g, red chillies powder 5 g, cumin seeds 20 g, garlic 100 g, chillies 20 in numbers, vinegar 300 mL.

Preparation technique

Fish → Cleaning and washing → Removal of undesirable parts → Cutting into 5 cm pieces → Mixing with turmeric red chilli powder and salt → Keeping the fish in a side for 30 min → Frying in 200 mL of gingelly oil till browning → Grinding of onion, garlic, cumin seeds, ginger in paste form and fried till it becomes light brown → Addition of vinegar with salt, chillies and turmeric powder to the mixture → Heating till vinegar is absorbed in fish → Cooling → Mixing with ground spices and preservative → Packing in air tight bottles → Storage/marketing

31.1.3.2 Prawn pickle

Ingredients

Prawns 1 kg, gingelly oil 1 L, vinegar 700 mL, green chillies 20 in number, cumin seed 15 g, mustard seed 15 g, ginger 10 g, garlic 100 g, salt 200 g, asafoetida 5 g.

Preparation technique

Fresh prawns → Cleaning and washing → Removal of undesirable parts and peeling → Blanching in 6% salt solution containing 0.02% citric acid at 100°C (for 15 min) → Draining → Cooling → Garlic and green chillies are cut longitudinally (cut pieces of lemons can also be used), grinding of asafoetida and mixed with vinegar, heating of edible oil at 200°C and frying of mustard in it → Mixing garlic, green chillies, lemon pieces with oil one after another → Stirring → Mixing of salt, ginger pieces and asafoetida → Addition of vinegar → Addition of liquid portion of blanched prawns slowly and mixed well → Heating the mixture at 100°C for 3 min → Cooling to 60°C → Mixing with preservatives → Packing of prawn pickle in air tight bottles → Storage/marketing

31.1.4 Fish paste

This is a staple food very popular in many countries large fish or other fishes can be used for production of fish paste. The technique used for preparation is as follows:

Fish → Clearing → Mixing with salt in ratio of 3:1 → Allow to ferment vats (proteolytic enzymes of fish start degrading the tissues) → Draining of excess liquids generated → Paste

31.1.5 Sauce

Sauce is prepared from small fish the technique used for preparation of sauce is as follows:

Small fish → Mashing or hand pressing → Putting in layer with salt in the earthen part (fish to salt ratio 3:2) → Pots burried in ground for 6–12 months → Supernatant formed is collected as first-grade sauce → The residue is extracted twice or thrice for production of second or third grade sauce

The method for preparation is time consuming; hence, the process can be accelerated by altering salt concentration and temperature and addition of enzyme source.

31.1.6 Prawn cracker

This is a delicious snack food. The product consists of wheat flour and starch seasoning and prawn fishes. The technique for preparation of prawn cracker is as follows:

Prawn fish → Mincing (mincing machine minces fresh plant to make ground prawn meat) → Addition of wheat flour, starch, water → Steaming → Kneading (dough containing 40% moisture) → Rolling (role into sheet with thickness of 2–2.5 mm and 300 mm wide) → Cooling in air under normal temperature → Leaving to mature (for about 10 h) → Drying in drier up to 20% moisture → Strip making (in strip making machine) → 1st drying → Conditioning (100 h) → 2nd drying up to 10% moisture → Baking → Seasoning → Addition of oil → Packaging (laminated film) → Storage/marketing

31.1.7 Smoked fish

The technique for the preparation of smoked fish is as follows:

Fresh fish → Cleaning and washing → Removal of slime, intestines, etc. → Dressed fish → Brining/salting → Hanging → Smoking (kiln temperature 80°C and fish temperature up to 60°C) → Packing → Storage/marketing

31.1.8 Sausages

The technique for the preparation of sausages is as follows:

Frozen fish → Thawing (uniformly at –5°C) → Mincing (keep fish at 4–10°C during mincing operation) → Kneading → Mixing with seasoning → Stuffing → Packing (casing) → Sterilizing → Cooling of casings → Drying (to prevent surface contamination) → Packing → Storage/marketing

31.1.9 Dried salted fish

The technique for preparation of dried salted fish is as follows:

Fish → Cleaning and washing → Dressing (splitting the fish open on the ventral side along with vertebral column with the dorsal side) → Removal of gills and entrails (in case of large fish fillets are prepared) → Salting of dressed fish with salt powder in the ratio of 1 part of salt to 3 parts of fish (salted powder contains sodium benzoate 0.02%, potassium sorbate 0.5% and acids sodium phosphate 0.5%. Salting is done at room temperature for 88 h) → Washing of salted fish with 5% salt solution to remove excess of salt sticking to the surface of the fish → Drying of salted fish in the sun or cabinet driers with inlet air temperature of 80°C and outlet air temperature of 45°C to a moisture content of about 25% → Packing → Dried fish in polythene bags which are further wrapped in wax papers and packed in wooden boxes/tins fitted with lever lids → Marketing

31.1.10 Frozen fish

Freezing extend the period of storage and can be kept similar in condition to that of fresh fish. The fishes are gutted and frozen down to –29°C within 2 h of its catch. Fin fish is frozen as tillets (lengthwise cuts), steaks (cross cut section) or sticks (lengthwise or cross wise cut). Large fish are frozen by the sharp freeze. Small fish, fillets and steaks are quick frozen. The storage life of quality frozen fish is very long.

31.1.11 Fish protein concentrate

This is an edible fish product suitable for human consumption. It is prepared from fresh fish. Fish protein concentrate is odourless, blend powder, light in colour and content low label of lipids that is less than 1%. Fish protein concentrate is very rich source of protein containing 70–80% and calcium. This can be prepared from any edible fish. The process for preparation of is as follows:

Dressed fish (gills, entails and viscera or internal organs) → Steam cooking → Press out water and lipids from cooked fish in a hydraulic press → Drying of material in cabinet drier → Fish protein concentrate → Packing → Storage/marketing

31.1.12 Fish liver oils

Fish oils are two types: liver oils and body oils. Fish liver oils is a natural source of vitamin A and fair source are vitamin D. Fishes which are good source of liver oils are tuna, cod, shark and halibut. The oil content varies with the fishes. Fishes which are good source of body oil are salmon, sardine and herring. The technique for preparation of liver oil is as follows:

Minced fish liver → Cooking at 35–95°C → Results in disintegration of liver cells and freeing of oil → Oil floating on the steam condensate, skimmed off by centrifugation → Packing → Marketing

Fisheries industry is gradually taking shapes but fish processing is still in its infancy in India. The kind of units which have come up in fish sectors is frozen and canned products mainly in fresh form. Apart from domestic market, there is good scope for export.

32
Processing waste and utilization

Food-processing industries generate, some amount of waste and causes serious problem of its disposal. This results environmental pollutions and reduces the economy in cost of production of products. Therefore, processing waste utilization is important for removing problem of pollution, achieving high per cent of raw material utilization and converting into value-added by-products for additional benefit or economy of the industry. Some of the by-products which can be manufactured from various processing waste are discussed in the following sections.

32.1 Plant-based processing waste

32.1.1 Fruits

Mango

Peel and kernel are the wastes from mango fruit. These are 30–35% of original raw material. Peel can be utilized for manufacture of pectin, ethanol and vinegar. Kernels can be used for making starch flour, oil and glucose syrup.

Guava

Cores and pomace are the wastes from guava fruits. These wastes are 40–45% of original raw material. These can be utilized for making cheese.

Citrus fruit

Peel seed and pomace are the wastes. These wastes constitute 50–55% of original raw material. Peel and seeds of citrus fruit can be used for making candy, essential oil and cattle field. Pomace is used for manufacture of pectin and cattle field. Citric acid can be prepared from lime and orange waste.

Banana

Peel and stem are the wastes from banana. These constitute 30–40% of original raw material. Pulpy portion of banana peel can be utilized for preparation of cheese. Stem of banana can be used in making pulp for paper.

Jackfruit

Rind and seed are the wastes from jackfruits. These are 50–55% of original raw material. Thick rind of jackfruit can be utilized for manufacture of pectin. Seed is used for making vegetable. Flour can also be prepared from seed which can be used in confectionary.

Pineapple

Peel, trimmings, core eyes, crown and pomace are the wastes. These are 45–50% of original raw material. Peel and trimming materials are used to recover the juice. Citric acid can be prepared from juice. Core is utilized for making candy. The pressed pomace from juice is dried and used for cattle feed. Crown leaves are used for fibre.

Papaya

Peels are the waste material in papaya. This can be used for manufacturing pectin and cattle feed.

Grapes

Stems, pomace, seed and skins are the wastes. These are 20–30% of original raw material. This can be used for cattle feed.

Apple

Peel, pomace, trimmings and core are the wastes from apple fruit. These are 30–35% of original raw material. These are utilized for making of pectin, cider, vinegar and cattle feed.

Apricot

Kernel/stone, core pit and peel are the waste from apricot fruit. These constitute 15–20% of original raw material. Kernel used for extraction of oil which is used in confectionary and cosmetic. Kernel oil cake is rich in protein and is used for cattle feeds.

Cherry

Kernel/stone is the waste in cherry fruit. This is utilized for extraction of edible oil.

Pear

Peels and cores are the wastes of pear fruits. These constitute 20–25% of original raw material. These can be fermented into perry and vinegar. It is also used for cattle feed.

Peach

Kernel/stone, peel and core pit are the wastes from peach fruit. These are 20–25% of original raw material. These can be utilized for extraction of edible oil.

32.1.2 Vegetables

Tomato

Trimmings, pomace, skin and seeds are the wastes from tomatoes. Trimmings are used for making juice/sauce/puree. Pomace is used for cattle feed and seed for edible oil.

Peas
Pods/shells and vines are the wastes of peas. These can be used as fresh cattle feed. Chlorophyll can also be extracted from these wastes.

Beans
Stalk and strings are the wastes at the harvesting time. These can be utilized for cattle feed.

Cauliflower
Leaves and stock are the wastes in cauliflower. Both can be used for making cattle feed.

Cabbage
Cabbage stalk is the waste in cabbage. This can be utilized for making cattle feed.

Potato
Stalk with leaves and trimmings are the wastes. These can be utilized for making cattle feed.

Sweet potato
Vines are the waste material. This can be used for cattle feed.

Carrot
Leaves and trimmings are the waste in carrot. This can be used for cattle feed.

Beetroot
Leaves and trimmings are the waste in beetroot. This can be used for cattle feed.

Turnip
Leaves and trimmings are the waste. These can be utilized for cattle feed.

Watermelon
Thick rind is the waste in watermelon. This can be used for making candy and pickle.

Ash gourd
Rind/peel is the waste. This can be used for cattle feed.

Onion
Onion skin is the waste. This can be utilized for the preparation of quercetin which is a flavouring material.

32.1.3 Plantation crops

Spices
Spent spice residue can be used as fuel, cattle feed and manure. Oils colour, starch, fibre and chemicals can be obtained from these residues.

Paper and paprika waste can be utilized for extraction of colour. Cinnamon leaves and twigs can be used for distillation to obtain essential oil. Nutmeg rind can be used for recovery of quality pectin.

Coconut

Coconut husk and coconut shell are the waste material from coconut. Husk is utilized in coir industry and shell can be used as a fuel and fancy articles.

Cashew nut

Cashew apple is the waste in cashew nut. Cashew apple utilized for preparation of fermented beverage fenny and non-fermented beverage such as RTS squash and syrup. Jam and chutney can also be prepared cashew apple.

Cocoa

Empty pods, cocoa shell, cocoa germ and shell nib are the wastes. Shell and germ can be utilized for economic extraction of theobromine. Shell is also used for manure and fuel. Shell nib mixture is utilized for recovery of fat.

Tea

Tea waste and tea seeds are the wastes. Tea waste can be utilized for production of caffeine, pectin, yellow and brown pigments. Seeds can be used for extraction of oil.

Coffee

Pulp, husk, caffeine and spent ground are the waste obtained from coffee. Pulp can be utilized for caffeine, protein, pectic enzymes and also as cattle feed. Husk can be used as fuel.

32.1.4 Cereals

Rice

Bran and broken are the wastes. Rice bran is utilized for making rice bran oil, deoiled cake and wax. Brokens are used for making rice flour and extruded food products.

Wheat

Germ is considered to be the waste in wheat-processing industry. It is utilized for making germ oil and cake.

Maize

Brokens are the processing waste in maize. This is utilized for making extruded food.

32.1.5 Pulses and oil seeds

In pulses, brokens are used for making extruded food products. In case of oil seeds, defatted cake is utilized for making extruded product and baking.

32.1.6 Sugarcane

Bagasse, molasses and press-mud are the processing waste of sugarcane. These products are rich in carbon compound and minerals. These products can be utilized for microbial fermentation to value-added products such as low calories sweeteners, energy option such as fuel/ethanol, medicines, pesticides, etc.

32.2 Animal-based processing waste

32.2.1 Milk

Whey is the major dairy waste. This is a liquid product obtained from milk in the preparation of paneer and cheese. The whey contains about 7% of total solids comprising about 70% of lactose, 0.9% of protein and trace amount of water soluble vitamins, minerals and fat. This can be utilized for preparation of soft drinks. Production of whey protein is also one of the ways for utilization of whey. Whey protein can be used for preparation of dairy products such as processed cheese, whey powder, ice–cream, infant food, etc.

32.2.2 Meat

Edible offal, blood, hair, skin and bones are the wastes from meat industry. Edible offal can be used for making comminuted meat products. Blood can be utilized in fertilizer industry. Hair is utilized for making over coat, hot tops and hand gloves for use in winter. Skin is utilized in leather industry. Bones are utilized for making gelatin and fertilizers such as calcium ammonium nitrate and calcium super phosphates.

32.2.3 Poultry

Feather, blood and intestine are the wastes from poultry industry. Feathers are utilized for making toys, shuttles and for pillow stuffing. Blood can be used as a source of protein which can be processed into products. It can also be used as source of lysine.

32.2.4 Fish

Fins, skin, air/swim bladder and chunk shells are the waste in fish industry. Fins are normally used for making of soup and gelatin. Skin is utilized in leather industry for making hand bags, shoes and other fancy articles. Air/swin bladder or fish maw is used for purification of wine and making soup. This has good export potential. Chunk shells are used for making bangles, amulets and buttons. Fish waste is also used for making oil, vitamin A and E. It can also be used as manure.

33

Food safety and standard

Food is the prime necessity of life. Food contains several chemical constituents which are known as nutrients including water, protein, carbohydrates, fats, vitamins, minerals and roughages. These are required to sustain life. Food directly affects human health and safety. The safety of food is utmost important and has gained a worldwide attention. The food safety crisis exists in several part of the world including India. Our food is devitalized, coloured, filled with chemicals, drugs and synthetic ingredients and polluted by agricultural and environmental chemicals.

Food safety can be defined as the practical certainty that injury or damage will not result from a food or ingredient used in a reasonable and customary manner and quantity. An understanding of food safety is developed by defining two basic concepts: toxicity and hazard. Toxicity is the capacity of a substance to produce harm or injury of any kind under any conditions. Hazard is the relative probability that harm or injury will result when the substance is used in proposed manner and quantity.

33.1 Food safety issues

Specific food safety concerns differ markedly. Food safety issues include:

- Additives, colours, flavours
- Antibiotics
- Fertilizers and other growing chemicals
- Irradiation
- Microbiological contamination
- Naturally occurring food toxicants
- Pesticides
- Pollutants
- Nutrition
- Processing, packaging and labelling
- Tampering

33.2 Food adulteration

Food adulteration is defined as the process by which the quality or the nature of food product is adversely affected through the addition of a foreign or inferior or deleterious substance or removal of vital component. Adulteration of food product may adversely affect health. Adulteration of foods is commonly practiced by the traders. The foods may be considered adulterated in following conditions:

- Contain a poisonous/deleterious substances which may render it injurious to health
- Contain any food or colour additives deemed unsafe
- Contain any filthy and decomposed substances
- Contain any residue in excess of the established tolerance
- Contain any substances, which increases weight or bulk
- Prepared and packed under unsanitary condition
- Taken from any part of diseased animal
- Packaging material which contains poisonous/injurious substance
- Prepared with omission of valuable constituents

33.2.1 Types of adulterants

There are three types of adulterants. These are intentional adulterants, incidental adulterants and metallic and chemical adulterants.

33.2.1.1 Intentional adulterants

Some adulterants added intentionally to food products to increase the margin of profit. Intentional substances used for adulteration are sands, marble chips, stones, mud, chalk powder, water to milk, mineral oil to edible oil, starch, salt, harmful colours, etc. The common intentional adulterants in various foods and their health hazards are as follows.

Sand, marble, chips, gravel and earth

These are added to grains, pulses, coriander seeds, rice, etc., and ingested they can upset the digestive system. These are carriers of infection. They are extremely unpleasant in the mouth and can hurt the teeth and gums.

Water

Water is used to adulterate milk. The source of water is generally not clean and therefore, it carriers infection.

Petroleum oils

Used for adulterating edible oils. Theses oils are toxic and cancer causing.

Mineral oil

Used for coating black pepper to prevent fungal growth. Some mineral oils are toxic for human and contain compounds causing cancer.

Argemone seeds and oil

Argemone seeds resemble mustard seeds and they are mixed with them during extraction of mustard oil. Both the seeds and oil are highly toxic and consumer can lose his eye sight and develop a condition called epidemic dropsy. Dropsy is a disease in which watery fluid collects in cavities of the body causing swelling, gastrointestinal disturbances and irregular fever. Death can occur due to cardiac arrest.

Khesari dal (Lathyrus sativus)

Khesari pulse is used to mix with Bengal gram to make Bengal gram flour. This can cause a form of crippling paralysis in boys and men. The disease is called lathyrism. The disease starts with stiffness of knee joints and legs with pain.

Papaya seeds

It is used to adulterate black pepper.

Talc

Talc is used to polish pulses. Talc has been linked to stomach cancer.

Washing soda

Washing soda is used to adulterate icing sugar.

Metanil yellow

Metanil yellow is used to give colour to turmeric and to *jalebies*. This is highly poisonous. Metanil yellow affects the reproductive organ and can cause sterility.

Used tea leaves

Used tea leaves are dried, powdered and coloured to adulterate tea leaves. Used tea leaves can be the cause of infection and food poisoning.

Coloured saw dust

Coloured saw dust is used to adulterate red chilli powder. This can upset digestion and cause infection.

Malachite

Used to colour dried peas a bright green so that, they look like fresh peas. This can be poisonous and cause cancer and abnormalities in kidney, spleen and liver.

The simple test to detect intentional adulterants in various foods is given in Table 33.1.

Table 33.1. Intentional adulterants and method of detection.

Food stuffs	Adulterants	Test to detect adulterants
Milk	Water	Lactometer measures specific gravity. The lactometer reading <1.026 indicates the adulteration of milk with water.
	Starch	Add tincture iodine and indication of blue colour shows the presence of starch.
Milk products		
Khoa	Starch	Add tincture of iodine, indication of blue colour shows the presence of starch.
Curds	Cane sugar	Add 0.1 g of resorcinol and 1 mL of concentrated HCl to 1 mL of sample and boil. A rose red colour indicates the presence of cane sugar.
Ghee and butter	Starch-mashed potato, sweet potato and other starch	Iodine solution is prepared by dissolving 2.5 g of iodine crystals and 3 g of potassium iodide in water to make the volume 100 mL. Add a drop of this iodine solution to a little sample of milk products. Formation of blue colour indicates added starch in any form.
	Vanaspati	Take about one teaspoonful of melted ghee or butter with equal quantity of concentrated hydrochloric acid in a test tube and add to it a pinch of cane sugar. Shake well for 1 min and observe it after 5 min. Appearance of crimson colour in lower (acidic) layer shows the presence of vanaspati.
Ice-cream	Metanil: it is a non-permitted coal tar dye	Extract colour with luke warm water from food article. Add few drops of commercial HCl. The development of magenta colour indicates the presence of metanil yellow.
Edible oil	Argemone oil	Add concentrated nitric acid to the sample and shake carefully. Red to reddish brown colour in acid layer would indicate the presence of argemone oil.
	Mineral oil	Mix 2 mL of oil with 2 mL of 3% alcoholic potassium hydroxide and heat in boiling water, wait for 15 min. Add 10 mL of water. Formation of any turbidity indicates mineral oil.

	Castor oil	Dissolve some oil in petroleum ether in a test tube and cool in ice salt mixture. Presence of turbidity with in 5 min, indicates the presence of castor oil.
Soft drinks	Mineral acid	Soak a strip of filter paper in a 0.1% solution of metanil yellow and then dry. Dip one end of paper into the soft drinks. The wetted portion terms violet and indicate the presence of mineral acid.
Coffee powder	Starch	Make decoction of the coffee. Decolorize it by adding potassium permanganate and then add a drop of iodine solution. Formation of blue colour indicates the presence of starch.
	Roasted dates and tamarinds seeds	Sprinkle the suspended coffee powder on white blotting paper and spray over it 1% sodium carbonate solution. Staining of blotting paper red indicates the presence of tamarind and dates seed powder.
	Chicory	Shake a small portion in cold water. Coffee will float while chicory will sink retaining the water brownish red.
Tea powder/ leaves	Exhausted tea or black gram or Bengal gram dal with colour	Sprinkle the powder on a wet white blotting paper. Spots of yellow and red colour appearing on paper indicate that is artificially coloured.
Sweetening agents		
Honey	Invert sugar	Fiehe's test. Mix about 5 g of honey with 10 mL ether in a mortar using a pestle. Decant off the ether extract in to a China dish. Repeat extraction twice with more ether and collect all the extracts in the same dish. Allow the ether to evaporate off at room temperature to the residue in the dish. Add a large drop of 1% solution of freshly sublimed resorcinol in concentrated hydrochloric acid. Appearance of cherry red colour immediately indicates invert sugar.
	Molasses (sugar and water)	A cotton wick dipped in pure honey burns when lighted with a matchstick. If adulterated, the presence of water will not allow the honey to burn, if it does, it will produce a crackling sound.
Sugar	Chalk powder	Dissolve in a glass of water, chalk will settle down at the bottom.

Jaggery powder	Chalk powder	Add few drops of HCl. Effervescence indicates adulteration. Stir a spoonful sample of sugar in a glass of water. The chalk powder settles down.
Cereal products (wheat flour, semolina, Bengal gram flour)	Sand, grit	At 5 mL of carbon tetrachloride to a little sample in a dry test tube and shake well. Sand and grit will settle at the bottom leaving flour on top.
	Chalk powder and lime powder	Treat sample with hot dilute HCl. The bubbling of gas indicates carbon dioxide from chalk or other carbonates.
Bengal gram flour	Yellow maize flour	Rubbing with fingers and roughness indicates the presence of maize flour.
	Metanil yellow	Shake portion of sample with cold or warm water. The water becomes yellowish and on treatment with few drops of concentrated HCl turns magenta red.
Food grains	Hidden insect infection	Take a filter paper impregnated with ninhydrine (1% in alcohol). Put some grains on it and then fold the filter paper and crush the grains with hammer. Spots of bluish purple colour indicate presence of hidden insect infestation.
Bajra	Infected with ergot fungus	Long irregular black grain indicates ergot. In 2% salt solution ergot floats.
Rice	Marble or other stones	Place a small quantity of rice on the palm of the hand and gradually immerse the same in water. The stone chips will sink.
Pulses (whole black, masoor and Bengal gram)	Khesari whole pulse	On visual examination, wedge-like shapes are seen. Brown colour appears with hydrochloric acid within 15-30 min.
Split and dehusked pulses (arhar dal and Bengal gram)	Khesari pulse	Khesari pulse can be detected by visual examination.
	Metanil yellow	Shake portion of sample with cold or warm water. The water becomes yellowish and on treatment with a few drops of concentrated hydrochloric acid terms magenta red colour.
Green peas	Colour, dye stuffs and dals	Sample is kept immersed in water for about half an hour and stirred. Colours separation indicates adulteration.

Tur dal	Lakh dal	Lakh dal is irregular in shape and of lighter colour than tur dal.
	Metanil yellow	Add concentrated HCl to moisten dal. Yellow colour will turn into magenta red if metanil yellow is present.
Black gram flour	Yellow maize flour	Rubbing with fingers and roughness indicates presence of maize flour.
	Metanil yellow	Shake portion of sample with cold or warm water. The water becomes yellowish and on treatment with few drops of HCl turns magenta red.
Spices		
Turmeric powder	Metanil yellow	Take a tea spoonful of turmeric powder in a test tube. Add few drops of concentrated HCl. Instant appearance of violet colour which disappears on dilution with water. If the colour persists, the presence of metanil yellow is indicated.
	Yellow clay	Mix powders with water and allow to stand for sometime. The yellow clay will settle down at the bottom leaving turmeric on the top.
Powder spices	Sand, grit, talk, colour	Shake a little of sample in a dry test tube with 5 mL of carbon tetrachloride. Allow to settle. Sand, talk and grit will sink to the bottom, leaving spice on top.
Chili powder	Stones/brick powder	Any grittiness that may be felt on tapping the sediment at the bottom of glass confirms the presence of brick powder or sand or stones.
Coriander powder	Common salt	Add a few drops of silver nitrate to 5 mL of sample. White precipitate indicates adulteration.
Black pepper whole	Papaya seeds	Papaya seeds are sunken, oval and greyish brown.
Cardamom	Oil is removed and parts are coated with talcum powder	On rubbing talcum will stick to the fingers. On tasting, there is hardly any aromatic flavour, which indicates removal of essential oil.
Cinnamon	Woodbark/cassiabark	Cinnamon barks are very thin and can be rolled. Cassiabark are thick and stiff or hard.

Cloves	Volatile oil extracted cloves	Exhausted cloves can be identified by small size and shrunken appearance. The characteristic pungent test of genuine cloves is less pronounced in exhausted cloves.
Saffron	Dyed tendrils of maize cobs	Genuine saffron will not break easily like artificial saffron which is prepared by soaking maize cob in sugar and colouring it with coal tar dye. The colour dissolves in water if artificially coloured. A bit of pure saffron when allowed to dissolve in water will continue to give its saffron colour so long as it lasts.
Cumin seeds	Grass seeds coloured with charcoal dust	Rub the cumin seeds on palms. If palms turn black, adulteration is indicated.
Asafoetida	Soap stone or other earthy matter	Shake with water. Soap, stone or other earthy matter will settle down.
	Starch	Add tincture of iodine. Appearance of blue colour indicates the presence of starch.
Mustard and rye seeds	Argemone seeds	Examination under magnifying glass shows small seeds resembling mustard but blacker, more rough and not uniformly smooth and round.
Mustard, rye, cumin seeds and khus-khus	Stones and foreign matter	This can be detected by visual examination.
Supari	Colour and saccharin	Colour dissolve in water. Saccharin gives excessive and lingering sweet taste.
Common salt	White powdered stones and chalk	Stir a sample of salt in a glass of water. The presence of chalk will make the solution white and other insoluble impurities will settle down.

The above tests of adulterants are in no way to replace the prescribed laboratory test; hence, adulteration detected as mentioned above needs to be confirmed by analysis by a recognized food testing laboratory.

33.2.1.2 Incidental adulterants

Incidental adulterants are pesticide residues, tin from can, dropping of rodents and larvae in foods. We are daily eating foods laced with some toxic pesticides. High degree of filth in the form of excreta, bodily secretions due to rodents, insects and microorganisms are responsible for food contamination and intoxification.

Food contamination with harmful microorganisms

Raw foods such as fruits, vegetables, milk, meat, fish, etc., grown on sewage are likely to be contaminated with harmful microorganisms. Though these are generally destroyed during cooking or processing of food yet some of the microorganisms survive due to low or inadequate heat processing. Some of the foods consumed in raw state which may cause food poisoning. Some foods such as food grains, legumes and oil seeds when stored in humid atmosphere are infected by pathogenic fungus which can cause serious illness. The pathogenic microorganisms are commonly found in the contaminated food, and the microorganisms responsible for causing serious illness are given in Table 33.2.

Table 33.2. Foodborne diseases caused by some pathogenic organisms.

Pathogenic organisms	Foods involved	Harmful effects of diseases
Bacterial		
Clostridium botulinum	Meat and fish processed defectively	Botulism or muscular paralysis, death due to respiratory failure
C. perfringens	Precooked meat defectively processed	Nausea, abdominal pain and diarrhoea
Bacillus cereus	Cereal products	Nausea, vomiting and abdominal pain
Salmonella	Fish, meat, egg products defectively processed and raw vegetables grown on sewage	Salmonellosis: vomiting, diarrhoea and fever
Shigella somel	Exposed food in unhygienic surroundings	Bacillary dysentery
Staphylococcus aureus	Exposed food in unhygienic surroundings	Increased salivation, vomiting, abdominal pain and diarrhoea
Streptococcus pyogenes	Exposed food in unhygienic surroundings	Scarlet fever, septic sore throat
Fungal		
Aspergillus flavus	Groundnut and corn	Liver damage and cancer
Claviceps purpurea	Ergot infected rye and pearl millet	Burning sensation in extremities and peripheral gangrene ergotism
Fusarium sporotrichiodes	*Fusarium*-infected cereals and millets	Alimentary toxic aleukia
Penicillium islandicum	Rice	Liver damage

Parasitic		
Ascaris lumbricoides	Vegetables grown on sewage farms	Ascariasis
Ancylostoma duodenale	Vegetables grown on sewage farms	Epigastric pain, loss of blood, anaemia
Entamoeba histolytica	Vegetables grown on sewage farms	Amoebic dysentery
Trichinella spiralis	Pork and pork products	Nausea, vomiting, diarrhoea, colic and muscular pain

Sequence of incidental adulteration in foods

- Contamination starts with the use of pesticides by farmers for crop protection. Health department spray pesticides to control malaria caused by mosquitoes.
- Residue remains long after spraying. Cattle fodder and chicken feeds are affected. Ground water is poisoned. Meat, fish, egg and milk get contaminated.
- Spray required to prevent fungus and rodents, damaging stored grains. This results in further increase of residue levels in food stuffs.
- Sellers dip vegetables in pesticides to look fresh and extend shelf life and used chemical such as carbide for fruit ripening. Oils and sweets are adulterated with prohibited substances.
- Vegetable washing and other food stuffs help but cooking rarely destroys toxic residues. Ingested pesticides are absorbed by the small intestine.
- Fatty tissues distributed throughout the body store this pesticide. These can damage vital organs such as kidney, liver, heart and brain.

Prevention of incidental poisoning

The followings points should be considered to prevent incidental poisoning:

- Warn people of dangerous build up of toxin in food through market survey.
- Educate farmers for integrated pest management programme against judicious use of pesticides. No spraying should be done a week before harvest.
- Promote pest control using their natural predators.
- Use safe pesticides.
- Washing of foods thoroughly before cooking to get rid of much of toxin.
- Prevent industries from dumping poisonous effluents.

33.2.1.3 Metallic and chemical contaminations

This type of adulterants are arsenic from pesticides, lead from water, mercury from effluents of chemical industry, tin from cans, mercuric salts from contaminated fish caught from water. The other elements toxic in small doses are arsenic antimony cobalt and cadmium. High level of pesticide residues in bovine milk and metals like arsenic, cadmium and lead are also found in some infant formula, canned products and turmeric (coated with lead chromate). Silver foil use for sweets and in pan masala contain carcinogenic nickel, lead, chromium and cadmium. Most of the metals and chemicals which generally gain entry in the foods are as incidental adulterants. The toxic effects of some common metals and chemicals are given in Table 33.3.

Table 33.3. Toxic effects of some metals and chemicals.

Contaminants	Foods involved	Toxic effects
Lead	Lead water pipes and some process food, turmeric coated with lead chromate	Nausea, abdominal pain, anaemia, muscular pain, paralysis and brain damage
Mercuric salt	Contaminated fish, seed grain, treated with mercury	Muscular paralysis, blindness, deaf and brain damage
Arsenic	Drinking water, fruits contaminated by lead arsenate spray	Dizziness, chills, crams, paralysis leading to death
Barium	Food contaminated by rat poison (barium carbonate)	Violent peristalsis, muscular twitching and convulsions
Cadmium	Fruit juices and soft drinks in contact of cadmium and plated vessels, crabs, oysters	Excessive salivation, liver, kidney damage prostrate cancer, multiple fractures
Cobalt	Water and beer	Cardiac failure
Copper	Acid foods in contact with tarnished copper ware	Vomiting, diarrhoea and abdominal pain
Tin	Canned foods	Colic, vomiting, photophobia
Zinc	Stored food in galvanised iron ware	Vomiting and dizziness
Pesticides	All types of food contaminated	Acute poisoning causing liver, kidney, brain and nerves damage leading to death
Antibiotics	Meat from animals fed with antibiotics	Drug resistance, hardening of arteries and heart disease

Tips to consumers for preventing food adulteration

At shopping

- Read label before purchase and purchase food articles from licensed shops with cash memo
- Prefer to purchase foods in packed containers
- Prefer to purchase foods certified by the government agencies like FSSA and ISI certification
- Avoid to purchase synthetic coloured foods like syrup, ice candy and sweet meats
- Do not purchase cut fruits and vegetables
- Do not use containers or package used for non-edible items like insecticides or chemicals
- Use only food-grade plastic packaging material for packed foods to avoid packaging hazards which create health hazards

At preparation and serving

- Wash hand properly before starts of preparing food.
- Cut nails short, keep them clean and cover cuts in hands by bandage.
- Wear clean over cloth and cover head with hair net or band.
- Wash food stuffs such as fruits, vegetables, eggs, fish, meat, etc., before cooking, eating or storage in refrigerator.
- Cook food at boiling temperature and avoid contact between cooked foods and raw foods.
- Serve hot cooked foods and store cooked food preferably below 10°C.
- Defrost and clean refrigerator every week.
- Stored food having off flavour, smell or rancidity should not be consumed.
- Clean or pure water should be used in preparing the food.

Misbranded food

Misbranding is also forbidden by law. A food may be considered misbranded under following conditions:

- Has false labelling which is misleading.
- Offered for sales under the name of another food.
- Imitates another food without the word imitation.
- Has container, which is made, formed or filled such which it is misleading.
- Had label, which does not contain the name of manufacturer, packer or distributor.
- Has label, which does not contain an accurate statement of the quantity or ingredients.

- Has label for, which makes a nutritional claim but does not contain nutritional labelling.
- Has a label, which does not contain the required information on the correct display panel or does not use the proper format for the nutritional label.

33.3 Consumer protection

Food products must be produced under strict hygienic conditions, free from contaminants, processed without much loss of nutritive value, packaged under sanitary conditions and marked with suitable labels. As buyers and consumers, it is over right of acquiring clean and wholesome food. Several laws have been promulgated to protect the interests of consumers in various countries. The Government of India also promulgated laws and standards regarding food quality and safety for a large number of food items.

33.3.1 Food laws

Food laws are very important to encourage the scientific development of the industry. Food laws and food control system help safe guard the interest of consumers in respect of safety that is health hazards which may arise due to adulteration, contamination, microbiological deterioration, decay and other factors. These have resulted in the passage of food laws in different countries of the world penalizing the sellers of diseased, unwholesome and corrupted food products. The laws define food, food products, preservative, artificial colour and debar the sale of food prepared under unsanitary conditions or containing any deleterious or unsafe substances. These also specify standards of quality for various classes of food. The main objectives of food laws are as follows:

- To protect the consumers against any health hazards arising out of adulteration
- To protect the consumer from unfair trade practices
- To ensure and enforce fair trade practices

33.3.2 Indian food laws

The Government of India has promulgated a number of laws to protect the interest of the consumers to ensure food safety. Some of food laws which are in operation are as follows.

33.3.2.1 Food Safety and Standard Act, 2006

The Food Safety and Standard Act received the assent of the president on 23 August 2006 and came into effect on 5 August 2011. The highlights of the Food Safety and Standard Act 2006 are as under the following laws.

(I) Repealed the previous laws

The act officially repealed the regulatory frame work established by the previous existing eight food laws by the Ministry of Health and Family Welfare. These central laws are Prevention of Food Adulteration Act 1954, the Fruit Products Order 1955, the Meat Food Products Order 1973, the Vegetable Oil Products (regulation) Order 1998, the Edible Oils Packaging (regulation) Order 1988, the Solvent Extracted Oil, Deoiled Meal and Edible Flour (control) Order 1967, Milk and Milk Products Order 1992 and any other order issued under the Essential Commodities Act 1955 relating to food.

(II) Consolidation of various laws into Food Safety and Standard Rules and Regulation 2011 under a single regulator

The act also aims to establish a single reference point for all matters relating to food safety and standards by moving from multi-level, multi-departmental control to a single line of command.

(III) Food Safety and Standards Regulation 2011

The Ministry of Health and Family Welfare published the final Food Safety and Standards Regulation 2011 in the Indian official gazette. The Food Safety and Standards Regulation 2011 came into force in August 2011. These regulations are as follows:

- Food Safety and Standard Regulation 2011 for licensing and registration of food business
- Food Safety and Standards Regulation 2011 for packaging and labelling
- Food Safety and Standards Regulation 2011 for food product standards and food additives
- Food Safety and Standards Regulation 2011 for prohibition and restriction on sales
- Food Safety and Standards Regulation 2011 for contaminants, toxins and residues
- Food Safety and Standards Regulation 2011 for laboratory and sampling analysis

(IV) Establishment of Food Safety and Standards Authority of India

The Food Safety and Standards Authority of India (FSSAI) has been established under the Food Safety and Standard Act 2006 as a statutory body for laying down science-based standards for articles of food and regulating manufacturing, processing, storage, distribution, sale and import of food so as to ensure safe and wholesome food for human consumption. FSSAI also consolidates various acts and orders related issue in various ministries and departments.

Ministry of Health and Family Welfare, Government of India is the administrative ministry for the implementation of FSSAI. The chairperson and chief executive officer of FSSAI are appointed by Government of India. The chairperson is in the rank of secretary to Government of India. FSSAI has been mandated by the Food Safety and Standard Act 2006 for performing the following functions:

- Framing of regulations to lay down the standards and guidelines in relation to articles of food and specifying appropriate system of enforcing various standards thus notified.
- Laying down mechanisms and guidelines for accreditation of certification bodies engaged in certification of food safety management system for food business.
- Laying down procedure and guidelines for accreditation of laboratories and notification of the accredited laboratories.
- To provide scientific advice and technical support to central government and state governments in the maters of framing the policy and rules in areas which have direct or indirect bearing of food safety.
- Collect and collate data regarding food consumption, incidence and prevalence of biological risk, contaminates in food, residues of various contaminates in food products, identification of emerging risks and introduction of rapid alert system.
- Creating and information network across the country so that the public, consumers, panchayats, etc., receive rapid, reliable and objective information about food safety and issues of concern.
- Provide training programmes for persons who are involved or intend to get involved in food business.
- Contribute to the development of international technical standards for food, sanitary and phytosanitary standards.
- Promote general awareness about food safety and food standards.
- The other laws relating to food-processing industry are legal metrology laws, physical laws, labour laws, foreign exchange laws, environmental laws and local laws.

33.3.3 Food standards

A wide range of processed foods are now being manufactured in various countries. Standardization and quality control of these processed foods for both domestic consumption and exports are essential from the view of safety, hygiene, nutrition, keeping quality and other aspect.

Food standards are of different types such as market standards (AGMARK), Bureau of Indian Standards (BIS), Codex, Hazard Analysis and Critical Control Point (HACCP) and ISO 9000.

33.3.3.1 Agricultural Produce (Grading and Marketing) Act 1937 (AGMARK)

The word AGMARK is a derivative of Agricultural Marketing. This act is commonly known as AGMARK. This is one of the oldest food laws enacted in the country. It is voluntary in nature. The act lays down the specification for various agricultural commodities including processed food. A number of grading standards of raw or processed agricultural or horticultural produce have been brought out by the AGMARK which include oils, fats, essential oil, spices, condiments, plantation products, etc. This act is administered by the directorate of marketing and inspection with agricultural marketing adviser to the Government of India. Any organization or packers who want to use AGMARK symbol on the level of the sample containers can apply to the authorities. The authorities after inspection and ensuring that the necessary facilities, like equipment, laboratory, etc., are available, allow them to use AGMARK symbol which ensures that the quality standard laid down for the product under AGMARK have been complied with.

33.3.3.2 Bureau of Indian Standards

Indian standards institution has been constituted under the act of parliament, which deals with standardization of various articles including food. Agriculture Food Division Council deals with the quality standards of various articles of foods. This organization prepares national standards for various articles of food in consultation with the experts in the country. The certification scheme under ISI is a voluntary one and any manufacturer who wants to use ISI on his food product may apply for the same to the authority. The authorities after inspection and other formalities permit the manufacturer to use ISI mark on their product. ISI symbol on any product ensures quality to the consumers. Recently ISI has been renamed as BIS. The bureau is responsible for facilitating harmonious development of standards, product certification, quality certification, quality system certification and environmental management systems certification.

33.3.3.3 The Codex Alimentarius Commission and FAO/WHO Food Standards Programme

The term Codex Alimentarius is a Latin word means food code. In 1962, the Food and Agriculture Organization (FAO) of the United Nation and the World Health Organization (WHO) formed Codex Alimentarius Commission (CAC). The commission implements the joint FAO/WHO food standards programme. The purpose of this is to protect health of consumer and to ensure fair practices in the food trade. The CAC is a collection of internationally adopted food standards for the safety and quality of food as well as codes of good manufacturing practice and other guidelines to protect the health of consumer and remove unfair practices in international trade.

The codex general principles of food hygiene are aimed for the following factors.

Identification

Essential principles of food hygiene application throughout food chain, that is, production to consumption.

Recommendation

The HACCP-based approach is a mean to enhance food safety.

Indication

How to implement these principles.

Guidance

For specific codes, guidance may be needed for sectors of food chain processes or commodities to amplify the hygiene requirements.

The controls described in this general principle documents are internationally recognized as essential to ensure the safety and suitability of food for consumption. The general principles are recommended to governments, industries and consumers.

Government role

- Provide, information, about, codex activities, to other government organizations, academia, industry and consumers.
- Participate in development of standards and other related issues.
- Circulate proposed documents to the appropriate organizations for review and comment.
- Assemble responses and submit by specified date to the codex secretariat for consideration.
- Ensure conformance to national standards and codes based on codex standard.

Industry role

- Participate in the development of food standards.
- Review draft standards before adoption by the CAC.
- Comply the codex and national standard in the manufacture, labelling, processing and shipment of food products.

Consumer role

- Consumer organizations participate in the review of draft standards before adoption.
- Submit consumer concerns and reactions to those standards that are not clear or address the needs of consumers.

33.3.3.4 *Sanitary and Phytosanitary Agreement*

The Sanitary and Phytosanitary (SPS) agreement is an agreement between nation agreed not to use SPS measures as artificial or unjustified barriers to trade.

Sanitary (human and animal health) and phytosanitary (plant health) measures are needed to ensure that food is safe and that pests/diseases of animal and plants are not to introduce into their countries. The SPS agreement confirms the right of nations to establish and use these measures to protect the consumers, their livestocks and wild life and their plants including important food crops. The SPS agreement uses CAC standards as a basis for decisions to be made in regard to food safety.

The SPS measures can be arbitrary and can be established not in the interest of consumers but as protectionist measures for national producers and industries. The SPS agreement brings the objective of these measures down to the baseline.

The SPS measures are fully justified to protect consumers' health and safety but they must not arbitrarily or unjustifiably discriminate between nations in favour of national producers or industries. Governments are required to notify other countries of their SPS requirement and maintain them in open and transparent manner.

33.3.3.5 *Agreement on Technical Barriers to Trade*

Any standards not directed for consumer health protection, for example, general labelling information is covered by the agreement on Technical Barriers to Trade (TBT) which also recommends the use of codex standards. Codex standards are reviewed frequently to ensure that SPS and TBT measures are based on up-to-date scientific data.

33.3.3.6 Hazard Analysis and Critical Control Point

The HACCP is a management system in which food safety is addressed through the analysis and control of biological, chemical and physical hazards from raw material production, procurement and handling to manufacturing, distribution and consumption of the finished product. The US Department of Agriculture has established HACCP for meat- and poultry-processing plants. FDA has developed regulation which has established

HACCP as the food safety standards throughout other areas of the food industry including both domestic and imported food products. HACCP has been endorsed by the National Academy of Science, the CAC (an international food standard setting organization) and the National Advisory Committee on microbiological criteria for foods. A number of US food companies already use the system in their manufacturing process and it is in use in other countries. This has been made mandatory for the most of the food-processing firms in the United States and the United Kingdom.

The HACCP is designed for use in all segments of the food industry from growing, harvesting, processing, manufacturing, distributing and merchandizing to prepare food for consumption. Pre-requisite programme such as current Good Manufacturing Practices is an essential foundation for the development and implementation of successful plans. Food safety system based on the HACCP principles has been successfully applied in food-processing plants, retail food stores and food service operations.

Principles of HACCP

The HACCP is based on seven principles which have been universally accepted by government agencies, trade association and the food industry around the world. These principle are as follows:

1. Analyze hazards: Biological such as microbe, chemical such as toxin, physical such as ground glass or metal fragments.
2. Identify critical control point: Points covering food production from raw state through processing and shipping to consumption such as cooking, cooling, packaging and metal detection.
3. Establish preventive measures with critical limits for each control point: For example, in cooked food, setting the minimum cooking temperature and time required to ensure the elimination or any harmful microbes.
4. Establish procedure to monitor the critical control points: The procedure may include determining how home cooking time and temperature should be monitored.
5. Establish corrective action to be taken when monitoring shows that critical limit has not been met. For example re-processing or disposing off food if minimum cooking temperature is not met.
6. Establish procedure to verify that the system is working properly. For example, testing time and temperature recording devices to verify that a cooking unit is working properly.
7. Establishing effective record keeping document at HACCP system: This may include records of hazards and their control methods, the monitoring of safety requirements and action taken to correct potential problems.

Each of these principles must be backed by sound scientific knowledge.

Need for HACCP

New challenges to the United States food supply have prompted for adopting a HACCP-based food safety system on wider basis. The need arised for HACCP are due to

- increasing number of new pathogens causing foodborne illness,
- increasing public health concern about chemical contamination,
- increasing the size of food industry and diversity of the products and processes,
- limited level of resources to ensure food safety and
- chemical and physical hazards in addition to other biological hazards.

Benefits of HACCP system

- Preventing hazards from contaminated food.
- Based on sound science.
- More efficient and effective monitoring.
- Ensuring food safety.
- Help food industry/company to compete more effectively in the world market.
- Reduce barriers to international trade.

33.3.3.7 ISO 9000 series standards

International organization for standardization (ISO) formed in 1946 and ISO 9000 standards were adopted in 1978 by the International organization of standards in Geneva, Switzerland, as a uniform standard of excellence in the European community. ISO 9000 standards established a standard frame work for a quality system. A quality system is a series of checks and balances which, when introduced and followed, ensures quality of output/product. This defined the quality system or model applicable to design, development, production, installation and servicing final inspection and test.

Models of ISO 9000 series

Three basic models/standards were developed covering different combinations of these discipline and a set of guidelines to assist in choosing the correct standard for application.

ISO 9001

Quality system models for quality assurance in design, development, production, installation and servicing. ISO 9001 is the super set of the contractual models for quality system. It contains 20 sections each of which specifies requirement for components of the quality system. ISO 9001 requires the development of quality manual and documented procedures which define the organization and operation of the quality system. It is the responsibility of a company to create and maintain these documents so that they are relevant and appropriate to the specific business operation.

ISO 9002

ISO 9002 is almost word for word equivalent to ISO 9001 except that it does not include requirements for design control. Hence, it contains 19 sections or requirements.

ISO 9003

Quality system models for quality assurance in final inspection and test. This is contractual model for quality system which does not include design or production. ISO 9003 contains about half of the requirements to suit the inspection and final test application. ISO 9003 requires the development of quality manual and documented procedures which define the organization and operation of the quality system. It is responsibility of a company to create and maintain these documents so that they are relevant and appropriate to the specific business operation.

ISO 9004

It is a set of guidelines including quality management in quality system.

Benefits with ISO quality system

The benefits associated with an ISO quality system are:

1. Error reduction from better systematic inspection and testing.
2. Error reduction resulting from increased employee participation and systematic employee training.
3. Better products resulting from better design control.
4. Improved productivity resulting from planning and team work.
5. Reduction in cost associated with failure.
6. Improved communication both internally and externally.
7. Recognition of compliance by an unbiased organization.

Achieving certification

Steps involved for achieving certification are as follows:

- Preparing quality system documents confirming to standards.
- Audit the quality system to discover inadequacies.
- Invite the certified third party auditor to assess the system.

The members involved in documenting and in implementing quality system of the company and achieving the quality system certification are

- *First party*: Company itself.
- *Second party*: Assisting the company in fulfilling the requirements of standards.
- *Third party*: Assisting the quality system documents, implementation and certification.

33.4 References

1. Anand, J.C. and Maini, S.B. 1997. Utilization of fruit and vegetable waste. *Indian Food Packer* 51(2), 45.
2. Anuj, M., Singh, G.P., Ahlawat, A.K., Shukla, R.B. and Yadav, R. 2011. *Value-Addition in Wheat Through Genetic Approaches and its Scope in India*. TB-ICN:86 IARI, New Delhi.
3. Barbutt, S. 2001. *Poultry Products Processing - An Industary Guide*. CRC Press, Boca Raton, FL, USA.
4. Cutting, C.L. 2008. *Fish Processing and Preservation*. Agrobios, Jodhpur.
5. Dhar, B.L. and Verma, R.N. 2001. *The Indian Mushroom Industry*. The International Society for Mushroom Science, pp. 3-6.
6. FAO Codex Alimentrius. 1997. *Volume IB Secretariat of Joint FAO/WHO*. Food Standard Programme Food and Agriculture Organization, Rome.
7. Jood, S. and Khetarpaul, N. 2002. *Food Preservation Agrotech Publishing Academy*. Udaipur, Rajasthan.
8. Jones, J.M. 1993. *Food Safety*. Eagan Press, St. Paul, MN, USA.
9. Hall, G.M.L. 1992. *Fish Processing Technology*. Blackie, New York.
10. Kapoor, J.N. 2014. *Mushroom Cultivation*. Indian Council of Agricultural Research, New Delhi.
11. Khader, V. 2013. *Text Book of Food Science and Technology*. Indian Council of Agricultural Research (ICAR), New Delhi.
12. Kumar, S. and Singh, I.S. 1998. *Studies on Processing of Papaya Fruits*. *Progressive Hort.* 30, 139-147.
13. Mead, G.C. 1989. *Processing of Poultry*. Chapman and Hall, London.
14. NIIR, 2000. *Modern Technology of Milk Processing and Dairy Products*. NIIR, New Delhi.
15. PPFPI, 2005a. *Oil Seed Based Products*. Enterpreneurship Development Institute of India, Ahmadabad.
16. PPFPI, 2005b. *Cereal and Pulse Based Products*. Enterpreneurship and Development Institute India, Ahmadabad.
17. Rathore, N.S., Mathur, G.K. and Chasta, S.S. 2012. *Post Harvest Management and Processing of Fruits and Vegetables*. Indian Council of Agricultural Research, New Delhi.
18. Satapathy, N. and Amla, B. L. 1967. Utilization of wastes and by products of some industrial as animal feed. *Indian Food Packer* 21, 16-19.
19. Setal, S.J. 1999. *Egg Nutrition and Biotechnology*. CABI Publishing, Wallingford, OX, UK.
20. Sethi, V. Sethi, S., Deka, B.C. and Meena, Y.R. 2005. *Processing of Fruits and Vegetables for Value Addition*. Indus, Publication Co. Pvt. Ltd., New Delhi.

21. Sharma, R.R. and Singh, D. 2010. Effect of different packaging material on shelf life and quality of apple during storage. *Indian J Hort.* 67, 94-101.

22. Skariyachan, S. and Abhilakh, M. 2012. *Introduction to Food Biotechnology*. CBS Publishers and Distributers Pvt. Ltd., New Delhi.

23. Shrivastava, R.P. and Kumar, S. 2002. *Fruit and Vegetable Preservation Principles and Practices*. International Distributing Co., Lucknow.

24. Shrivastava, R.K. and Singh, S. 1987. *Utilization of Mushroom for Preparation of Different Types of Preserved Products.* Government Fruit Preservation and Canning Institute, Lucknow.

25. Singh, I.S. 2000. Mahua - an oil bearing tree. Bulletin, ND, University of Agriculture and Technology, Faizabad.

26. Singh, I.S. 2011. *Food Processing*. Westville Publishing House, New Delhi.

27. Singh, I.S. 2014. *Aonla - Production, Handling and Processing*. Westville Publishing House, New Delhi.

28. Singh, I.S. and Singh, V. 2014. Post Harvest Handling and Processing of Fruits and Vegetables. West Ville Publishing House, New Delhi.

29. Singh, I.S. and Kumar, S. 2015. *Vegetable Crops: Production Handling and Processing*. West Ville, New Delhi.

30. Singh, A. and Singh, I.S. 1991. Chemical evaluation of mahua (*Madhuca indica*) seed. *Food Chemistry* 4, 221-228.

31. Singh, I.S. and Singh, V. 2015a. *Fruit Crops: Production Handling and Processing.* West Ville Publishing House, New Delhi.

32. Singh, I.S. and Singh, V. 2015b. *Production Handling and Processing of Spices*. West Ville Publishing House, New Delhi.

33. Singh, J. and Singh, R.D. 2008. *Processing, Handling and Storage of Sugarcane Jaggery*. Indian Institute of Sugarcane Research, Lucknow, India.

34. Solomon, S., Grewal, S.S., Li, Y.R., Magarey, R.C. and Rao, G.P. 2004. *Sugarcane Production Management and Agro-Industrial Imperatives*. International Book Distribution Co., Lucknow, India.

35. Srilakshmi, B. 2013. *Food Science*. New Age International (P) Ltd Publishers, New Delhi.

36. Subbulakshmi, G. and Udipy, S.A. 2001. *Food Processing and Preservation*. New Age International (P) Ltd. Publishers, New Delhi.

37. Swaminathan, M. 1987. *Food Science Chemistry and Experimental Foods*. The Bangalore Printing and Publishing Co. Ltd, Bangalore.

38. Varnam, A.H. 1994. *Milk and Milk Products: Technology, Chemistry and Micro Biology*. Chapman and Hall, London.

39. Verma, L.R. and Joshi, V.K. 2000. *Post Harvest Technology of Fruits and Vegetables. Handling, Processing, Fermentation and Waste Management*. Vols. I and II. Indus Publication Co. Pvt. Ltd., New Delhi.

40. Warris, P.D. 2000. *Meat Science. An Introductory Text*. CABI Publishing, Wallingford, OX, UK.

41. Wilson, K. 2007. *A Hand Book of Poultry Practices*. Agrobios, Jodhpur.

42. Winton, A.L. and Wintom K.B. 2006. *Milk and Milk Products*. Agrobios, Jodhpur.

Index

C

D

E

F

G

H

I

J

K

Q

R

S

T

U

V

W

Y

Z